# Natural Toxicants in Food

# Sheffield Food Technology

*Series Editor:* P.R. Ashurst

A series which presents the current state of the art of chosen sectors of the food and beverage industry. Written at professional and reference level, it is directed at food scientists and technologists, ingredients suppliers, packaging technologists, quality assurance personnel, analytical chemists and microbiologists. Each volume in the series provides an accessible source of information on the science and technology of a particular area.

*Titles in the Series:*

**Chemistry and Technology of Soft Drinks and Fruit Juices**
Edited by P.R. Ashurst

**Natural Toxicants in Food**
Edited by D.H. Watson

**Technology of Bottled Water**
Edited by D.A.G. Senior and P.R. Ashurst

# Natural Toxicants in Food

Edited by

DAVID WATSON
Joint Food Safety and Standards Group,
Ministry of Agriculture, Fisheries and Food / Department of Health
Smith Square, London

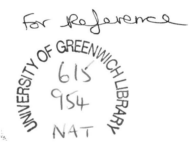
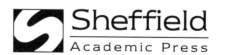

Sheffield
Academic Press

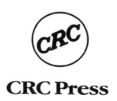

**CRC Press**

First published 1998
Copyright © 1998 Sheffield Academic Press

Published by
Sheffield Academic Press Ltd
Mansion House, 19 Kingfield Road
Sheffield S11 9AS, England

ISBN 1-85075-862-X

Published in the U.S.A. and Canada (only) by
CRC Press LLC
2000 Corporate Blvd., N.W.
Boca Raton, FL 33431, U.S.A.
Orders from the U.S.A. and Canada (only) to CRC Press LLC

U.S.A. and Canada only:
ISBN  0-8493-9734-0

This book contains information obtained from authentic and highly regarded sources. Reprinted
material is quoted with permission, and sources are indicated. Reasonable efforts have been
made to publish reliable data and information, but the author and the publisher cannot assume
responsibility for the validity of all materials or for the consequences of their use.

**Trademark Notice:** Product or corporate names may be trademarks or registered trademarks,
and are used only for identification and explanation, without intent to infringe.
No claim to original U.S.A. Government works.

Printed on acid-free paper in Great Britain by
Bookcraft Ltd, Midsomer Norton, Bath

**British Library Cataloguing-in-Publication Data:**
A catalogue record for this book is available from the British Library

**Library of Congress Cataloging-in-Publication Data:**
A catalog record is available from the Library of Congress

# Preface

This book is intended to guide readers with at least a basic understanding of chemistry through the currently important areas of work on naturally occurring toxicants in food. It covers a broader range of topics than in Watson, D. (1987) *Natural Toxicants in Food: Progress and Prospects*, Ellis Horwood. As editor, I have adopted the same general approach as was used in a book on a related subject (Watson, D. [1993] *Safety of Chemicals in Food: Chemical Contaminants*, Woodhead Publishing/Ellis Horwood).

The intended audience for this book includes scientists, technologists and managers. Since this audience is international, every effort has been made to adopt a global perspective in marshalling the facts, figures and issues. However, it is an unavoidable fact that scientific work on some natural toxicants—for example those in plants—is carried out mainly in the USA, Australasia and Europe. This has been something of a constraint in presenting a truly global picture. Nevertheless I hope that this book will encourage wider interest in natural toxicants in food. Because scientific work on natural toxicants in food can be complex, every effort has been made to spell out the main points (and abbreviations!).

I would like to emphasise that those contributing to this book are expressing their own views, not those of the organizations that employ them. My thanks go to them for all their hard work, and to my colleagues and friends for their considerable understanding whilst this book was causing me the usual birth pangs.

I hope readers find this book interesting and stimulating. It was fun to compile!

David Watson

# Contributors

| | |
|---|---|
| **Dr Daphne Aldridge** | c/o Dr C. Tahourdin, Food Contaminants Division, Room 209, Joint Food Safety and Standards Group, Ergon House, 17 Smith Square, London SW1P 3JR, UK |
| **Dr Fiona Angus** | Scientific and Technical Information, Leatherhead Food Research Association, Randalls Road, Leatherhead, Surrey KT22 7RY, UK |
| **Dr Raymond Coker** | Process Quality Management Group, National Resources Institute, Central Avenue, Chatham Maritime, Chatham, Kent ME4 4TB, UK |
| **Mr Colin Crews** | MAFF Central Science Laboratory, Food Science Laboratory, Norwich Research Park, Colney Lane, Norwich, Norfolk NR4 7UQ, UK |
| **Dr Matthijs Dekker** | Department of Food Technology and Nutrition Sciences, Integrated Food Science Group, Agricultural University Wageningen, PO Box 8129, 6700 EV Wageningen, The Netherlands |
| **Dr David Gray** | Food Research Centre, The Robert Gordon University, St Andrew Street, Aberdeen AB25 1HG, UK |
| **Dr Fiona Hannah** | University Marine Biological Station, Millport, Isle of Cumbrae KA28 0EG, UK |
| **Professor Wim M.F. Jongen** | Department of Food Technology and Nutrition Sciences, Integrated Food Science Group, Agricultural University Wageningen, PO Box 8129, 6700 EV Wageningen, The Netherlands |
| **Dr Helen Kay** | Food Research Centre, The Robert Gordon University, St Andrew Street, Aberdeen AB25 1HG, UK |

**Dr John Leftley**            Scottish Association for Marine Science, Dunstaffnage Marine Laboratory, PO Box 3, Oban, Argyll PA34 4AD, UK

**Dr Ian Millar**             Food Research Centre, The Robert Gordon University, St Andrew Street, Aberdeen AB25 1HG, UK

**Mr Andrew Moore**           Room 415, Joint Food Safety and Standards Group, Ergon House, 17 Smith Square, London SW1P 3JR, UK

**Dr G.E. Neal**              MRC Toxicology Unit, Hodgkin Building, Lancaster Road, University of Leicester, Leicester LE1 9HN, UK

**Mr Keith Scudamore**        KAS Mycotoxins, 6 Fern Drive, Taplow, Maidenhead, Berks SL6 0JS, UK

**Dr Caroline Tahourdin**     Food Contaminants Division, Room 209, Joint Food Safety and Standards Group, Ergon House, 17 Smith Square, London SW1P 3JR, UK

**Dr David Tennant**          TAS International, 31 Dover Street, London W1X 3RA, UK

**Dr Ruud Verkerk**           Department of Food Technology and Nutrition Sciences, Integrated Food Science Group, Agricultural University Wageningen, PO Box 8129, 6700 EV Wageningen, The Netherlands

**Dr David Watson**           Room 212, Joint Food Safety and Standards Group, Ergon House, 17 Smith Square, London SW1P 3JR, UK

**Dr Roger Wood**             Food Labelling and Standards Division, Joint Food Safety and Standards Group, CSL Food Science Laboratory, Norwich Research Park, Colney Lane, Norwich NR4 7UQ, UK

# Contents

**4 Natural oestrogenic compounds**      **55**

## D. ALDRIDGE AND C. S. M. TAHOURDIN

**5 Nut allergens**      **84**

## F. ANGUS

**8  Phycotoxins in seafood**      **182**

J. W. LEFTLEY AND F. HANNAH

**9    The control of natural toxicants**                               **227**
     A. MOORE

     9.1   Introduction                                               227
     9.2   The regulation of aflatoxins in the UK                     227
     9.3   Other national and international control of aflatoxins     229
     9.4   Control of other mycotoxins                                231
     9.5   Other natural toxicants                                    232
     9.6   Problems with legislation                                  233
     9.7   UK regulations on inherent toxicants                       234
     9.8   Regulations in other countries                            234
     9.9   Consequences of legislation                                234
           9.9.1   Changes in practices                               234
           9.9.2   Changes to the properties of foodstuffs            234
     9.10  The future of regulation in this area                      235
     9.11  Conclusions                                                235

**10  Quality assurance**                                               **236**
     R. WOOD

     10.1  Introduction                                               236
           10.1.1  European Union - Food Control Directives           236
           10.1.2  Codex Alimentarius Commission                      237
     10.2  Accreditation                                              239
     10.3  Internal Quality Control: harmonised guidelines for internal quality
           control in analytical chemistry laboratories               240
           10.3.1  Basic concepts                                     240
           10.3.2  Scope of the guidelines                            241
           10.3.3  Internal Quality Control and uncertainty           242
           10.3.4  Recommendations in the guidelines                  243
     10.4  Proficiency testing                                        245
           10.4.1  What is proficiency testing?                       245
           10.4.2  Why proficiency testing is important               245
           10.4.3  ISO/IUPAC/AOACI harmonised protocol for proficiency
                   testing of (chemical) analytical laboratories      246
     10.5  Methods of analysis                                        250
           10.5.1  AOAC International                                 251
           10.5.2  The European Union                                 251
           10.5.3  The Codex Alimentarius Commission                  252
           10.5.4  European Committee for Standardization (CEN)       254
           10.5.5  Requirements of official bodies for methods of analysis 255
           10.5.6  Collaborative trials                               256
           10.5.7  Assessment of the acceptability of the precision characteristics
                   of a method of analysis                            259
           10.5.8  Summary of requirements for a collaborative trial  260
     10.6  Recovery factors: development of an internationally agreed protocol for the 260
           use of recovery factors
           10.6.1  Introduction                                       260

# 1 Introduction

David Watson

## 1.1 What are natural toxicants?

Surprisingly for such a large and important group of substances, there is no standard definition of natural toxicants. They are generally understood to be chemicals with potentially toxic effects on human beings as a result of their natural occurrence in food. The natural occurrence of these toxicants arises from their production by living organisms.

Natural toxicants in food can originate in plants, bacteria, algae, fungi and, arguably, animals. Taking those in plants first, they can reach our plates from the harvesting of crops that are then sold to us direct or in processed form, or are fed to food-producing animals. Farm animals can in some cases act as a biological barrier between natural toxicants in animal feed and meat-eating or milk-drinking consumers. This generally depends on whether or not the animal's own metabolism can detoxify the natural toxicant or the animal can excrete the toxicant. If neither of these processes remove the toxicant, it is likely to occur in food.

It is not generally considered that animals themselves produce natural toxicants, although some of the substances produced by animals may have effects on our health. One can rationalise this scientifically: substances in animals that might harm our health are produced by primary metabolism, i.e. the processes necessary for life. Natural toxicants in plants, fungi, algae and bacteria are produced in another way, by secondary metabolism, which gives the organism its particular characteristics. Although this difference between substances produced by animals and those formed by other living organisms is useful it really only identifies differences in the origins of two different types of natural toxicant. Nevertheless it is convention that animal metabolites are not considered to be natural toxicants. This approach is followed in this book, except in one place: there is mention of hormone-disrupting substances from food-producing animals in Chapter 4. Scientific work on these substances is crossing many traditional scientific barriers in its search to identify the main sources of exposure to hormone-disrupting substances in our diet.

The routes by which we are exposed to bacterial toxins are quite direct— these natural toxicants are generated by bacteria in food or in our gastro-intestinal tracts. Bacterial toxins produced in food are reviewed in this book.

Toxicants produced by algae contaminate our food by one main route, directly up the food chain, for example from toxigenic (toxin-producing) algae that are consumed by some filter-feeding molluscs which we in turn eat.

Of all the potential sources of natural toxicants in our diet, fungi are probably the most ubiquitous. The natural toxicants that are produced by some fungi are called mycotoxins. These toxicants can contaminate our food at virtually any stage in its production.

Research on natural toxicants in the diet is carried out across the world. For example there are extensive data in the scientific literature on the presence of some mycotoxins, particularly aflatoxins, in food in very many countries. However, much scientific work is still needed, particularly on the toxicology of many natural toxicants. For example cycasin, which is produced by cycads, a source of food starch in some parts of the tropics, appears to be both neurotoxic (toxic to the nervous system) and carcinogenic (a cause of cancer). This is one example among many where more is known about the presence in food of a natural toxicant than about whether that toxicant is actually toxic to man. This makes it difficult to define what the risk is, if any, of eating cycad starch or the many other foods across the world that contain natural toxicants of unknown potency.

## 1.2   What is the effect of natural toxicants in food on us?

The possible effects of natural toxicants, as a group of substances, include most of the common chronic (long-term) illnesses such as cancer. It is not surprising that these effects have been suggested since they are the ones that are most commonly looked for in experimental work on the toxicity of chemicals. The difficulty is in relating information about the presence of natural toxicants in the diet to us as consumers. The objective is to determine the likely incidence of illness from exposure to known amounts of a given natural toxicant in the diet. It is less difficult to estimate exposure and hence risk for the relatively few natural toxicants, such as bacterial and algal toxins, that have fairly immediate effects on us. This is because the time between eating contaminated food and the onset of illness is relatively short, so there is more chance of finding out which food caused the illness. However, even for these toxicants it can sometimes be difficult to establish the link between cause and effect. Where an illness might have arisen as a result of consuming a particular foodstuff from time to time over a period of years, establishing the exact cause is extremely difficult.

## 1.3   Scientific work on natural toxicants in food

A lot of scientific work has been done on a few natural toxicants and much less on others. There are several reasons for this, not least history. The idea that a natural chemical present in food or feed might cause illness was given credence about 30 years ago when aflatoxins were found to be the cause of a major outbreak of illness in turkeys. This stimulated a lot of research on mycotoxins. However, most of the work was done on only a few of the many fungal toxins that might be found in the food chain. Much of this effort was on the mycotoxins' chemistry rather than on their toxicology (which as a discipline often requires considerably more resources than chemistry to establish a scientific finding). It is still not known whether many of the mycotoxins are likely to be toxic to man or farm animals. Much the same can be said about many toxicants from food plants: there is a shortage of toxicological information compared with information about their chemistry.

The application of chemical methodology to scientific work on natural toxicants in food has certainly become widespread. In particular, methods of chemically separating and purifying natural toxicants have become widely used over the last 20 years. The main methods used are: high performance liquid chromatography, gas chromatography and mass spectrometry, which were originally developed for use in chemistry and immunoassay techniques, which were originally used in biochemical research. Using these methods in research on natural toxicants has helped to reduce detection limits to parts per million or better for many toxicants in food. There has also been a growth in the application of analytical quality assurance to ensure the quality of the scientific results. The use of quality assurance is considered in Chapter 10. These developments have also occurred in many other areas of food analysis, for example in work on the chemical contamination of food.

Some of the most important work still to be done on the effects of natural toxicants in food is in the investigation of possible links between localised high incidences of diet-related diseases and their possible origins in natural toxicants in food. At the moment the evidence for such links is at best speculative. For example, a high incidence of oral cancer in central and south-east Asia appears to be related to chewing betel quid (a mixture of betel nut, betel leaf and lime). The toxicants responsible have not been identified, however. Indeed the cancer may be caused by tobacco, which is often used in conjunction with betel quid. Current ways of quantifying exposure to natural toxicants in food are described in Chapter 11.

There has been limited progress in developing methods of removing natural toxicants from food. Given the emphasis on chemistry as opposed to toxicology in research on natural toxicants in food, this is perhaps not surprising. Both of these disciplines need to be applied before risk can be identified and the need established for methods of detoxification. The use of chemical methods of detoxification has been primarily explored to reduce aflatoxin contamination (Chapter 12), where the use of ammonia and steam has been applied on an industrial scale to degrade aflatoxins in some subtropical crops. The use of biological methods of control, for example removing or disabling genes that code for toxicants from the respective food-producing plants, has not progressed as far as one might perhaps have expected, given the rapid progress in the development of genetic engineering in recent years.

## 1.4   Key examples of natural toxicants

The choice of natural toxicants to review in detail in this book has not been easy. Few books on the subject cover even similar sets of toxicants. However, in the last three decades it has become clear that in addition to the foodborne toxicants that are widely accepted as potential risks to the consumer, i.e. bacterial and algal toxins (Chapters 6 and 8), risk may also arise from some fungal toxins (Chapter 7) and some toxicants produced by some food plants. The picture has become particularly clear on two groups of toxicants from plants: the glucosinolates (Chapter 3) and the pyrrolizidine alkaloids (Chapter 2). There has also been progress in research and a considerable growth in interest in hormone-disrupting natural toxicants (Chapter 4) and nut allergens (Chapter 5).

## 1.5   Some examples of other natural toxicants in food

As the science of natural toxicants is still developing, one or more of the substances that are briefly reviewed below may prove to be as important as the natural toxicants reviewed in subsequent chapters of this book. The examples described below are natural toxicants in plants. The many mycotoxins that might be of importance, but which do not warrant detailed description at present in a book of this type, are listed at the end of Chapter 7. The bacterial and algal toxins are relatively few in number; all the relevant substances are reviewed in detail in Chapters 6 and 8, respectively.

### 1.5.1   Psoralens
These substances have been found in many plants, including members of three plant families: the Umbelliferae (e.g. celery), the Leguminosae (legumes) and the Rutaceae (citrus fruits).

Three psoralens have been studied in detail: xanthotoxin, bergapten and psoralen itself. Until recently relatively little was known about the levels of these compounds in most of the food plants in which they might occur, with the exception of parsnips and celery. However, a major survey in the UK (Ministry of Agriculture, Fisheries and Food, 1996) found high levels in limes as well as in parsnips and celery. Levels were reduced by cooking, particularly boiling.

The toxicology of these compounds has been studied quite extensively in relation to the use of xanthotoxin and bergapten, in conjunction with exposure to ultra-violet A radiation, to treat psoriasis and other skin diseases. Whilst this is clearly not of direct relevance to the possible effects of oral exposure to these substances in the diet, it forms a useful reference point. In their consideration of the UK survey, the Committee on Toxicity of Chemicals in Food, Consumer Products and the Environment concluded that the likelihood of any risk to health from dietary intakes of such substances is very small (Ministry of Agriculture, Fisheries and Food, 1996). More recently the psoralens have been implicated in adverse reactions to some antihistamine preparations.

### 1.5.2 Cyanogenic and other glycosides

Cyanogenic glycosides (cyanogen[et]ic glycosides) have been found in stone fruit kernels and lima beans (Liener, 1966). These substances are not themselves toxic, but on hydrolysis hydrocyanic acid (HCN) is released. This process takes places in two steps (Figure 1.1): hydrolysis leading to the release of two glucose molecules, and decomposition of the α-hydroxynitrile formed to give a carbonyl compound and free hydrocyanic acid. HCN produced by cyanogenic glycosides in edible plants may enter the organism via the lungs, gastro-intestinal tract and skin. In humans the lethal dose after oral administration lies between 0.5 and 3.5 mg HCN/kg body weight. Consumption of foods containing cyanogenic glycosides by humans has very rarely resulted in cyanide poisoning. However, major livestock losses have occurred due to their consuming cyanogenic glycosides. Cattle and other ruminants are more sensitive to these glycosides because the near-neutral pH in their stomachs favours the release of HCN. Incidents of livestock losses typically involve the consumption of forage sorghums and wild cherries.

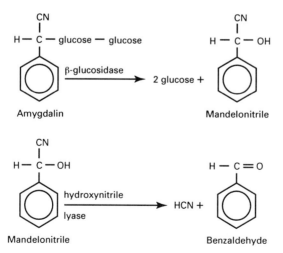

**Figure 1.1**

There are many other glycosides in plants (Table 1.1), but there is too little information about their toxicology to judge whether any of these substances in plants used for food or feed is a potential risk to consumers or animals.

**Table 1.1** Some plant glycosides

| Glycoside | Family | Species | Common name |
|---|---|---|---|
| Acacipetalin | Leguminosae | *Acacia* species | Acacias |
| Cyanolipids | Sapindaceae | Many species | |
| Dhurrin | Graminae | *Sorghum* species | Sorghum |
| Linamarin | Euphorbiaceae | *Manihot esculentum* | Cassava |
| | Linaceae | *Linum usitatissimum* L. | Flax |
| | Leguminosae | *Lotus corniculatus* L. | Bird's foot trefoil |
| | | *Trifolium repens* L. | White clover |
| Lotaustralin | Leguminosae | *Lotus australis* L. | Clover |
| Prunasin | Rosaceae | *Prunus* species | Cherries |

### 1.5.3 Bracken carcinogen

Bracken (*Pteridium aquilinum*) is consumed in Japan. The young fern is boiled in water before consumption. This is believed to remove the toxic principles. There have been many observations that bracken may cause cancer in some farm animals, notably cattle, but these were mainly where very large amounts of the plant were consumed. There are limited human epidemiological data (Ministry of Agriculture, Fisheries and Food, 1996) but nevertheless there has been an extensive search for the carcinogenic principle in bracken and many candidate compounds have been identified (Table 1.2). Despite this considerable effort it is not known which substance in bracken is carcinogenic. The UK Committee on Toxicity of Chemicals in Food, Consumer Products and the Environment has concluded that the risk to the population is very low (Ministry of Agriculture, Fisheries and Food, 1996).

### 1.5.4 Glycoalkaloids

These toxicants are found in greened potatoes and at lower levels in normal potatoes (*Solanum tuberosum*). Although the glycoalkaloids are often described as Solanum alkaloids they are found only at very low levels, if at all, in another Solanum, the tomato.

High levels of these alkaloids cause gastro-enteritis. Although a tolerance of 20 mg of alkaloids per 100 g fresh tuber weight has been generally accepted, there are continuing doubts about whether this value is too low. However, it has proved an effective guide to the suitability of new varieties of potato. Indeed if this standard had been in place in 1968, the new variety *Lenape* would not have been put on the market in North America (Morgan and Coxon, 1987). Two years after its introduction this variety was withdrawn because glycoalkaloids made the potatoes taste bitter (Morgan and

**Table 1.2**  The search for the carcinogenic principle in bracken

| Extract | Test | Result |
|---|---|---|
| Acidic fraction of urine from cattle fed on bracken fern | Implantation of pellets containing the fraction into the urinary bladder of mice | + |
| Methanol extract of bracken fern | Implantation of pellets containing the fraction into the urinary bladder of mice | + |
| Shikimic acid | Intraperitoneal injection or intragastric administration in mice | + |
| Pterosin and pteroside Pteridolactam | Feeding experiment in rats Urinary bladder implantation in mice, feeding or intragastric administration in rats | – – |
| Tannin Shikimic acid | Urinary bladder implantation in mice Feeding experiment in rats | + – |
| Tannin and tannin-free fraction of bracken fern | Subcutaneous injection of tannin fraction Diet containing tannin fraction Chloroform fraction Tannin-free fraction given to rats | + – + + |
| Quercetin | Feeding experiment     Rats     Mice | +/– – |

Coxon, 1987). This is one of several examples of natural toxicants, psoralens are another (Soborg et al., 1996), which act as a form of defence for the plant that produces them. Where defence is not the reason it is usually unclear why natural toxicants are produced. Not knowing why they are produced is one of several difficulties in controlling them in food. Current controls in western Europe are described in Chapter 9.

## 1.6  Summary

Natural toxicants are generally understood to be chemicals with potentially toxic effects on human beings as a result of their natural occurrence in food. These toxicants can originate in plants, bacteria, algae, fungi and, arguably, animals, and have been found in food across the world.

There has been a considerable amount of scientific work carried out on a few natural toxicants in food and much of this research has been on their chemistry. Whilst the application of chemical methodology to scientific work on natural toxicants in food has become widespread, there has been less progress on the toxicology of many natural toxicants and in developing methods of removing them from food.

In the last three decades it has become clear that in addition to the food-borne toxicants that are widely accepted as potential risks to the consumer (bacterial and algal toxins), risk may also arise from some fungal toxins in food and a limited range of toxicants in some food-producing plants. There has also been a considerable growth in interest in hormone-disrupting natural toxicants and nut allergens. As the science of natural toxicants is still developing, one or more of the following substances in plants may also prove to be important to food safety: psoralens, cyanogenic glycosides, bracken carcinogen and glycoalkaloids.

## Dedication and Acknowledgement

To A.E.W.


## References

Liener, I.E. (1966) Cyanogenetic glycosides, in *Toxicants Occurring Naturally in Foods* (eds. J.M. Coon and J.L. Powers), National Academy of Sciences/National Research Council Publication 1354, Washington DC, pp. 58-61.

Ministry of Agriculture, Fisheries and Food (1996) Inherent natural toxicants in food, Food Surveillance Paper No. 51, HMSO, London.

Morgan, M.R.A. and Coxon, D.T. (1987) Tolerances: glycoalkaloids in potatoes, in *Natural Toxicants in Food: Progress and Prospects* (ed. D.H. Watson), Ellis Horwood, Chichester, pp. 221-30.

Soborg, I., Andersson, C. and Gry, J. (1996) Furocoumarins in plant food—exposure, biological properties, risk assessment and recommendations. *TemaNord* **600**, available from HMSO, London, and UNIPUB, Lanham, Maryland.

# The Chemistry and Toxicology
# of Natural Toxicants in Food

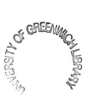

# 2  Pyrrolizidine alkaloids

Colin Crews

## 2.1  Introduction

Among the many chemical compounds ingested when plants are consumed, the alkaloids perhaps have the most potent action on bodily function. These effects are often harmful, but sometimes beneficial or desired, leading to the intentional ingestion of many alkaloid-containing plants as medicines or intoxicants. Consumption of toxic alkaloids in some plants elicits a response that may be delayed by years and in this circumstance the toxicity of the plant might be unobserved or denied by the subject.

Alkaloids are basic nitrogenous compounds in which the nitrogen is usually contained within a heterocyclic ring system. Most are derived from amino acids by biosynthesis, although others are derived from triterpenes. Their functions in the plant are relatively poorly understood but are possibly linked to a protective function as they appear to act as feeding deterrents to a wide range of animals, from insects to herbivorous mammals. The potent pharmacological action of the alkaloids has led to intensive study and a wealth of literature has been established; recent reviews include those of Cooper-Driver (1983), Cheeke (1989), Rizk (1991a), Hartmann (1991) and Huxtable (1992).

The alkaloids are widely distributed, occurring in some 20% of flowering plants, however, this chapter will concentrate on the group of alkaloids that is perhaps of greatest significance to humans, the pyrrolizidine alkaloids, which occur in a wide variety of food plants. With the exception of the ubiquitous caffeine these are the naturally occurring alkaloids most likely to be ingested in foodstuffs. Some other alkaloids present in a narrower range of foods or food raw materials are the lupines, tropanes, berberine and the ergot alkaloids.

Many alkaloids, such as berberine, atropine, lobeline, sparteine, hydrastine and the pyrrolizidines, occur in plants prepared as medicines, which often are dried tissues or tinctures that could provide dangerously high dosages. In Europe and the USA consumer demand and commercial promotion have led to a large increase in the consumption of potentially dangerous plants that are usually described as beneficial herbs.

## 2.2 The pyrrolizidine alkaloids

Pyrrolizidine alkaloids are toxic secondary metabolites of a wide variety of plants found in various environments throughout the world, from the colder temperate climates to sparsely vegetated hot dry regions. Plants containing pyrrolizidines have been responsible for numerous outbreaks of poisoning of livestock on several continents and continue to cause serious economic damage. Although most of the respective pasture-contaminating plants are unpalatable to grazing animals, they may be foraged in times of food shortage or ingested via contaminated silage. In recent years pyrrolizidine alkaloids have been identified as causing human deaths in less developed countries as a result of contamination of cereal crops and harvested seed, and they have been suspected of causing illness following intentional ingestion as vegetables and in the form of herbal remedies. Several authors have described specific aspects of pyrrolizidine chemistry and toxicity or have given overviews: some of the more comprehensive reviews have been presented by Bull *et al.* (1968), Peterson and Culvenor (1983), Mattocks (1986), World Health Organisation (1988) and Rizk (1991b).

### 2.2.1 Structures

The pyrrolizidine structure is based upon two fused five-membered rings that share a bridgehead nitrogen atom, forming a tertiary alkaloid. In nature the rings are most frequently substituted with a hydroxymethylene group at position C-1 and a simple hydroxyl group at position C-7, forming a structure known as a necine base. The bases most commonly encountered are heliotridine and retronecine, which differ only in their configuration about C-7 as shown in Figure 2.1.

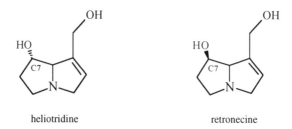

heliotridine                    retronecine

**Figure 2.1**   The pyrrolizidine bases heliotridine and retronecine.

The necine base alcohols are normally esterified with any of a series of characteristic (necic) acids to form pyrrolizidine alkaloids. The esterification may be in the form of C-1 mono-esters, open-chain diesters or, more frequently, a macrocyclic diester. The substituting acids are mostly highly branched chains of five to ten carbon atoms substituted with methyl, methylene, hydroxyl and/or keto groups, producing several isomeric alkaloids. Summaries of the structures of many of the pyrrolizidine alkaloids, especially those most commonly associated with human toxicity, have been assembled by Rizk (1991b), Hartmann and Witte (1995) and Roeder (1995).

Over 250 pyrrolizidine alkaloids have so far been identified and characterised. Examples of two important representatives are shown in Figure 2.2.
These share the base retronecine but differ in their esterification. In senecionine, which is one of the more widespread pyrrolizidine alkaloids [found for
example in ragworts (*Senecio* spp.)] the base is esterified with the cyclic ten-
carbon senecic acid. In acetyllycopsamine, which is a major alkaloid of the
comfreys (*Symphytum* spp.), the C-7 alcohol is esterified with acetic acid
and the C-9 alcohol with viridifloric acid.

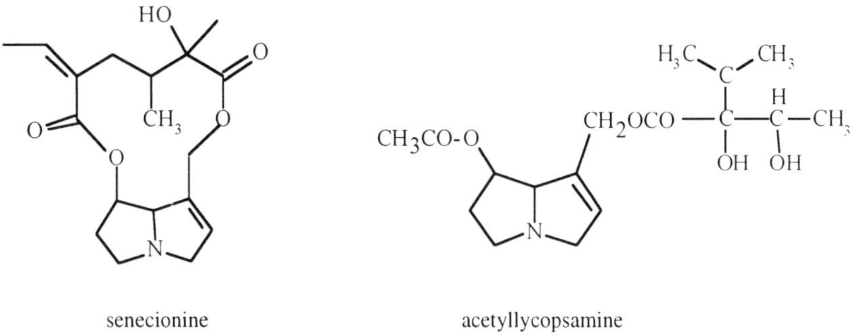

senecionine                              acetyllycopsamine

**Figure 2.2**   Two typical pyrrolizidine alkaloids: senecionine and acetyllycopsamine.

Many pyrrolizidine alkaloid structures have been synthesised, particularly with a view to the study of antimitotic effects of some compounds that
have potential as antitumour agents. Recent developments in this field have
been summarised in publications by Robins (1995) and Liddell (1996).

### 2.2.2 Occurrence

Pyrrolizidines are found mainly in the families Compositae (Asteraceae),
Boraginacea and Leguminosae, but also in Apocyanacae, Ranunculacae and
Scrophulariacae. The genera *Senecio, Eupatorium, Symphytum, Cynoglossum, Heliotropium* and *Crotalaria* contain the species most frequently associated with human illness. These genera are widely distributed throughout
different climates and their pyrrolizidine alkaloid-containing species could
comprise as much as 3% of the world's flowering plants (Smith and
Culvenor, 1981). Comprehensive lists of plants containing unsaturated
pyrrolizidine alkaloids have been published (Smith and Culvenor, 1981;
Mattocks, 1986; Rizk, 1991b; Hartmann and Witte, 1995). Each species has
an unusually specific range of pyrrolizidine alkaloids and a specific ratio of
free base to N-oxide (Molyneux and James, 1990). Some may contain
essentially only a single pyrrolizidine alkaloid but most contain between
five and eight.

Alkaloid content varies between species, plant organ and season, but can be up to several per cent of the plant's dry weight. In general, levels are considerably higher in roots than in leaves and they are higher in buds, inflorescences and young leaves than in older leaves. In some species, notably *Crotalaria*, high levels (up to 5% dry weight) have been found in the seed (Johnson and Molyneux, 1984; Johnson *et al.*, 1985), presenting a serious threat to health in cases of contamination of grain intended for human consumption. Several necine bases lack the 1,2 unsaturation and their alkaloids are relatively non-toxic. These saturated pyrrolizidine alkaloids may be found associated with their toxic counterparts in particular species, but they are much less widespread.

### 2.2.3 Formation and function

The biosynthetic routes of some of the major pyrrolizidine alkaloids have been elucidated, largely by means of radiotracer experiments (Robins, 1989). In the biosynthesis of the base retronecine, depending on plant species, either L-ornithine or L-arginine or both are combined to form two molecules of putrescine. The biosynthesis proceeds via homospermidine as shown in Figure 2.3.

The necic acids are synthesised from the α-amino acids L-valine, L-leucine, L-isoleucine and L-threonine by the route compiled by Roeder (1995) and illustrated in Figure 2.4. These reactions occur in the roots of the plant where the primary product in most species studied is the N-oxide (Hartmann and Toppel, 1987; van Dam *et al.*, 1994). This is much more water-soluble than the base and can be transported within the plant. The mechanism and purpose of pyrrolizidine alkaloid transport are not yet well understood, but the alkaloids are specifically channelled via the phloem to the younger leaves and flowering parts of the plant, where they accumulate. The purpose of this is possibly to provide important tissues with a deterrent towards herbivores. Many grazing animals avoid eating plants that contain pyrrolizidine alkaloids, although sheep and goats have some tolerance. Some insects, particularly certain moths and butterflies, accumulate the toxins, which they can then use as a defence against predators or as intermediates in the production of substituted carbonyl pyrrolizidines that act as pheromones. Concise and informative reviews have been published describing the varied functions and uses of pyrrolizidine alkaloids by insects (Boppré, 1990; Hartmann and Witte, 1995).

### 2.2.4 Human exposure

The two most significant sources of exposure of humans to pyrrolizidine alkaloids are the accidental contamination of foodstuffs and the intentional ingestion of plants containing pyrrolizidine alkaloids in the form of culinary vegetables or herbal medicines. The incidence of pyrrolizidine poisoning of

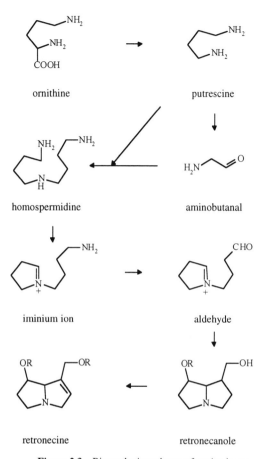

ornithine                                        putrescine

homospermidine                                   aminobutanal

iminium ion                                      aldehyde

retronecine                                      retronecanole

**Figure 2.3**  Biosynthetic pathway of necine bases.

humans has probably been underestimated owing to the lack of association between plants and disease, poor recognition of chronic effects, and the time lag between ingestion and the appearance of symptoms in sub-acute poisoning (Roitman, 1983).

Serious and wide-scale incidents of illness have been reported through contamination of cereal grains with the seeds of pyrrolizidine alkaloid-containing plants. In 1976 in Afghanistan over 20% of a population of 7200 villagers who had consumed wheat contaminated with the seed of *Heliotropium* showed signs of liver disease (Mohabbat *et al.*, 1976). The wheat had been consumed over a period of two years with an estimated minimum intake of 1.5 g of the alkaloid in the form of the N-oxide. In the previous year contamination of local grain heavily contaminated with seeds of *Crotalaria* species was responsible for the death of 28 patients from 67 people affected in four villages in India (Tandon *et al.*, 1976).

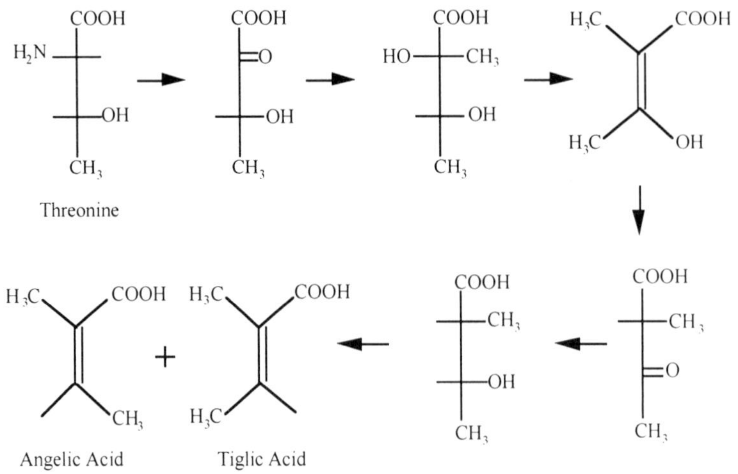

**Figure 2.4** Biosynthetic pathway of necic acids.

Contamination of foods on a smaller scale occurs where there is an intermediate agent between the plant source and the foodstuff. Examples of this are the transfer of pyrrolizidine alkaloids from plants into milk by herbivores and into honey by bees. Both of these routes have been established but have caused little concern due to the low levels of alkaloid involved. The transfer of pyrrolizidines from plants into animal tissue that might be consumed by humans has not been convincingly demonstrated. The carcinogenic nature of some pyrrolizidine alkaloids means, however, that there might be risk to those populations who consume low levels of pyrrolizidine alkaloids over extended periods.

The proportion of pyrrolizidine alkaloids passed into milk from goats fed *Senecio jacobaea* (ragwort) was determined to be about 0.1% of that ingested (Deinzer *et al.*, 1982). Radiotracer studies using *Senecio* alkaloids fed to lactating mice showed similar levels with the bulk of the remainder being excreted in the urine (Eastman *et al.*, 1982). With the pooling of milk samples being widespread practice, any risk to health is probably confined to the consumption of milk from individual animals and particularly species such as goats, which are comparatively willing to eat pyrrolizidine-containing plants (Molyneux and James, 1990).

Relatively high concentrations (up to 4 mg/kg) of pyrrolizidines have been measured in honey produced from *S. jacobaea* (Deinzer and Thompson, 1977; Crews *et al.*, 1997) and *Echium plantagineum* (Culvenor *et al.*, 1981). Ragwort is avoided by most grazing animals and has become a prolific weed in many climates. It can sometimes be the predominant nectar source in some localities during its flowering season (Figure 2.5). There is therefore considerable potential for the localised contamination of honey. Although honey from individual hives in areas of high ragwort density might accumulate high levels of alkaloids, beekeepers can usually recognise ragwort contamination of the honey and take action to remove it from the food chain. Honey containing high levels of nectar from *S. jacobaea* is unpalatable due to a strong butyric odour, but at lower levels of contamination the product is sometimes blended with uncontaminated honey.

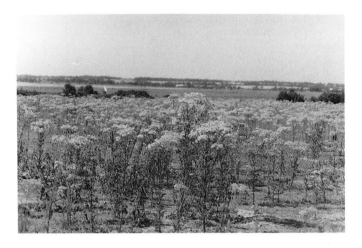

**Figure 2.5** Ragwort (*Senecio jacobaea*).

Honeys produced in study hives situated adjacent to sites in the UK where ragwort flowered were found to contain ragwort pollen and ragwort alkaloids (senecionine, seneciphylline, jacobine, jacoline and jacozine). The alkaloid concentrations ranged from 0.01 to 0.06 mg/kg but were not correlated to the pollen levels (Crews *et al.*, 1997). Honeys produced and sold in a region of ragwort growth in the UK did not contain detectable levels of pyrrolizidine alkaloids and the alkaloid contribution of honey to the diet does not cause concern (Ministry of Agriculture, Fisheries and Food, 1995). Results from the analysis of honeys from study hives near ragwort sites, ragwort-contaminated honey and retail honey produced in areas of ragwort growth are shown in Table 2.1.

Many plants that contain pyrrolizidine alkaloids are deliberately consumed as food or herbal remedies in all parts of the world and reports of such use have been assembled (Mattocks, 1986; Hirono, 1993). In Japan plants of *Petasites*, *Symphytum* and *Tussilago* are eaten as vegetables, although in other countries the major uses are medicinal. Increasing interest in 'alternative' therapies and herbal medicines in Europe and the USA has led to preparations of pyrrolizidine-alkaloid-containing plants being made

**Table 2.1**  Concentrations of pyrrolizidine alkaloids and ragwort pollen in honeys from study hives, ragwort-contaminated honey and retail honey.

| Honey source | Date | Ragwort pollen (%) | Alkaloid concentration (mg/kg) | | | | | |
|---|---|---|---|---|---|---|---|---|
| | | | Jacoline | Jacozine | Jacobine | Seneciphylline | Senecionine | Total |
| Study hive | 071394 | 0.1 | —[a] | — | — | — | — | — |
| Study hive | 072094 | 0 | — | — | — | — | — | — |
| Study hive | 073094 | 5.5 | — | 0.009 | 0.0025 | 0.009 | 0.013 | 0.056 |
| Study hive | 080594 | 8.9 | — | 0.006 | 0.019 | 0.007 | 0.008 | 0.040 |
| Study hive | 081094 | 6.3 | — | — | 0.005 | 0.003 | 0.003 | 0.001 |
| Study hive | 081794 | 3.5 | — | 0.003 | 0.010 | 0.004 | 0.005 | 0.022 |
| Ragwort | 1990 | 4.4 | 0.006 | 0.020 | 0.031 | 0.260 | 1.160 | 1.477 |
| Ragwort | 1994 | 2.0 | 0.003 | 0.012 | 0.025 | 0.070 | 0.310 | 0.420 |
| Retail | 1994 | 1.1 | — | — | — | — | — | — |
| Retail | 1994 | 0 | — | — | — | — | — | — |

[a] — = less than 0.002 mg/kg.

widely available commercially and publicised for their health-giving properties. Comfrey (*Symphytum officinale*) in particular has long been a popular herb in Europe and the USA. Preparations of comfrey in the form of
dried leaves, dried root and root powder tablets and capsules, often mixed
with other herbs, have been sold with active promotion of the plant's sup-
posed healing and digestive properties. Figure 2.6 shows dried preparations
of comfrey leaf and root intended for consumption as teas.

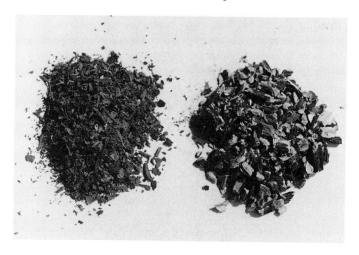

**Figure 2.6**   Comfrey herbal teas: leaf (left) and root (right).

Numerous reports of poisonings directly related to herbal teas and similar products have been published (Weston *et al.*, 1981; Kumana *et al.*, 1985;
Ridker *et al.*, 1985; Margalith *et al.*, 1985; Culvenor *et al.*, 1986; Ridker and
McDermott, 1989). The practice in Jamaica of brewing teas from unculti-
vated plants for medicinal purposes (bush teas) has been associated with
epidemics of pyrrolizidine poisoning (Bras *et al.*, 1954). However, government campaigns there have led to a reduction in the frequency of these incidents.

Herbal preparations of *Symphytum*, *Tussilago*, *Borago* and *Eupatorium*,
in the form of leaf, root powders, tablets and root extract tinctures, sold in
the UK in 1994 were surveyed for pyrrolizidine alkaloid content (Ministry
of Agriculture, Fisheries and Food, 1994). Comfrey (*Symphytum*) tablets
contained up to 5000 mg/kg and root powders up to 8300 mg/kg of
pyrrolizidine alkaloids, giving estimated potential intakes in excess of 35
mg/day. The alkaloids were present mainly as lycopsamine, its isomer intermedine and their 7-acetyl esters. Comfrey and borage (*Borago*) leaf preparations intended for consumption as teas contained less than 100 mg/kg total
pyrrolizidine alkaloids. Experiments to estimate the dose delivered by brew-

ing comfrey leaf teas indicated an extraction into the water of about 50% of the total acetyllycopsamine and symphytine but only about 5% of the lycopsamine. This unexpected effect was possibly due to binding of the more polar lycopsamine to the plant tissue.

A survey of comfrey leaf and root products sold in the USA in 1989 showed them to contain up to 1200 mg/kg of pyrrolizidine alkaloids (Betz *et al.*, 1994). Teas prepared from comfrey root and leaf showed preferential extraction of acetyllycopsamine and acetylintermedine over lycopsamine and intermedine. In the USA at least seven cases of veno-occlusive disease have recently been associated with pyrrolizidine-containing herbal products (Kessler, 1993). Concerns about the safety of comfrey have led to the publication of warnings in the more responsible herbalist literature (Foster, 1992) and industry action to remove the more potent root preparations from sale (Ministry of Agriculture, Fisheries and Food, 1995).

The misidentification of plants is an additional risk to consumers of vegetables and herbs. This is particularly likely to occur where the intended plant is closely related to a more toxic species. For example, Sperl *et al.* (1995) reported a poisoning case in which *Adenostyles* had been gathered and consumed in place of the less toxic *Tussilago*, and a commercial preparation sold in the UK as 'Life root' (*Senecio aureus*) was found to contain pyrrolizidine alkaloids not present in that species (Ministry of Agriculture, Fisheries and Food, 1994). Similar and additional problems of herbal products have been described by Huxtable (1990a).

### 2.2.5 Toxicity and metabolism

The toxicity and metabolism of pyrrolizidine alkaloids have been studied and reviewed (McLean, 1970; Mattocks, 1986; Winter and Segall, 1989; Huxtable, 1990b; Segall *et al.*, 1991; Cheeke and Huan, 1995). The main details are given here.

Early experimental work involved the feeding of isolated alkaloids and pyrrolizidine-alkaloid-containing plants to sheep, cattle and horses. This has been complemented by more recent experiments on isolated organs and tissues. The relative toxicity of pyrrolizidine alkaloids towards different animals varies dramatically between animal species. Guinea pigs, hamsters, gerbils and quails show considerable resistance (Cheeke and Pierson-Goeger, 1983; Cheeke, 1994).

Pyrrolizidine N-oxides have the same toxicity in principle as their bases but as these are considerably more hydrophilic they are mainly excreted. However, there is evidence of some reabsorption in the small intestine after reduction by bacteria (Mattocks, 1971). It is clear that the N-oxides can play a major role in experimental or accidental toxicity (Moore *et al.*, 1989). Hepatotoxicity was produced in cattle by isolated riddelline N-oxide or by vegetable parts of the plant Riddell groundsel (*Senecio riddellii*) which contains predominantly riddelline N-oxide, whereas feeding of the free base alone produced no symptoms (Molyneux *et al.*, 1991).

Ingestion of pyrrolizidine alkaloids has long been associated with severe damage to the liver. The hepatic veins become blocked by a build up of connective tissue, a condition known as veno-occlusive disease. Giant cells, which are dysfunctional, develop in the liver through the intense antimitotic activity of pyrrolizidine alkaloids preventing the completion of cell division. The condition frequently leads to death. The symptoms have been shown to be identical to those of Budd–Chiari syndrome, an illness characterised by thrombosis of the hepatic veins that leads to enlargement of the liver, ascites and portal hypertension (Bull *et al.*, 1968; McLean, 1970).

Several other organs (principally the lungs) are affected by many, but not all, pyrrolizidine alkaloids as a result of the release of toxic metabolites from the liver. Monocrotaline, for example, is solely pneumotoxic. The effects on these organs become particularly apparent when the dose received is insufficient to cause rapid death through liver damage. Long-term, sublethal doses of pyrrolizidine alkaloids are usually associated with cattle exposed during grazing to plants containing them or with humans who habitually take herbal medicines or regularly consume pyrrolizidine-containing plants as vegetables. Long-term exposure to low levels of pyrrolizidine alkaloids may cause cumulative damage to body organs and cancer, but even exposure to high levels is not necessarily fatal.

*2.2.5.1 Metabolism.*    Many studies into the hepatic metabolism of pyrrolizidine alkaloids have been carried out on rats but the trend is towards using cultured organ cells where the administration and monitoring of the parent alkaloids and their metabolites can be more easily monitored and controlled.

It is well established that bioactivation of pyrrolizidine alkaloids is required to produce toxicity. Activation of toxins in the liver results from the formation of polar compounds that are conjugated to glutathione. This produces hydrophilic compounds that can be readily excreted, the intended effect being detoxification. In the case of pyrrolizidine alkaloids some of these metabolites are highly reactive and toxic. This toxicity can be demonstrated by the administration to animals of metabolites produced *in vitro*, when necrosis is produced at the injection site. Where this site is a vein, toxicity is also manifested in the lung.

The metabolism of pyrrolizidine alkaloids takes place primarily in the parenchymal cells of the liver. These reactions are hydrolysis to the parent base and acids, and oxidation to form the N-oxide and pyrroles. Additional minor reactions have been postulated or identified for various pyrrolizidine alkaloids. Pyrrole formation is considered to be responsible for toxicity. The pyrrolizidine base is converted by microsomal oxygenases into a short-lived dehydro pyrrolizidine alkaloid that either undergoes hydrolysis to form a dihydronecine pyrrole, 6,7-dihydro-7-hydroxy-1-hydroxymethyl-5H-pyrrolizine (DHP), or binds to tissue nucleophiles such as glutathione and DNA. The dihydronecine pyrrole formed from retronecine-based alkaloids is dehydroretronecine. The structures of a dehydro pyrrolizidine alkaloid and DHP are shown in Figure 2.7. Both of these metabolites have an alkylating structure and there is some controversy as to which is responsible for pyrrolizidine toxicity.

dehydrosenecionine                    dihydropyrrolizine, DHP

**Figure 2.7**  Two significant pyrrolizidine alkaloid metabolites.

Pyrrole and N-oxide formation are activated mainly by P450 cytochromes in the presence of NADPH, but the pathways appear to be independent (Mattocks and Bird, 1983a). The P450 enzymes are induced by phenobarbital and by pregnelone-16α-carbonitrile and other steroids, but the *in vitro* action of these inducers is not easily explained in terms of effects observed *in vivo* in different species and with different alkaloids (Miranda *et al.*, 1991, 1992).

The toxicity of pyrrolizidine alkaloids is related to a reactive allyl structure present in both the dehydropyrrolizidine and DHP. This can form stable carbonium ions at positions that react with OH, SH, or NH groups of proteins and nucleotides or low molecular weight species such as glutathione (Mattocks and Bird, 1983b). The reactivity depends on the stability of the leaving group, esterified pyrroles being stronger alkylating agents than dehydroretronecine because the ester is a better leaving group (Huxtable, 1990b). The necine base must have 1:2 unsaturation, esterified hydroxyl groups at C7 and/or C9, and branching of at least one of the esterifying acids in order to form toxic products (McLean, 1974).

The rates of the metabolic reactions, and the proportions of their products, depend on the type of esterification of the necine base. More lipophilic alkaloids undergo faster reaction and the non-cyclic diesters form proportionately more N-oxide (Mattocks and Bird, 1983a). Branching of the necic acid chains impairs hydrolysis through steric hindrance. The greater proportion of N-oxides formed from monoesters and open diesters might account for the lesser toxicity of these compounds compared to the cyclic diester pyrrolizidine alkaloids. The considerable toxicity shown by N-oxides possibly results from conversion to the pyrrolizidine alkaloid base in the liver (Mattocks, 1971; Couet *et al.*, 1996) rather than microbial action in the gut.

Experiments showing that metabolic detoxification pathways vary according to the animal species and the alkaloid involved have been summarised by Cheeke (1994). These variations are most likely to be due to differences between the animals' P450 enzyme systems, which catalyse the pyrrole production reactions and the conjugation reactions at different relative rates in different species (Cheeke and Huan, 1995).

Other potentially toxic pyrrolizidine alkaloid metabolites produced in the liver include unsaturated short-chain carbonyl compounds, such as hexenal products of the breakdown of senecionine (Segall *et al.*, 1985) and monocrotaline (Lanfranconi *et al.*, 1985).

### 2.2.5.2 *Extra-hepatic effects.*

Pyrrole production in the liver results in the release of reactive compounds into the bloodstream and hence to other organs, notably the lungs, which are incapable of metabolising pyrrolizidine alkaloids (Mattocks and White, 1971). The effects on the lung have been comprehensively reviewed (Huxtable, 1990b). The major effects are pulmonary arterial hypertension and right ventricular hypertrophy (Chesney *et al.*, 1974; Lanfranconi and Huxtable, 1981). Morphological changes include thickening of the arteries, an increase in tissue mass, platelet accumulation and microthrombi formation leading to occlusion. Restriction of the pulmonary artery increases blood pressure and consequently the workload on the right chambers of the heart, causing damage to that organ.

Fewer pyrrolizidine alkaloids cause damage to the lung than affect the liver, although monocrotaline is particularly active. Lung tissue damage becomes evident after a delay of 9 to 12 days from exposure to the alkaloid. Unmetabolised pyrrolizidine alkaloids appear to be excreted rapidly following administration by injection, but symptoms of activity against the lung continue to develop. This suggests that the alkaloids initiate reactions within the lung. This is supported by the finding that the same degree of damage is induced by any dose of pyrrolizidine alkaloid that is in excess of a threshold.

There is strong evidence that dehydroalkaloids, rather than DHP, are responsible for extra-hepatic toxicity. The short-lived, alkylating pyrrolic ester dehydromonocrotaline has been trapped from liver perfusions of rats given monocrotaline, suggesting that this is the metabolite released from the liver that can damage other organs (Mattocks, 1990). The corresponding hydrolysis product, dehydroretronecine, was not trapped. Thiol adducts of

DHP have been found in perfused rat livers exposed to monocrotaline. However, the dehydroalkaloid appears to be the primary cause of extra-hepatic toxicity in the rat (Yan and Huxtable, 1995). That thiol compounds have a significant role in pneumotoxicity is supported by the fact that high glutathione binding to the alkaloid metabolites reduces the toxic effect. Glutathione adduct formation, and oxidation and hydrolysis reactions are more rapid in the guinea pig than in the rat (Dueker *et al.*, 1994). This animal clearly has an effective detoxification system.

In other organs such as the kidneys and pancreas of animals intoxicated with certain pyrrolizidine alkaloids, megalocytosis and associated symptoms also occur, the most extensive studies having been made on pigs (Hooper, 1978).

Pyrrolizidine alkaloid metabolism is affected by the presence in the diet of certain minerals, particularly copper, which accumulates in excess by sheep poisoned by the alkaloids. Zinc exerts a protective effect by promoting synthesis of sulphydryl-rich proteins such as metallothionein, which can immobilise pyrroles. The nutritional interactions of pyrrolizidines with minerals and vitamins have been reviewed by Cheeke (1991).

*2.2.5.3 Genotoxic effects.*   The antimitotic effect of pyrrolizidine alkaloid metabolites is caused by binding to proteins and DNA or between separate strands of DNA. The ability of pyrrolizidine metabolites to alkylate DNA in the same position as the known carcinogen aflatoxin B1 (Chapter 7) has been shown (Niwa *et al.*, 1991). This suggests carcinogenicity and mutagenicity but in practice it has been difficult to demonstrate in animal experiments because of the alkaloids' toxicity (Roitman, 1983). Limited evidence for genotoxicity in animals of some pyrrolizidines has been described (International Agency for Research on Cancer, 1983; Hirono, 1993) but more detailed evidence has emerged from *in vitro* investigations carried out on human cell lines and on eucaryotes such as *Drosophila*.

Comparative studies on the mutagenicity of various types of pyrrolizidine alkaloid have been carried out using wing spot tests on *Drosophila melangosta*. The macrocyclic alkaloids senkirkine, monocrotaline and senecionine exhibited the strongest mutagenicity. Increasing the degree of hydroxyl substitution of the cyclic necic acid reduced the activity, which was lower still in the open chain esters acetyllycopsamine and acetylintermedine, and lowest in the alcohols lycopsamine and intermedine (Frei *et al.*, 1992).

Studies comparing the mutagenicity of individual alkaloids do not necessarily give a clear indication of the action of the mixtures of alkaloids and oxides normally encountered in the plant. Mutagenicity of the p53 tumour suppressor gene of human cell lines has been demonstrated for extract of comfrey (*Symphytum officinale*), but some of the isolated components, symphytine and its N-oxide, did not show this effect (Couet *et al.*, 1996).

## 2.3 Conclusions

Despite our increasing knowledge of their chemistry and toxicity, pyrrolizidine alkaloids continue to be a significant threat to human health. Their plant sources flourish through their diversity and lack of palatability to grazing animals. Education of people in the developing countries has reduced their exposure to harmful traditional herbal medicines. Conversely, a revival of interest in natural and alternative therapies has led to the commercial sale of toxic plant preparations in the more developed countries. The scale of the threat caused by the consumption of pyrrolizidine-containing herbs and vegetables will only be realised fully once the genotoxic action and chronic low-dose toxicity of the major alkaloids are known. The risk of large-scale poisoning through cereal contamination, however, remains serious in view of the continuing practice of consuming poor quality grain in times of drought and famine.

Investigations into the metabolism of pyrrolizidine alkaloids, the mechanism of their toxicity and their genotoxic activity proceed apace, driven by an increased awareness of their potential for causing disease and the availability of ever more sophisticated techniques for studying the action of toxic chemicals at the cellular and sub-cellular level. Because of the great variety of pyrrolizidine alkaloid structures and the diversity of their effects in different species such studies will continue for a long time.

## References

Betz, J.M., Eppley, R.M., Taylor, W.C. and Andrzejewski, D. (1994) Determination of pyrrolizidine alkaloids in commercial comfrey products (*Symphytum* sp.). *Journal of Pharmaceutical Sciences*, **83** (5) 649-53.

Boppré, M. (1990) Lepidoptera and pyrrolizidine alkaloids, exemplification of complexity in chemical ecology. *Journal of Chemical Ecology*, **16** (1) 165-85.

Bras, G., Jellife, D.B. and Stuart, K.L. (1954) Veno-occlusive disease of the liver with non-portal type of cirrhosis, occurring in Jamaica. *Archives of Pathology*, **57** 285-300.

Bull, L.B., Culvenor, C.C.J. and Dick, A.T. (1968) *The Pyrrolizidine Alkaloids: Their Chemistry, Pathogenicity and other Biological Properties*, North-Holland, Amsterdam.

Cheeke, P.R. (1989) *Toxicants of Plant Origin, Volume 1 Alkaloids*, CRC Press, Boca Raton, FL.

Cheeke, P.R. (1991) Nutritional implications of pyrrolizidine alkaloids as contaminants of foodstuffs, in *Poisonous Plant Contamination of Edible Plants* (ed. A.-F.M. Rizk), CRC Press, Boca Raton, FL, pp. 163-75.

Cheeke, P.R. (1994) A review of the functional and evolutionary roles of the liver in the detoxification of poisonous plants, with special reference to pyrrolizidine alkaloids. *Veterinary and Human Toxicology*, **36** (3) 240-47.

Cheeke, P.R. and Huan, J. (1995) Metabolism and toxicity of pyrrolizidine alkaloids, in *Phytochemicals and Health. Current Topics in Plant Physiology, 15* (eds. D.L. Gustine and H.E. Flores), American Society of Plant Physiologists, Rockville, MD, pp. 155-64.

Cheeke, P.R. and Pierson-Goeger, M.L. (1983) Toxicity of *Senecio jacobaea* and pyrrolizidine alkaloids in various laboratory animals and avian species. *Toxicological Letters*, **18** (3) 343-50.

Chesney, C.F., Allen, J.R. and Hsu, I.C. (1974) Right ventricular hypertrophy in monocrotaline pyr-role treated rats. *Experimental Molecular Pathology*, **20**.257-68.

Cooper-Driver, G.A. (1983) Chemical substances in plants toxic to animals, in *Handbook of Naturally Occurring Food Toxicants* (ed. M. Rechcigl), CRC Press, Boca Raton, FL, pp. 213-40.

Couet, C.E., Crews, C. and Hanley, A.B. (1996) Analysis, separation and bioassay of pyrrolizidine alkaloids from comfrey (*Symphytum officinale*). *Natural Toxins*, **4** 163-67.

Crews, C., Startin, J.R.S. and Clarke, P.A. (1997) Determination of pyrrolizidine alkaloids in honey from selected sites by solid phase extraction and HPLC-MS. *Food Additives and Contaminants*, **14** (5) 419-28.

Culvenor, C.C. J., Edgar, J.A. and Smith, L.W. (1981) Pyrrolizidine alkaloids in honey from *Echium plantagineum* L. *Journal of Agricultural and Food Chemistry*, **29** 958-60.

Culvenor, C.C.J., Edgar, J.A. and Smith, L.W. (1986) *Heliotropium lasiocarpum* Fisch and Mey identified as cause of veno-occlusive disease due to a herbal tea. *Lancet*, 978.

Deinzer, M.L. and Thompson, P.A. (1977) Pyrrolizidine alkaloids: their occurrence in honey from Tansy Ragwort (*Senecio jacobaea* L.). *Science*, **195** 497-99.

Deinzer, M.L., Arbogast, B.L. and Buhler, D.R. (1982) Gas chromatographic determination of pyrrolizidine alkaloids in goat's milk. *Analytical Chemistry*, **54** 1811-14.

Dueker, S.R., Lamé, M.W., Jones, A.D., Morin, D. and Segall, H.J. (1994) Glutathione conjugation with the pyrrolizidine alkaloid jacobine. *Biochemical and Biophysical Research Communications*, **198** (2) 516-22.

Eastman, D.F., Dimenna, G.P. and Segall, H.J. (1982) Covalent binding of two pyrrolizidine alka-loids, senecionine and seneciphylline, to hepatic macromolecules and their distribution, excre-tion, and transfer into milk of lactating mice. *Drug Metabolism and Disposition*, **10** 236-40.

Foster, S. (1992) Comfrey: a fading romance. *The Herb Companion*, **4** (3) 50-55.

Frei, H.J., Luthy, J., Brauchili, J., Zweifel, U., Wuergler, F.E. and Schlatter, C. (1992) Structure/activity relationships of the genotoxic potencies of sixteen pyrrolizidine alkaloids assayed for the induction of somatic mutation and recombination in wing cells of *Drosophila melangoster*. *Chemico-Biological Interactions*, **83** 1-22.

Hartmann, T. (1991) Alkaloids, in *Herbivores, their Interactions with Secondary Plant Metabolites, vol. 1, The Chemical Participants*, 2nd edn (eds. G.A. Rosenthal and M.R. Berenbaum), Academic Press, San Diego, pp. 79-121.

Hartmann, T. and Toppel, G. (1987) Senecionine N-oxide, the primary product of pyrrolizidine alka-loid biosynthesis in root cultures of *Senecio vulgaris*. *Phytochemistry*, **26** (6) 1639-43.

Hartmann, T. and Witte, L. (1995) Chemistry, biology and chemoecology of the pyrrolizidine alka-loids, in *Alkaloids: Chemical and Biological Perspectives, vol. 9* (ed. S.W. Pelletier), Pergamon Press, Oxford, pp. 156-233.

Hirono, I. (1993) Edible plants containing naturally occurring carcinogens in Japan. *Japanese Journal of Cancer Research*, **84** 997-1006.

Hooper, P.T. (1978) Pyrrolizidine alkaloid poisoning—pathology with particular reference to dif-ferences in animal and plant species, in *Effects of Poisonous Plants on Livestock* (eds. R.F. Keeler, K.R. van Kampen and L.F. James), Academic Press, New York, pp. 161-76.

Huxtable, R.J. (1990a) The harmful potential of herbal and other plant products. *Drug Safety*, **5** (suppl. 1) 126-36.

Huxtable, R.J. (1990b) Activation and pulmonary toxicity of pyrrolizidine alkaloids. *Pharmacological Therapeutics*, **47** 371-89.

Huxtable, R.J. (1992) The toxicology of alkaloids in food and herbs, in *Handbook of Natural Toxins, vol. 7, Food Poisoning* (ed. A.T. Tu), Marcel Dekker, New York, pp. 237-62.

International Agency for Research on Cancer (1983) *IARC Monographs on the Evaluation of the Carcinogenic Risk to Humans, vol. 31, Some food additives, feed additives and naturally occur-ring substances*, IARC, Lyon, pp. 207-46.

Johnson, A.E. and Molyneux, R.J. (1984) Variation in pyrrolizidine alkaloid content of plants, asso-ciated with site, stage of growth and environmental conditions. *Plant Toxicology, Proceedings of the Australia–USA Poisonous Plants Symposium, Brisbane May 14–18, 1984*, pp. 209-18.

Johnson, A.E., Molyneux, R.J. and Merrill, G.B. (1985) Chemistry of toxic range plants. Variation in pyrrolizidine alkaloid content of *Senecio, Amsinkia* and *Crotalaria* species. *Journal of Agricultural and Food Chemistry*, **33** (1) 50-57.

Kessler, D.A. (1993) Regulating the marketing and use of dietary supplements. Statement to the Congress Committee on Labor and Human Resources 21/10/93 CON00083.

Kumana, C.R., Ng, M., Lin, H.J., Ko, W., Wu, P.-C. and Todd, D. (1985) Herbal tea induced hepatic veno-occlusive disease: quantification of toxic alkaloid exposure in adults. *Gut*, **26** 101-104.

Lanfranconi, W.M. and Huxtable, R.J. (1981) Pyrrolizidines and the pulmonary vasculature. *Reviews of Drug Metabolism and Drug Interactions*, **3** 271-315.

Lanfranconi, W.M., Ohkuma, S. and Huxtable, R.J. (1985) Biliary excretion of novel pneumotoxic metabolites of the pyrrolizidine alkaloid monocrotaline. *Toxicon*, **23** 983-92.

Liddell, J.R. (1996) Pyrrolizidine alkaloids. *Natural Product Reports*, **13** 187-94.

Margalith, D., Heraief, E., Schindler, A.M., Birchler, R., Mosimann, F., Aladjem, D. and Gonvers, J.J. (1985) Veno-occlusive disease of the liver due to the use of tea made from Senecio plants. A report of two cases. *Journal of Hepatology*, **1** (suppl. 2) S280.

Mattocks, A.R. (1971) Hepatotoxic effects due to pyrrolizidine alkaloid N-oxides. *Xenobiotica*, **1** 563-65.

Mattocks, A.R. (1986) *Chemistry and Toxicology of Pyrrolizidine Alkaloids*, Academic Press, London, New York.

Mattocks, A.R. (1990) Pyrrolizidine alkaloids: what metabolites are responsible for extrahepatic tissue damage in animals? *Proceedings of the 3rd International Symposium on Poisonous Plants*, Iowa State University, pp. 192-97.

Mattocks, A.R. and Bird, I. (1983a) Pyrrolic and N-oxide metabolites formed from pyrrolizidine alkaloids by hepatic microsomes *in vitro*: relevance to *in vivo* hepatotoxicity. *Chemico-Biological Interactions*, **43** (2) 209-22.

Mattocks, A.R. and Bird, I. (1983b) Alkylation by dehydroretronecine, a cytotoxic metabolite of some pyrrolizidine alkaloids. An *in vitro* test. *Toxicology Letters*, **16** (1-2) 1-8.

Mattocks, A.R. and White, I.N.M. (1971) The conversion of pyrrolizidine alkaloids to N-oxides and to dihydropyrrolizine derivatives by rat liver microsomes *in vitro*. *Chemico-Biolological Interactions*, **3** 393-96.

McLean, E.K. (1970) The toxic actions of pyrrolizidine (*Senecio*) alkaloids. *Pharmacological Reviews*, **22** (4) 429-83.

McLean, E.K. (1974) *Senecio* and other plants as liver poisons. *Israeli Journal of Medical Science*, **10** 436-40.

Ministry of Agriculture, Fisheries and Food (1994) Naturally occurring toxicants in food, Food Surveillance Paper No. 42, HMSO, London.

Ministry of Agriculture, Fisheries and Food (1995) Surveillance for pyrrolizidine alkaloids in honey, Food Surveillance Information Sheet No. 52, HMSO, London.

Miranda, C.L., Reed, R.L., Guengerich, F.P. and Buhler, D.R. (1991) Role of cytochrome 50IIIA4 in the metabolism of the pyrrolizidine alkaloid senecionine in human liver. *Carcinogenisis*, **12** 515-19.

Miranda, C.L., Rawson, C., Reed, R.L., Zhao, X., Barnes, D.W. and Buhler, D.R. (1992) C3H/10T1/2 Cells: a model to study the role of metabolism in the toxicity of the pyrrolizidine alkaloid retrorsine. *In Vitro Toxicology*, **5** (1) 21-32.

Mohabbat, O., Younos, S.M., Merzad, A.A., Srivastava, R.N., Sediq, G.G. and Aram, G.N. (1976) An outbreak of hepatic veno-occlusive disease in north-western Afghanistan. *Lancet*, 269-71.

Molyneux, R.J. and James, L.F. (1990) Pyrrolizidine alkaloids in milk: thresholds of intoxication. *Veterinary and Human Toxicology*, **32** (suppl.) 94-103.

Molyneux, R.J., Johnson, A.E., Olsen, J.D. and Baker, D.C. (1991) Toxicity of pyrrolizidine alkaloids from Riddell groundsel (*Senecio riddelli*) to cattle. *American Journal of Veterinary Medicine*, **52** (1) 146-51.

Moore, D.J., Batts, K.P., Zalkow, L.L., Fortune, G.T. and Powis, G. (1989) Model systems for detecting the hepatotoxicity of pyrrolizidine alkaloids and pyrrolizidine alkaloid N-oxides. *Toxicology and Applied Pharmacology*, **101** (2) 271-84.

Niwa, H., Ogawa, T., Okamoto, O. and Yamada, K. (1991) Alkylation of nucleosides by dehydromonocrotaline, the putative toxic metabolite of the carcinogenic pyrrolizidine alkaloid monocrotaline. *Tetrahedron Letters*, **32** (7) 927-30.

Peterson, J.E. and Culvenor, C.C.J. (1983) Hepatotoxic pyrrolizidine alkaloids, in *Handbook of Natural Toxins: Plant and Fungal Toxins* (eds. R.F. Keeler and A.T. Tu), Marcel Dekker, New York, pp. 637-71.

Ridker, P.M. and McDermott, W.V. (1989) Comfrey herb tea and veno-occlusive disease. *Lancet*, 657-58.

Ridker, P.M., Ohkuma, S., McDermott, W.V., Trey, C. and Huxtable, R.J. (1985) Hepatic veno-occlusive disease associated with the consumption of pyrrolizidine containing dietary supplements. *Gastroenterology*, **88** 1050-54.

Rizk, A.-F.M. (1991a) *Poisonous Plant Contamination of Edible Plants*, CRC Press, Boca Raton, FL.

Rizk, A.-F.M. (1991b) *Naturally Occurring Pyrrolizidine Alkaloids*, CRC Press, Boca Raton, FL.

Robins, D.J. (1989) Biosynthesis of pyrrolizidine alkaloids. *Chemical Society Reviews*, **18** 375-408.

Robins, D.J. (1995) Pyrrolizidine alkaloids. *Natural Product Reports*, **12** 413-18.

Roeder, E. (1995) Medicinal plants in Europe containing pyrrolizidine alkaloids. *Pharmazie*, **50** 83-98.

Roitman, J.N. (1983) Ingestion of pyrrolizidine alkaloids: a health hazard of global proportions, in *Xenobiotics in Foods and Feed* (eds. J.W. Finley and D.E. Schwass), American Chemical Society, Washington, DC, pp. 345-78.

Segall, H.J., Wilson, D.W., Dallas, J.L. and Haddon, W.F. (1985) Trans 4-hydroxy-2-hexenal: a reactive metabolite from the macrocyclic pyrrolizidine alkaloid senecionine. *Science*, **229** 472-75.

Segall, H.J., Wilson, D.W., Lamé, Morin, D. and Winter, C.K. (1991) Metabolism of pyrrolizidine alkaloids, in *Handbook of Natural Toxins*, vol. 6 (R.F. Keeler and A.T. Tu), Marcel Dekker, New York, pp. 3-26.

Smith, L.W. and Culvenor, C.C.J. (1981) Plant sources of hepatotoxic pyrrolizidine alkaloids. *Journal of Natural Products*, **44** 129-52.

Sperl, W., Stuppner, H., Gassner, I., Judmaier, W., Dietze, O. and Vogel, W. (1995) Reversible hepatic veno-occlusive disease in an infant after consumption of pyrrolizidine-containing herbal tea. *European Journal of Pediatrics*, **154** 112-16.

Tandon, B.N., Tandon, H.D., Tandon, R.K., Narndranathan, M. and Joshi, Y.K. (1976) An epidemic of veno-occlusive disease of liver in Central India. *Lancet*, **2** 271-72.

van Dam, N.M., Witte, L., Theuring, C. and Hartmann, T. (1994) Distribution, biosynthesis and turnover of pyrrolizidine alkaloids in *Cynoglossum officinale*. *Phytochemistry*, **39** (2) 287-92.

Weston, C.F., Cooper, B.T., Davies, J.D. and Levine, D.F. (1981) Veno-occlusive disease of the liver secondary to ingestion of comfrey. *British Medical Journal*, **44** 129-44.

Winter, C.K. and Segall, H.J. (1989) Metabolism of pyrrolizidine alkaloids, in *Toxicants of Plant Origin* (ed. P.R. Cheeke), CRC Press, Boca Raton, FL, pp. 1-22.

World Health Organisation (1988) International Programme on Chemical Safety. *Environmental Health Criteria 80: Pyrrolizidine Alkaloids*, WHO, Geneva.

Yan, C.C. and Huxtable, R.J. (1995) The relationship between the concentration of the pyrrolizidine alkaloid monocrotaline and the pattern of metabolites released from the isolated liver. *Toxicology and Applied Pharmacology*, **130** 1-8.

# 3  Glucosinolates

Ruud Verkerk, Matthijs Dekker and Wim M.F. Jongen

## 3.1  Introduction

Glucosinolates are secondary plant metabolites found exclusively in cruciferous plants. These sulphur-containing glycosides occur at highest concentrations in the families Resedaceae, Capparaceae and Brassicaceae.

The majority of cultivated plants that contain glucosinolates belong to the family of Brassicaceae. Mustard seed, used as a seasoning, is derived from *B. nigra*, *B. juncea* (L.) Coss and *B. hirta* species. Vegetable crops include cabbage, cauliflower, broccoli, Brussels sprouts and turnip of the *B. oleracea* L., *B. campestris* L. and *B. napus* L. species. Kale of the *B. oleracea* species is used for forage, pasture and silage. *Brassica* vegetables such as Brussels sprouts, cabbage, broccoli and cauliflower are the major source of glucosinolates in the human diet. They are frequently consumed by humans from Western and Eastern cultures (Fenwick and Heaney, 1983) as well as by animals. In The Netherlands, the amounts consumed by humans are not known exactly, but more than 36 g brassica per person per day is available (Godeschalk, 1987). The typical flavour of brassicas is largely due to glucosinolate-derived volatiles.

Glucosinolates and their breakdown products are of particular interest in food research because of their nutritive and antinutritional properties (Fenwick *et al.*, 1983), the adverse effects of some glucosinolates on health, their anticarcinogenic properties and finally because they are responsible for the characteristic flavour and odour of many vegetables. The versatility of these compounds is also demonstrated in the fact that glucosinolates are quite toxic to some insects and therefore could be included as one of many natural pesticides. However, a small number of insects, such as the cabbage aphids, use glucosinolates to locate their favourite plants as feed and to find a suitable environment to deposit their eggs (Harborne, 1989). Furthermore, glucosinolates show antifungal and antibacterial properties (Chew, 1988).

Currently more than 100 different glucosinolates have been characterized, of which only a few have been investigated thoroughly. A considerable amount of data on levels of total and individual glucosinolates is now available. The levels of total glucosinolates in plants may depend on variety, cultivation conditions, climate and agronomic practice, while the levels in a particular plant vary between the parts of the plant. Generally the same glucosinolates occur in a particular subspecies regardless of genetic origin, and in most species only between one and four glucosinolates are found in relatively high concentrations.

Glucosinolates appear to have little biological impact themselves, but are converted to biologically active products such as isothiocyanates, organic cyanides, oxazolidinethiones and ionic thiocyanate on enzymatic degradation by myrosinase in the presence of water. The anticarcinogenic mechanisms (section 3.6.1) by which these compounds may act include the induction of detoxification enzymes and the inhibition of activation of promutagens/procarcinogens (Wattenberg, 1992; Dragsted *et al.*, 1993; Jongen, 1996).

The toxic effects (section 3.6.2) are mainly due to the goitrogenic effects of certain breakdown products of glucosinolates (Paik *et al.*, 1980). In most animal studies performed in the past, goitrogenicity induced by glucosinolate breakdown products appeared to be limited to situations of iodine deficiency.

Tiedink *et al.* (1990, 1991) investigated the role of indole compounds and glucosinolates in the formation of N-nitroso compounds in vegetables. These studies revealed that the indole compounds present in brassica vegetables can be nitrosated and thereby become mutagenic. However, the nitrosated products are stable only in the presence of large amounts of free nitrite.

## 3.2 Chemistry

The chemistry and occurrence of glucosinolates and their breakdown products have been reviewed extensively by Rosa *et al.* (1997).

Very few glucosinolates are isolated in the pure state. The first crystalline glucosinolate was isolated from the seed of white mustard in 1830 and since then the elucidation of their structures and chemistry has continued (Gildemeister and Hofmann, 1927). The common structure of glucosinolates is shown in Figure 3.1. The side chain determines the chemical and biological nature of glucosinolates. They are considered to be (Z)-*cis*-N-hydroximinosulfate esters possessing a side chain R and a sulphur-linked D-glucopyranose moiety. Natural glucosinolates contain exclusively a β-D-glucopyranosyl linkage (Blanc-Muesser *et al.*, 1990).

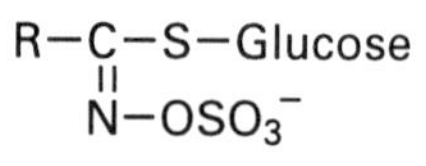

$$R-\underset{\underset{N-OSO_3^-}{\|}}{C}-S-Glucose$$

**Figure 3.1** General structure of glucosinolates

The side chain of the glucosinolates is variable and is the basis for their structural heterogenity and for the biological activity of the enzymatic and chemical breakdown products. The side chains can be divided into three main groups: aliphatic, heterocyclic (indolyl) and aromatic. Table 3.1 gives an overview of the glucosinolates commonly found in brassica vegetables.

**Table 3.1** Glucosinolates commonly found in brassica vegetables

| Trivial name | Chemical name (cf. Side chain (R) |
| --- | --- |
| Aliphatic glucosinolates | |
| Glucoiberin | 3-Methylsulphinylpropyl |
| Progoitrin | 2-Hydroxy-3-butenyl |
| Sinigrin | 2-Propenyl |
| Gluconapoleiferin | 2-Hydroxy-4-pentenyl |
| Glucoraphanin | 4-Methylsulphinylbutyl |
| Glucoalyssin | 5-Methylsulphinylpentyl |
| Glucocapparin | Methyl |
| Glucobrassicanapin | 4-Pentenyl |
| Glucocheirolin | 3-Methylsulphonylpropyl |
| Glucoiberverin | 3-Methylthiopropyl |
| Gluconapin | 3-Butenyl |
| | |
| Indole glucosinolates | |
| 4-Hydroxyglucobrassicin | 4-Hydroxy-3-indolylmethyl |
| Glucobrassicin | 3-Indolylmethyl |
| 4-Methoxyglucobrassicin | 4-Methoxy-3-indolylmethyl |
| Neoglucobrassicin | 1-Methoxy-3-indolylmethyl |
| | |
| Aromatic glucosinolates | |
| Glucosinalbin | *p*-Hydroxybenzyl |
| Glucotropaeolin | Benzyl |
| Gluconasturtiin | 2-Phenethyl |

## 3.3 Biosynthesis

Kjaer and Conti (1954) suggested that amino acids may be natural precursors of the aglycone moiety of glucosinolates based on the similarities between the carbon skeletons of some amino acids and the glucosinolates. This hypothesis was confirmed by studies of the different biosynthetic stages. Most of these studies involved the administration of variously labelled compounds ($^3$H, $^{14}$C, $^{15}$N or $^{35}$S) to plants and the assessment of their relative efficiencies as precursors on the basis of the extent of incorporation of isotope into the glucosinolate. The classification of glucosinolates as shown in Table 3.1 depends on the amino acid from which they are derived; aliphatic glucosinolates derive from methionine, indole glucosinolates derive from tryptophan and aromatic glucosinolates derive from phenylalanine and tyrosine (Sørensen, 1990).

The biosynthesis of glucosinolates was reviewed extensively by Rosa *et al.* (1997). The biosynthesis of glucosinolates from amino acids starts with modification of the amino acids (or chain-extended derivatives of amino acids) via an aldoxime intermediate. The same modifications also take place in the biosynthetic route of cyanogenic glycosides (Chapter 1). However, the co-occurrence of glucosinolates and cyanogenic glycosides in the same plant is very rare (an example is *Carica papaya*). The biosynthesis of the cyanogenic glycosides has been elucidated recently in more detail by Halkier and Lindberg-Møller (1991) and by Koch *et al.* (1992). Following the formation of the aldoxime, the glucosinolate is formed by S-insertion, glucosylation and sulphation. Further modification of the side chain can occur in the formed glucosinolate by, for example, oxidation and/or elimination reactions. The different steps in the synthesis are discussed below in more detail.

### 3.3.1 Amino acid modification

Kutáček *et al.* (1962) demonstrated that [3-$^{14}$C]tryptophan was converted into 3-indolylmethylglucosinolate (glucobrassicin). Similarly Underhill *et al.* (1962) and Benn (1962) showed that phenylalanine was incorporated into benzylglucosinolate (glucotropaeolin) with great efficiency. The glucosinolates can be divided into two groups by origin: those derived from common amino acids and those derived from modified amino acids.

Not all of the common amino acids lead to corresponding glucosinolates being found in nature. For instance, the glucosinolate from glycine is probably chemically unstable and has therefore never been found in plants (Kjaer, 1976). The glucosinolate from alanine (methyl glucosinolate) is apparently absent in brassicas but is the most widely distributed glucosinolate within the Capparaceae. Valine and isoleucine glucosinolates (isopropyl and sec-butyl glucosinolates) are widely distributed in brassicas. Phenylalanine and tyrosine can be transformed into benzyl- and *p*-hydroxybenzyl glucosinolates respectively. The glucosinolate from tryptophan (indol-3-ylmethyl glucosinolate) appears to occur only in seedlings and young vegetative tissue in various families, including the Brassicaceae.

The modification of common amino acids is mainly in the form of side chain elongation. A general route for this was proposed by Kjaer (1976). Various enzymes are involved in these steps. The elongation of the side chain from the amino acid methionine gives rise to a large family of glucosinolates that occur in brassicas. Their side chains can be generally expressed as $MeS(CH_2)_n$ with *n* ranging from 3 to 11 (Dawson *et al.*, 1993). At a later stage these glucosinolates can be oxidized to the corresponding sulphoxides or sulphones. Aromatic amino acids may also undergo homologization, for example phenylalanine is metabolized to 2-phenethyl glucosinolate (Dawson *et al.*, 1993).

### 3.3.2 Aldoxime formation

Aldoxime formation systems have been elucidated in cassava and sorghum (Halkier and Lindberg-Møller, 1991; Koch *et al.*, 1992). In these plants aldoxime formation is involved in the synthesis of cyanogenic glycosides. In Chinese cabbage the formation of indole-3-aldoxime is by another system (Ludwig-Muler and Hilgenberg, 1988). Both systems are membrane bound. Koch *et al.* (1992) proposed the recent pathway for aldoxime biosynthesis. Dawson *et al.* (1993) showed homophenylalanine to be effectively converted to 3-phenylpropanaldoxime when added to rapeseed (*Brassica napus*) leaf microsomal preparations. Lykkesfeldt and Lindberg-Møller (1993) observed that extracts of *Tropaeolum majus* inhibit glucosinolate formation in microsomal systems. The extracts also inhibited cyanogenic glycoside formation in a sorghum microsomal preparation. The authors suggested benzyl isothiocyanate to be the (partly) inhibiting compound.

### 3.3.3 Glucosylation and sulphation

Formation of the aldoxime is followed by conjugation reactions that introduce sulphur to form thiohydroximic acid. Sulphur from cysteine is most effectively incorporated (Underhill *et al.*, 1973). The subsequent S-glucosylation is catalyzed by thiohydroximate S-glucosyltransferase. This enzyme has been purified and characterized by Groot Wassink *et al.* (1994). Sulphation of the desulphoglucosinolate is effected by 3'-phosphoadenosine-5'-phosphosulphate. After this formation of the overall glucosinolate skeleton, modification can occur by stereospecific insertion of oxygen and elimination of methylthiols. The simplified biosynthetic pathway for glucosinolates is shown in Figure 3.2 (based on Rosa *et al.*, 1997).

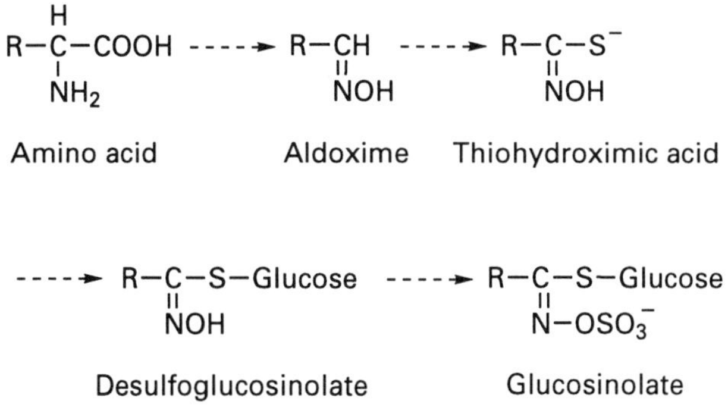

**Figure 3.2** The simplified biosynthetic pathway for glucosinolates.

## 3.4 Occurrence

The occurrence of glucosinolates is limited to dicotyledonous angiosperms. They occur in the families Capparaceae, Brassicaceae, Koebliniaceae, Moringaceae, Resedaceae and Toceriaceae (Kjaer, 1974). Glucosinolates are prevalent in the brassicas. These species are cultivated mainly as vegetables, seasonings and sources of oil and feed. Generally, plant species contain up to four different glucosinolates in significant amounts. The highest concentrations are usually found in the seeds, except for indol-3-ylmethyl and N-methoxyindol-3-ylmethyl glucosinolates, which are rarely found in seeds (Tookey *et al.*, 1980). The same glucosinolates usually occur in a particular subspecies regardless of genetic origin (Rosa *et al.*, 1997). Several reports have given the results of the glucosinolate composition of cabbages and rapeseed varieties. These reports have been reviewed extensively by Rosa *et al.* (1997). The data are summarized in Table 3.2. The differences in the levels of these substances are large even in the same studies, and are even larger in different studies. Reasons for these different findings are the use of different varieties, growing conditions and the analytical methods used.

**Table 3.2**   Principal glucosinolates occurring in the main brassica vegetables (From Rosa *et al.*, 1997)

| Species/glucosinolate | Concentration (μmol/100 g of fresh wt) | | Reference |
|---|---|---|---|
| | Average | Range | |
| White cabbage | | | |
| (*B. oleracea* L., Capitata group) | | | |
|    2-Propenyl | 36.3 | 4.3–147.4 | VanEtten *et al.* (1976) |
| | 26.4 | 8.8–148.6 | VanEtten *et al.* (1980) |
| | 57.2 | 18.6–104.3 | Sones *et al.* (1984a) |
| | 66.2 | 18.6–162.7 | Sones *et al.* (1984c) |
|    3-Methylsulphinylpropyl | 34.7 | 13.0–70.9 | VanEtten *et al.* (1976) |
| | 28.3 | 10.0–58.6 | VanEtten *et al.* (1980) |
| | 72.7 | 5.0–193.1 | Sones *et al.* (1984a) |
| | 97.6 | 5.0–279.8 | Sones *et al.* (1984c) |
|    Indole glucosinolates | 49.4 | 28.0–106.4 | VanEtten *et al.* (1976) |
| | 31.2 | 10.5–104.9 | VanEtten *et al.* (1980) |
|    Indol-3-ylmethyl | 39.3 | 9.3–129.8 | Sones *et al.* (1984a) |
| | 60.7 | 9.3–200.0 | Sones *et al.* (1984c) |
|    *Total* | 143.8 | 66.4–236.7 | VanEtten *et al.* (1976) |
| | 117.3 | 57.5–234.5 | VanEtten *et al.* (1980) |
| | 68.6 | 17.7–112.8 | Mullin and Sahasrabudhe (1977) |
| | 200.9 | 93.8–348.2 | Sones *et al.* (1984a) |
| | 238.3 | 78.8–602.6 | Sones *et al.* (1984c) |
| (*B. oleracea* L., Sabauda group) | | | |
|    2-Propenyl | — | 35.8 | VanEtten *et al.* (1976) |
| | 14.2 | 0.1–39.7 | VanEtten *et al.* (1980) |
| | 93.2 | 31.5–162.7 | Sones *et al.* (1984a) |
| Savoy cabbage | | | |
|    3-Methylsulphinylpropyl | — | 100.7 | VanEtten *et al.* (1976) |
| | 46.7 | 15.2–91.1 | VanEtten *et al.* (1980) |
| | 169.8 | 72.5–279.8 | Sones *et al.* (1984a) |

**Table 3.2** (continued)

| Species/glucosinolate | Concentration (μmol/100 g of fresh wt) | | Reference |
|---|---|---|---|
| | Average | Range | |
| Indole glucosinolates | — | 111.3 | VanEtten *et al.* (1976) |
| | 80.5 | 61.7–108.2 | VanEtten *et al.* (1980) |
| Indol-3-ylmethyl | 123.0 | 70.2–199.8 | Sones *et al.* (1984a) |
| 2-Hydroxybut-3-enyl | — | 1.6 | VanEtten *et al.* (1976) |
| | 0.5 | 0.0–1.3 | VanEtten *et al.* (1980) |
| | 13.8 | 5.6–29.5 | Sones *et al.* (1984a) |
| *Total* | — | 275.6 | VanEtten *et al.* (1976) |
| | 164.5 | 100.4–265.0 | VanEtten *et al.* (1980) |
| | 461.3 | 267.1–653.4 | Sones *et al.* (1984a) |
| Red cabbage | | | |
| (*B. oleracea* L., Capitata group) | | | |
| 2-Propenyl | 12.6 | 11.1–14.1 | VanEtten *et al.* (1976) |
| | 10.5 | 1.5–25.7 | VanEtten *et al.* (1980) |
| 3-Methylsulphinylpropyl | 16.1 | 12.4–19.7 | VanEtten *et al.* (1976) |
| | 14.5 | 4.8–31.0 | VanEtten *et al.* (1980) |
| 4-Methylsulphinylbutyl | 56.8 | 46.7–66.9 | VanEtten *et al.* (1976) |
| | 52.3 | 31.6–82.1 | VanEtten *et al.* (1980) |
| Indole glucosinolates | 72.8 | 42.6–102.9 | VanEtten *et al.* (1976) |
| | — | 31.9–67.9 | VanEtten *et al.* (1980) |
| But-3-enyl | 15.1 | 13.9–16.3 | VanEtten *et al.* (1976) |
| | 9.9 | 4.6–15.6 | VanEtten *et al.* (1980) |
| 2-Hydroxybut-3-enyl | 12.2 | 10.1–14.3 | VanEtten *et al.* (1976) |
| | 8.3 | 4.4–5.5 | VanEtten *et al.* (1980) |
| *Total* | 204.3 | 150.5–258.1 | VanEtten *et al.* (1976) |
| | 163.4 | 88.2–234.4 | VanEtten *et al.* (1980) |
| | 68.8 | 34.4–98.9 | Mullin and Sahasrabudhe (1977) |
| Brussels sprouts | | | |
| (*B. oleracea* L., Gemmifera group) | | | |
| 2-Propenyl | 136.0 | 27.7–392.9 | Heaney and Fenwick (1980) |
| | 10.7 | 3.9–22.7 | Carlson *et al.* (1987a) |
| | 112.1 | 4.0–280.6 | Sones *et al.* (1984c) |
| 3-Methylsulphinylpropyl | 76.6 | 0.0–154.2 | Sones *et al.* (1984c) |
| | 11.8 | 2.4–18.9 | Carlson *et al.* (1987a) |
| 4-Methylsulphinylbutyl | 8.2 | 0.4–22.6 | Carlson *et al.* (1987a) |
| Indol-3-ylmethyl | 113.2 | 45.3–228.4 | Heaney and Fenwick (1980) |
| | 128.4 | 54.3–326.3 | Scones *et al.* (1984c) |
| | 391.8 | 327.8–469.4 | Carlson *et al.* (1987a) |
| 1-Methoxyindol-3-ylmethyl | 21.3 | 1.9–34.3 | Sones *et al.* (1984c) |
| But-3-enyl | 36.5 | 7.3–121.7 | Heaney and Fenwick (1980) |
| | 61.3 | 6.1–221.2 | Sones *et al.* (1984c) |
| | 4.2 | 0.5–12.2 | Carlson *et al.* (1987a) |
| 2-Hydroxybut-3-enyl | 67.9 | 93.7–231.9 | Heaney and Fenwick (1980) |
| | 111.9 | 29.3–303.5 | Sones *et al.* (1984c) |

**Table 3.2** (continued)

| Species/glucosinolate | Concentration ($\mu$mol/100 g of fresh wt) | | Reference |
|---|---|---|---|
| | Average | Range | |
| | 8.3 | 1.0–25.4 | Carlson *et al.* (1987a) |
| Total | 367.2 | 330.3–406.5 | Mullin and Sahasrabudhe (1977) |
| | 461.9 | 138.6–900.7 | Heaney and Fenwick (1980) |
| | 495.0 | 318.4–861.9 | Sones *et al.* (1984c) |
| | 553.0 | 465.6–600.6 | Carlson *et al.* (1987a) |
| **Collards** | | | |
| (*B. olefacea* L., Acephala group) | | | |
| 2-Propenyl | 20.7 | 12.6–28.7 | Carlson *et al.* (1987a) |
| 3-Methylsulphinyl-propyl | 38.6 | 8.4–69.3 | Carlson *et al.* (1987a) |
| Indol-3-ylmethyl | 55.5 | 44.2–69.5 | Carlson *et al.* (1987a) |
| | 47.3 | — | VanEtten and Tookey (1979) |
| Total | 220.4 | 64.4–306.7 | Carlson *et al.* (1987a) |
| **Kale** | | | |
| (*B. oleracea* L., Acephala group) | | | |
| 2-Propenyl | 97.0 | 62.5–197.3 | Carlson *et al.* (1987a) |
| 3-Methylsulphinylpropyl | 11.7 | 0.0–49.9 | Carlson *et al.* (1987a) |
| Indol-3-ylmethyl | 107.5 | 67.2–165.3 | Carlson *et al.* (1987a) |
| But-3-enyl | 21.3 | 5.8–38.1 | Carlson *et al.* (1987a) |
| 2-Hydroxybut-3-enyl | 70.1 | 16.8–130.3 | Carlson *et al.* (1987a) |
| Total | 439.1 | 316.1–600.0 | Carlson *et al.* (1987a) |
| **Broccoli** | | | |
| (*B. oleracea* L., Italica group) | | | |
| 3-Methylsulphinylpropyl | 74.1 | 0.0–327.2 | Lewis *et al.* (1991) |
| 4-Methylsulphinylbutyl | 63.9 | 28.9–88.3 | Carlson *et al.* (1987a) |
| | 97.5 | 54.0–190.2 | Lewis *et al.* (1991) |
| Indol-3-ylmethyl | 59.4 | 42.2–71.7 | Carlson *et al.* (1987a) |
| | 56.0 | 22.8–101.0 | Lewis *et al.* (1991) |
| 1-Methoxyindol-3-ylmethyl | 8.6 | 2.4–18.4 | Lewis *et al.* (1991) |
| Total | 161.9 | 98.5–323.9 | Mullin and Sahasrabudhe (1977) |
| | 188.2 | 102.2–262.7 | Carlson *et al.* (1987a) |
| | 248.4 | 152.2–448.6 | Lewis *et al.* (1991) |
| **Cauliflower** | | | |
| (*B. oleracea* L., Botrytis group) | | | |
| 2-Propenyl | 37.8 | 1.3–157.9 | Sones *et al.* (1984b) |
| | 35.8 | 1.3–157.9 | Sones *et al.* (1984c) |
| | 10.0 | 2.9–16.5 | Carlson *et al.* (1987a) |
| 4-Methylsulphinylbutyl | 63.8 | 1.8–190.1 | Lewis *et al.* (1991) |
| 3-Methylsulphinylpropyl | 41.0 | 0.0–90.9 | Sones *et al.* (1984b) |
| | 37.5 | 1.3–90.9 | Sones *et al.* (1984c) |
| | 5.2 | 0.0–22.8 | Carlson *et al.* (1987a) |

**Table 3.2** (continued)

| Species/glucosinolate | Concentration (μmol/100 g of fresh wt) | | Reference |
|---|---|---|---|
| | Average | Range | |
| | 51.0 | 0.0–327.2 | Lewis *et al.* (1991) |
| Indol-3-ylmethyl | 50.0 | 14.8–162.3 | Sones *et al.* (1984b) |
| | 46.7 | 13.6–162.3 | Sones *et al.* (1984c) |
| | 60.6 | 18.8–104.7 | Carlson *et al.* (1987a) |
| | 42.1 | 21.0–101.0 | Lewis *et al.* (1991) |
| 1-Methoxyindol-3-ylmethyl | 10.0 | 1.1–32.0 | Sones *et al.* (1984b) |
| | 9.3 | 1.2–32.0 | Sones *et al.* (1984c) |
| | 7.3 | 2.3–17.4 | Lewis *et al.* (1991) |
| *Total* | 105.0 | 59.1–180.6 | Mullin and Sahasrabudhe (1977) |
| | 161.9 | 30.2–520.4 | Sones *et al.* (1984b) |
| | 135.7 | 30.2–455.8 | Sones *et al.* (1984c) |
| | 94.6 | 41.1–160.6 | Carlson *et al.* (1987a) |
| | 178.2 | 57.1–448.6 | Lewis *et al.* (1991) |
| Turnip tops | | | |
| (*B. campestris* L., and *B. rapa* L., Rapifera group) | | | |
| But-3-enyl | — | 294.0 | Carlson *et al.* (1981) |
| | 103.0 | 38.0–181.0 | Carlson *et al.* (1987b) |
| Pent-4-enyl | — | 151.0 | Carlson *et al.* (1981) |
| | 58.0 | 20.0–112.0 | Carlson *et al.* (1987b) |
| *Total* | — | 586.0 | Carlson *et al.* (1981) |
| | 186.0 | 80.0–292.0 | Carlson *et al.* (1987b) |
| Rapeseed | | | |
| (*B. napus* L.) | | | |
| But-3-enyl | 3187 | — | Fenwick *et al.* (1983) |
| 2-Hydroxybut-3-enyl | 10937 | — | Fenwick *et al.* (1983) |
| Pent-4-enyl | 824 | — | Fenwick *et al.* (1983) |
| 2-Hydroxypent-4-enyl | 522 | — | Fenwick *et al.* (1983) |
| *Total* | | | |
| Summer rape | 8031 | 8425–17002 | Fenwick *et al.* (1983) |
| Spring rape | — | 8140–12582 | Fenwick *et al.* (1983) |
| | 2175 | 1000–2700 | Sang and Salisbury (1988) |
| Rapeseed | | | |
| (*B. campestris* L.) | | | |
| But-3-enyl | 13455 | 10706–16107 | Fenwick *et al.* (1983) |
| | 3863 | 1302–10281 | Sang and Salisbury (1988) |
| | 14207 | 11960–15698 | Sang and Salisbury (1988) |
| | 23450 | — | Davis *et al.* (1991) |
| 2-Hydroxybut-3-enyl | 1836 | 1050–2387 | Sang and Salisbury (1988) |
| | 209 | 0–520 | Sang and Salisbury (1988) |
| | 250 | — | Davis *et al.* (1991) |
| Pent-4-enyl | 1704 | 1092–2941 | Sang and Salisbury (1988) |
| | 240 | 0–334 | Sang and Salisbury (1988) |

**Table 3.2** (continued)

| | Concentration (μmol/100 g of fresh wt) | | |
|---|---|---|---|
| Species/glucosinolate | Average | Range | Reference |
| 2-Hydroxypent-4-enyl | 322 | 234–385 | Sang and Salisbury (1988) |
| | 161 | 0–334 | Sang and Salisbury (1988) |
| 4-Hydroxyindol-3-ylmethyl | 396 | 294–475 | Sang and Salisbury (1988) |
| | 261 | 0–474 | Sang and Salisbury (1988) |

## 3.5  Hydrolysis

### 3.5.1  Myrosinase

Myrosinase (thioglucoside glucohydrolase EC 3.2.3.1) is the trivial name for the enzyme (or group of enzymes) responsible for the hydrolysis of glucosinolates. It is located in cellular compartments separate from glucosinolates in the plant and is released when plant cells are damaged by cutting or chewing (Fenwick and Heaney, 1983).

The glucosinolate/myrosinase system may have several functions in the plant: (i) plant defence against fungal diseases and pest infestation; (ii) sulphur and nitrogen metabolism; and (iii) growth regulation. Myrosinase has been found in the seed, leaf, stem and roots of glucosinolate-containing plants and the activity appears to be higher in the young tissues of the plant. The complexity of the glucosinolate/myrosinase system indicates an important role in cruciferous plants (Bones and Rossiter, 1996).

Plant breeding strategies over past decades have concentrated on reducing the glucosinolate content of rapeseed to improve the acceptability of rapeseed meal and meet the increasingly stringent requirements of the rapeseed processing industry. One approach to reducing the undesired breakdown products of glucosinolates would be to change the amount of myrosinase available for hydrolysis of the glucosinolates.

Myrosinase exists in multiple forms in many plants. By analytical gel electrophoresis various studies have demonstrated the presence of several myrosinase isoenzymes (MacGibbon and Allison, 1970; Buchwaldt et al., 1986). Different patterns were found depending on whether the extracts were made from the leaf, stem, root or seed. Little is known about the substrate specificity of myrosinase isoenzymes. There are two myrosinases isolated by James and Rossiter (1991) that degrade different glucosinolates at different rates. However, both isoenzymes show highest activity against aliphatic glucosinolates and least activity against indole glucosinolates. Members of a given class of glucosinolates are degraded at approximately the same rate *in vitro*. It is also possible that the specificity is affected by

associated factors like epithiospecifier protein, myrosinase-binding protein
or other myrosinase-associated proteins or components

Ascorbic acid has been shown to modulate myrosinase activity in some
species; it inhibits at high concentrations and activates at low levels.
Activation appears to be the result of a conformational change in the protein
structure, leading to an enhanced reaction rate when the effector binding
sites are occupied (Ohtsuru and Hata, 1973).

### 3.5.2 Hydrolysis products

Hydrolysis products of glucosinolates contribute significantly to the typical
flavour of brassica vegetables. Myrosinase catalyses the hydrolysis of glucosinolates by splitting off the glucose. The unstable aglucone (thiohydrox-
ymate-O-sulphonate) then eliminates sulphate by a Lossen rearrangement
(Figure 3.3). The structure of the resulting products depends on a variety of
factors. Whether isothiocyanates or nitriles are formed depends on the
specific glucosinolates, the part of the plant where they are located, the treatment of plant material before the hydrolysis of glucosinolates and conditions during hydrolysis, especially pH. Isothiocyanates are usually produced
at neutral pH while nitrile production occurs at lower pH.

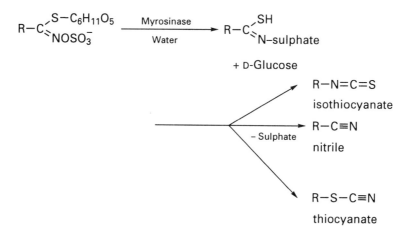

**Figure 3.3**   Hydrolysis of alkenyl glucosinolates and the breakdown products formed

Indole glucosinolates such as glucobrassicin undergo enzymatic hydrolysis to give 3-indolemethanol, 3-indoleacetonitrile and 3,3' diindolyl-
methane (Labague et al., 1991). Hanley et al. (1990) isolated an indole
isothiocyanate from neoglucobrassicin degradation under specific experimental conditions. Less volatile compounds such as epithionitriles and oxa-
zolidine-2-thiones are formed from glucosinolates with a hydroxyl group at

*3.6.2  Toxicity*

Vegetables and seeds of the Cruciferae family, such as crambe, kale, mustard, rape, cabbage and turnips, are rich in glucosinolates. Many feeds containing a high concentration of rape or crambe seed meal have been shown to decrease feed intake and growth rate and to cause goitrogenicity, enlarged livers, kidneys, thyroid and adrenal glands in different animal species. These adverse effects were attributed to the high content of glucosinolates and their derivatives, which include goitrin, isothiocyanates and nitriles. In man, epidemiological surveys show a correlation between endemic goitre and the consumption of cruciferous vegetables, whereas experimental studies are unambiguous. Langer *et al.* (1971) demonstrated the goitrogenic properties of cruciferous vegetables and purified glucosinolates and their derivatives. However, the findings of McMillan *et al.* (1986) are not in agreement with these results.

Among the problems associated with the consumption of these compounds, those affecting the thyroid have been studied most extensively (VanEtten, 1969). The breakdown product 5-vinyloxazolidine-2-thione (OZT) was found to be the predominant product from heat-treated rape meal regardless of the source of myrosinase enzyme. This may explain the ability of rapeseed to induce thyroid hypertrophy (McKinnon and Bowland, 1979). In certain parts of the world the consumption of excessive amounts of brassicas may contribute to hypothyroidism, particularly when natural iodine in the diet is limited. Furthermore, the extent to which the thyroid function is impaired by glucosinolates is related to species, intake, duration of feeding and the nature of the compound. In addition, the mechanisms involved seem to be different. Thiocyanate ions are considered to behave as iodine competitors and therefore cause goitrogenicity only in cases of iodine deficiency, while oxazolidine-2-thiones interfere with thyroxine synthesis and therefore will be goitrogenic irrespective of iodine status (Fenwick *et al.*, 1983). In addition, isothiocyanates of the parent glucosinolates sinigrin, glucocheirolin, glucotropaeolin and nitriles have also shown goitrogenic effects, depending on the iodine content of the diet.

Most studies on the physiological properties of glucosinolates and their breakdown products have been carried out with feeding experiments using rapeseed and *Crambe abyssinica*. These studies showed considerable enlargement of the thyroid, adrenal gland, kidney and liver.

The levels of glucosinolates consumed by humans are not usually a problem but animals can suffer if they are fed too much rapeseed meal used as a protein supplement in livestock and poultry feeds. Unfortunately the use of this meal for feeding purposes can result in various manifestations of toxicity. These problems have led to the introduction of double zero varieties of rape, which are low in both erucic acid (less than 2% of the total fatty acids) and glucosinolates (less than 1% w/w). These double zero varieties are common in Canada and are given the general name Canola (Bell, 1993).

During seed processing most glucosinolate breakdown products are formed. The degree of degradation depends on seed properties and on processing conditions such as moisture level, pressure and temperature. A reduction in glucosinolate content can be obtained by autoclaving meal for 1.5 h (Mansour et al., 1993), treatment of meal with $Cu^{2+}$ and the use of ammonia in conjugation with other processing (Keith and Bell, 1982).

The use of rapeseed meal containing glucosinolates as a feedstuff and its antinutritional effects have been extensively studied. Although there is some controversy about the quantity of glucosinolates that is tolerated by various animal species, threshold levels for glucosinolates in diets have been suggested (Hill, 1991; Bell, 1993; Mawson et al., 1993).

## 3.7   Food quality and glucosinolates

The typical flavour and odour of brassicas are largely due to glucosinolate-derived volatiles (isothiocyanates, thiocyanates, nitriles). It has been shown that the glucosinolates sinigrin and progoitrin are involved in the bitterness observed in Brussels sprouts (Fenwick et al., 1983). Van Doorn et al. (1997) confirmed the role of sinigrin and progoitrin in taste preference by using taste trials with samples of Brussels sprouts. It appeared that consumers preferred Brussels sprouts with a low sinigrin and progoitrin content. In cabbage sinigrin is an abundant glucosinolate that gives a pungent and bitter flavour. The stronger flavour in the heart of the cabbage is consistent with the presence of greater amounts of sinigrin found in cabbage heads. Low levels of 2-propenyl isothiocyanates formed from sinigrin result in a flat and dull product (Rosa et al., 1997). Pungency and bitterness caused by glucosinolate breakdown products play a role in the taste preference of consumers and are therefore important quality factors for brassicas.

Improvement in the flavour and nutritional properties of brassicas can be achieved by using molecular markers in selecting specific glucosinolate lines in breeding programmes (Campos-De Quiroz and Mithen, 1996). Developing brassicas less susceptible to diseases, less attractive to insects and with desirable agronomic storage and sensory characteristics by manipulating the glucosinolate levels can result in crops with greater commercial value (Borek et al., 1994; Brown and Morra, 1995).

The positive effects against cancer can be considered as another notable quality factor of glucosinolates and their derivatives. Brassicaceous vegetables or glucosinolate derivatives have been shown to modify endogenous detoxification processes and thus they may interfere in a positive way with the metabolism of chemical carcinogens (McDanell et al., 1988; Jongen,

1996). Enhancement of these effects by increasing the levels of specific glucosinolates is of importance in obtaining protective effects at normal consumption levels.

## 3.8   Responses to stress factors

Glucosinolates and their breakdown products are considered to function as part of the plant's defence against insect attack and to act as phagostimulants (Chew, 1988).

There is now considerable information on the importance of glucosinolates in insect–plant interactions. However, less is known about the influence of biotic factors on glucosinolate metabolism in plants. It has been demonstrated that attack by aphids (Lammerink et al., 1984), root flies (Birch et al., 1990, 1992) and flea beetles (Koritsas et al., 1991), changes both the total concentration of glucosinolates in different plant tissues and the relative proportions of aliphatic and aromatic compounds.

Other examples of stress-induced increases in levels of glucosinolates are mechanical wounding and infestation (Koritsas et al., 1991), methyl jasmonate exposure (Doughty et al., 1995), and grazing (Macfarlane Smith et al., 1991) for intact plants or UV-irradiation (Monde et al., 1991) and chopping (Verkerk et al., 1997a) for vegetables after harvesting. Apparently, besides a breakdown mechanism for glucosinolates, an induction mechanism of glucosinolate biosynthesis by stress factors is present in brassica vegetables.

## 3.9   Effects of processing

The effects of processing on glucosinolate levels in vegetables have been reviewed by De Vos and Blijleven (1988). Processes such as chopping for raw consumption, cooking and fermentation damage plant cells and bring myrosinase into contact with glucosinolates. This influences the levels of glucosinolates, the extent of hydrolysis and the composition, flavour and aroma of the final products. In addition, low-temperature storage processes such as freezing and refrigerating can alter the metabolism of glucosinolates. Freezing without previous inactivation of myrosinase results in an almost complete decomposition of glucosinolates after thawing (Quinsac et al., 1994). During sauerkraut fermentation of white cabbage all glucosinolates were hydrolyzed within two weeks according to Daxenbichler et al. (1980). The breakdown products investigated were the thiocyanate ion, isothiocyanates, goitrin and the nitriles 1-cyano-3-methylsulphinylpropane (from glucoiberin) and 1-cyano-2,3-epithiopropane (from sinigrin). Isothiocyanates, goitrin and cyano-2,3-epithiopropane were not detectable throughout fermentation.

The effects of cooking on glucosinolates have received a relatively large amount of attention. Cooking reduces glucosinolate levels by approximately 30 to 60%, depending on the type of compound. Thermal degradation and wash-out also occur, leading to large losses of intact glucosinolates. Degradation products are hardly detectable after cooking, with the exception of the thiocyanate ion and ascorbigen (MacLeod and MacLeod, 1968; McMillan *et al.*, 1986). Pulping of plant tissues results in the complete breakdown of glucosinolates by autolysis.

Chopping of vegetables is necessary prior to many other processing steps. Chopping of fresh plant tissues creates optimal conditions for myrosinase and a high degree of glucosinolate hydrolysis can be expected. In contrast to these expectations and reported findings, Verkerk *et al.* (1997a) observed elevated levels of all indole and some aliphatic glucosinolates after chopping and prolonged exposure of brassica vegetables to air of different kinds. In white cabbage the largest increase they found was for 4-methoxyglucobrassicin, which increased 15-fold (Figure 3.4).

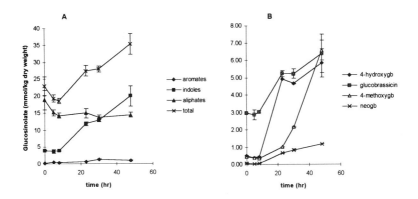

**Figure 3.4**    Levels of glucosinolates in white cabbage after chopping and prolonged exposure at room temperature (Verkerk *et al.*, 1997b)

Increasing the amount of indole glucosinolates can have a great influence on the quality factors, such as flavour, and anticarcinogenicity of brassica vegetables. Koritsas *et al.* (1991) mention the parallels with the induction of indole glucosinolates by infestation or mechanical wounding of brassica plants.

## 3.10 Analytical methods

The large amounts of different glucosinolates in brassicas and the fact that each glucosinolate can produce different breakdown products makes their analysis very complicated. The analytical methodology was extensively reviewed by McGregor *et al.* (1983). A brief overview is presented here.

Analytical methods can be divided into those for total glucosinolates, individual glucosinolates and the breakdown products. Over the past four decades, increased knowledge of the diversity of the glucosinolates, their enzymatically released products and factors influencing their release have led to a multiplicity of analytical methods.

Since glucosinolates coexist with myrosinase in the plant, processes like grinding or cutting of fresh tissue in the presence of water will initiate a rapid hydrolysis of these compounds. For analysis of intact glucosinolates, inhibition of myrosinase activity is therefore essential. Before disruption of the material, samples should be completely dried by freeze-drying or freezing in liquid nitrogen. The use of aqueous methanol for extraction, in combination with high temperatures, also inhibits myrosinase (Heaney and Fenwick, 1993).

### 3.10.1 Total glucosinolates

Glucosinolates yield equimolar amounts of glucose on hydrolysis with myrosinase. This is true for almost all glucosinolates and methods based on the measurement of enzymatically released glucose are relatively rapid and simple to apply (Heaney *et al.*, 1988). The total glucosinolate content of a food sample can be measured by determining the quantity of glucose released after treatment with the enzyme, but this takes no account of endogenous glucose. Alternatively, extraction of glucosinolates can be performed, followed by selective clean-up that eliminates free glucose and other interfering compounds, after which the controlled enzymatic release of bound glucose is possible.

Myrosinase hydrolysis of glucosinolates gives rise to an unstable aglucone, which after a Lossen rearrangement produces an equimolar amount of bisulphate. Several methods have been described for the quantification of this bisulphate ion using titrimetry and gravimetry. Schnug (1987) described a method in which the bisulphate liberated after sulphation is precipitated with barium chloride and the residual barium is measured by X-ray emission spectroscopy.

### 3.10.2 Individual glucosinolates

Gas liquid chromatography (GLC) of derivatized glucosinolates is the traditional method for identifying and quantifying individual glucosinolates (Underhill and Kirkland, 1971). Initially glucosinolates were extracted with boiling water, and derivatized and separated by isothermal chromatography. Substantial improvements to this method have been made by Thies (1976). Ion-exchange purification of glucosinolate extracts to remove carbohydrates and other impurities before derivatization increases the sensitivity. A major breakthrough in glucosinolate analysis was achieved with the introduction of enzymatic on-column desulphation using aryl sulphatase. The introduction of a desulphation step before derivatization was performed to eliminate sulphate that interfered with gas chromatographic analysis. Desulphation was elegantly carried out on the ion-exchange column using a commercially available sulphatase isolated from an edible snail (*Helix pomatia*). Free sulphate in the glucosinolate extract, which could inhibit the sulphatase, was precipitated by addition of barium acetate and removed by centrifugation before addition of the extract to the ion-exchange column.

Some indole glucosinolates are thermally unstable, therefore high performance liquid chromatography (HPLC) has become a preferred method of analysis. HPLC has the advantage of direct determination of glucosinolates. The first successful application of the technique was described by Helboe *et al.* (1980). Glucosinolates were purified and desulphated on-column and then separated by ion-exchange chromatography (Olsen and Sørensen, 1979) or reverse phase ion-pairing chromatography using a $C_{18}$ Nucleosil column (with gradient elution using acetonitrile–water mixtures as the mobile phase and tetraoctylammonium bromide as the source of counterion). By avoiding the use of buffer solutions and ion-pairing reagents, glucosinolates could be collected in a pure form suitable for identification by mass spectrometry. With the aid of this method, two new glucosinolates were separated and identified, 4-hydroxy-3-indolylmethyl glucosinolate and 4-methoxy-3-indolylmethyl glucosinolate (Truscott *et al.*, 1982).

Several mass spectrometric techniques have been investigated for structure elucidation of the various (desulpho-)glucosinolates (e.g. direct probing electron impact, chemical ionization and fast atom bombardment). Considerable structural information can be obtained with these techniques.

One of the major problems in the analysis of glucosinolates has been the lack of suitable standards. The only commercially available glucosinolates are benzylglucosinolate (glucotropaeolin) and 2-propenylglucosinolate (sinigrin). Sinigrin is not a suitable internal standard because of the presence of this compound in most brassicaceous plants. Glucotropaeolin is not normally present in brassicas and has been used as an internal standard.

### 3.10.3 Breakdown products

The application of HPLC to the investigation of glucosinolate breakdown products has been limited due to the volatility of many compounds. Furthermore, thiocyanates and nitriles are not detectable spectrometrically. Isothiocyanates and nitriles can be analyzed by GLC. HPLC with UV detection may be used for analysis of oxazolidinethiones and indoles. Quinsac *et al.* (1992) developed a method for analyzing oxazolidinethiones in biological fluids with a high degree of selectivity. However, HPLC finds most use in the analysis of intact glucosinolates or desulphoglucosinolates. For identification and confirmation of structures both techniques can be coupled to mass spectrometry. Mass spectroscopy has proved to be an important tool in the identification and structural elucidation of glucosinolates and their breakdown products. Positive ion fast atom bombardment mass spectrometry (FAB) (Fenwick *et al.*, 1982) has yielded mass spectra characterized by abundant protonated and cationized molecular ions with relatively little fragmentation. In the negative ion mode, FAB produces an abundant molecular ion (of the glucosinolate anion). This has proved especially advantageous in the analysis of crude plant extracts and mixtures of purified glucosinolates.

Zhang *et al.* (1992b) developed a spectroscopic quantitation of organic isothiocyanates. Under mild conditions nearly all organic isothiocyanates react quantitatively with an excess of vicinal dithiols to give rise to five-membered cyclic condensation products, with release of the corresponding free amines. The method can be used to measure 1 nmol or less of pure isothiocyanates or isothiocyanates in crude mixtures.

### 3.11  Conclusions

Glucosinolate research is expanding from toxicological areas into more health-promoting areas. Much of this research nowadays is focused on the potential effects of glucosinolates, and their breakdown products, on biological processes associated with cellular damage and cancer development. The role and mechanisms of glucosinolates and their products in protecting plants against fungal and insect attack and the allelochemical affects on behaviour, health and growth of other species is another important area of research.

It is clear that the factors inducing and directing indole glucosinolate metabolism in plants need to be studied in much greater detail as the evidence concerning the biological activities of these compounds in relation to man increases.

### References

Bell, J.M. (1993) Factors affecting the nutritional value of canola meal: a review. *Canadian Journal of Animal Science*, **73** 679-97.

Benn, M.H. (1962) Biosynthesis of the mustard oils. *Chemistry and Industry*, **12** 1907.

Birch, A.N.E., Griffiths, D.W. and MacFarlane-Smith, W.H. (1990), Change in forage and oilseed rape (*B. napus*) root glucosinolates in response to attack by turnip root fly (*Delia floralis*) larvae. *Journal of the Science of of Food and Agriculture*, **51** 309-20.

Birch, A.N.E., Griffiths, D.W., Hopkins, R.J., Macfarlane-Smith, W.H. and McKinlay, R.G. (1992) Glucosinolate responses of swede, kale, forage and oilseed rape to root damage by turnip root fly (*Delia floralis*) larvae. *Journal of the Science of Food and Agriculture*, **60** 1-9.

Blanc-Muesser, M., Drigues, H., Joseph, B., Viaud, M.C. and Rollin, P. (1990) First synthesis of *alpha*-glucosinolates. *Tetrahedron Letters*, **31** 3867-68.

Bones, A.M. and Rossiter, J.T. (1996) The myrosinase–glucosinolate system, its organisation and biochemistry. *Physiologia Plantarum*, **97** 194-208.

Borek, V., Morra, M.J., Brown, P.D. and McCaffrey, J.P. (1994) Allelochemicals produced during sinigrin decomposition in soil. *Journal of Agricultural Food Chemistry*, **42** 1030-34.

Brown, P.D. and Morra, M.J. (1995) Glucosinolate-containing plant tissues as bioherbicides. *Journal of Agricultural Food Chemistry*, **43** 3070-74.

Buchwaldt, L., Melchior Larsen, L., Ploger, A. and Sørensen, H. (1986) Fast polymer liquid chromatography isolation and characterization of plant myrosinase, β-thioglucoside glucohydrolase isoenzymes, *Journal of Chromatography*, **363** 71-80.

Campos-De Quiroz, H. and Mithen, R. (1996) Molecular markers for low-glucosinolate alleles in oilseed rape (*Brassica napus* L.). *Molecular Breeding*, **2** (3) 277-81.

Carlson, D.J., Daxenbichler, M.E., VanEtten, C.H., Tookey, H.L. and Williams, P.H. (1981) Glucosinolates in crucifer vegetables: turnips and rutabagas. *Journal of Agricultural Food Chemistry*, **29** 1235-39.

Carlson, D.J., Daxenbichler, M.E., VanEtten, C.H., Kwolek, W.F. and Williams, P.H. (1987a) Glucosinolates in crucifer vegetables: broccoli, brussels sprouts, cauliflower, collards, kale, mustard greens and kohlrabi. *Journal of the American Society for Horticultural Science*, **112** 173-78.

Carlson, D.J., Daxenbichler, M.E., Tookey, H.L., Kwolek, W.F., Hill, C.B. and Williams, P.H. (1987b) Glucosinolates in turnip tops and roots: cultivars grown for greens and/or roots. *Journal of the American Society for Horticultural Science*, **112** 179-83.

Chew, F.S. (1988) Biological effects of glucosinolates, in *Biologically Active Natural Products for Potential Use in Agriculture* (ed. H.G. Cutler), American Chemical Society, Washington, DC, pp. 155-81.

Davis, J.B., Auld, D.L. and Erickson, D.A. (1991) Glucosinolate content and composition of eight Brassicaceae species. *Cruciferae Newsletters*, **14/15** 118-19.

Dawson, G.W., Hick, R.N., Bennett, R.N., Donald, A., Pickett, A. and Wallsgrove, R.M. (1993) Synthesis of glucosinolate precursors and investigations into the biosynthesis of phenylalkyl- and methylthioalkylglucosinolates. *Journal of Biological Chemistry*, **268** 27154-59.

Daxenbichler, M.E., VanEtten, C.H. and Williams, P.H. (1980) Glucosinolate products in commercial sauerkraut. *Journal of Agricultural Food Chemistry*, **28** 809-11.

De Vos, R.H. and Blijleven, W.G.H. (1988) The effect of processing conditions on glucosinolates in cruciferous vegetables. *Zeitschrift für lebensmittel Untersuchung und Forschung*, **187** 525-29.

Doughty, K.J., Kiddle, G.A., Pye, P.J., Wallsgrove, R.M. and Pickett, J.A. (1995) Selective induction of glucosinolates in oilseed rape leaves by methyl jasmonate. *Phytochemistry*, **38** (2), 347-50.

Dragsted, L.O., Strube, M. and Larsen, J.C. (1993) Cancer-protective factors in fruits and vegetables: biochemical and biological background. *Pharmacology and Toxicology*, **72** (suppl. 1) 116-35.

Fenwick, G.R. and Heaney, R.K. (1983) Glucosinolates and their breakdown products in cruciferous crops, foods and feedingstuffs. *Food Chemistry*, **11** 249-71.

Fenwick, G.R., Eagles, J. and Self, R. (1982) The fast atom bombardment mass spectra of glucosinolates and glucosinolate mixtures. *Organic Mass Spectrometry*, **17** 544-46.

Fenwick, G.R., Griffiths, N.M. and Heaney, R.K. (1983) Bitterness in Brussels sprouts (*Brassica oleracea* L. var gemmifera): the role of glucosinolates and their breakdown products. *Journal of the Science of Food and Agriculture*, **34** 73-80.

Gildemeister, E. and Hofmann, F. (1927) *Die Aetherische Ole*, 3rd edn, vol. 1, Schimmel and Co., Leipzig, p. 145.

Godeschalk, F.E. (1987) Consumptie van voedingsmiddelen in Nederland in 1984 en 1985. Periodieke rapportage **64**, LEI, The Hague.

GrootWassink, J.W.D., Reed, D.W. and Kolenovsky, A.W. (1994) Immunopurification and immunocharacterisation of the glucosinolate biosynthetic enzyme thiohydoximate S-glucotransferase. *Plant Physiology*, **105** 425-33

Halkier, B.A. and Lindberg-Møller, B. (1991) Involvement of cytochrome P-450 in the biosynthesis of dhurrin in *Sorghum bicolor* (L.) Moench. *Plant Physiology*, **96** 10-17.

Hanley, A.B., Parsley, K.R., Lewis, J.A. and Fenwick, G.R. (1990) Chemistry of indole glucosinolates: intermediacy of indol-3-ylmethylisothiocyanates in the enzymic hydrolysis of indole glucosinolates. *Journal of the Chemical Society Perkin Transactions*, **1** 2273-76.

Harborne, J.B. (1989) Biosynthesis and functions of anti-nutritional factors in plants. *Aspects of Applied Biology*, **19** 21-28.

Heaney, R.K. and Fenwick, G.R. (1980) Glucosinolates in brassica vegetables: analysis of 22 varieties of Brussels sprouts. *Journal of the Science of Food and Agriculture*, **31** 785-93.

Heaney, R.K. and Fenwick, G.R. (1993) Methods for glucosinolate analysis, in *Methods in Plant Biochemistry*, vol. 6 (ed. P.G. Waterman), Academic Press, London, pp. 531-50.

Heaney, R.K., Spinks, E.A. and Fenwick, G.R. (1988) Improved method for the determination of the total glucosinolate content of rapeseed by determination of enzymatically released glucose. *Analyst*, **113** 1515-18.

Helboe, P., Olson, O. and Sørensen, H. (1980) Separation of glucosinolates by HPLC. *Journal of Chromatography*, **197** 199-205.

Hill, R. (1991) Rapeseed meal in the diets of ruminants. *Nutrition Abstracts and Reviews*, **61** 139-55.

James, D. and Rossiter, J.T. (1991) Development and characteristics of myrosinase in *Brassica napus* during early seedling growth. *Plant Physiology*, **82** 163-70.

Jongen, W.M.F. (1996) Glucosinolates in brassica: occurrence and significance as cancer-modulating agents. *Proceedings of the Nutrition Society*, **55** 433-46.

Keith, M.O. and Bell, J.M. (1982) Effects of ammoniation on the composition and nutritional quality of low glucosinolate rapeseed (canola) meal. *Canadian Journal of Animal Science*, **62** 547-55.

Kjaer, A. (1974) The natural distribution of glucosinolates: a uniform class of sulphur containing glucosides, in *Chemistry in Botanical Classification* (eds. G. Bendz and J. Santesson), Academic Press, London, pp. 229-34.

Kjaer, A. (1976) Glucosinolates in the cruciferae, in *The Biology and Chemistry of the Cruciferae* (eds. J.G. Vaughan, A.J. MacLeod and B.M.G. Jones), Academic Press, London, pp. 207-19.

Kjaer, A. and Conti, J. (1954) Isothiocyanates, VII: a convenient synthesis of erysoline. *Acta Chemica Scandinavica*, **8** 295-98.

Koch, B. Nielson, V.S. and Halkier, B.A. (1992) Biosynthesis of cyanogenic glucosides in seedlings of cassava. *Archives of Biochemistry and Biophysics*, **292** 141-50.

Koritsas, V.M., Lewis, J.A. and Fenwick, G.R. (1991) Glucosinolate responses of oilseed rape, mustard and kale to mechanical wounding and infestation by cabbage stem fleabeetle (*Psylliodes chrysocephala*). *Annual Applied Biology*, **118** 209-21.

Kutácek, M., Prochazka, Z. and Veres, K. (1962) Biogenesis of glucobrassicin, the *in vitro* precursor of ascorbigen. *Nature*, **194** 393-94.

Labague, L., Gardrat, G., Coustille, J.L., Viaud, M.C. and Rollin, P. (1991) Identification of enzymatic degradation products from synthesised glucobrassicin by GC-MS. *Journal of Chromatography*, **586** 166-70.

Lammerink, J., MacGibbon, D.B. and Wallace, A.R. (1984) Effect of cabbage aphid on total glucosinolate in the seed of oilseed rape. *New Zealand Journal of Agricultural Research*, **27** 89-92.

Langer, P., Michajlovskij, N., Sedlak, J. and Kutka, M. (1971) Studies on the antithyroid activity of naturally occurring L-5-vinyl-2-thiooxazolidone. *Endokrinologie*, **57** 225-29.

Lewis, J.A., Fenwick, G.R. and Gray, A.R. (1991) Glucosinolates in brassica vegetables: green-curded cauliflowers and purple-headed broccoli. *Lebensmittel-Wissenschaft Technology*, **24** 361-63.

Ludwig-Muler, J. and Hilgenberg, W. (1988) A plasma membrane-bound enzyme oxidizes L-tryptophan to indole-3-acetaldoxime. *Plant Physiology*, **74** 240-50.

Lykkesfeldt, J. and Lindberg-Møller, B. (1993) Synthesis of benzylglucosinolate in *Tropaeolum majus* L.: isothiocyanates as potent enzyme inhibitors. *Plant Physiology*, **102** 609-13.

Macfarlane-Smith, W.H., Griffiths, D.W. and Boag, B. (1991) Overwinter variation in glucosinolate content of green tissue of rape (*Brassica napus*) in response to grazing by wild rabbit (*Oryctolagus cuniculus*). *Journal of the Science of Food and Agriculture*, **56** 511-21.

MacGibbon, D.B. and Allison, R.M. (1970) A method for the separation and detection of plant glucosinolases (myrosinases). *Phytochemistry*, **9** 541-44.

MacLeod, A.J. and MacLeod, G. (1968) Volatiles of cooked cabbage. *Journal of the Science of Food and Agriculture*, **19** 273-77.

Mansour, E.H., Dworschák, E., Lugasi, A., Gaál, Ö., Barna, É. and Gergely, A. (1993) Effects of processing on the antinutritive factors and nutritive value of rapeseed products. *Food Chemistry*, **47** 247-52.

Mawson, R., Heaney, R.K., Piskula, M. and Kozlowska, H. (1993) Rapeseed meal glucosinolates and their antinutritional effects, 1: rapeseed production and chemistry of glucosinolates. *Die Nahrung*, **37** 131-40.

McDanell, R., McLean, A.E.M., Hanley, A.B., Heaney, R.K. and Fenwick, G.R. (1988) Chemical and biological properties of indole glucosinolates (Glucobrassicins): a review. *Food and Chemical Toxicology*, **26** (1) 59-70.

McGregor, D.I., Mullin, W.J. and Fenwick, G.R. (1983) Analytical methodology for determining glucosinolate composition and content. *Journal of the American Official Analytical Chemists*, **66** 825-49.

McKinnon, P.J. and Bowland, J.P. (1979) Effects of feeding low and high glucosinolate rapeseed meals and soybean meals on thyroid function of young pigs. *Canadian Journal of Animal Science*, **59** 589-96.

McMillan, M., Spinks, E.A. and Fenwick, G.R. (1986) Preliminary observations on the effect of dietary Brussels sprouts on thyroid function. *Human Toxicology*, **5** 15-19.

Monde, K., Takasugi, M., Lewis, J.A. and Fenwick, G.R. (1991) Time-course studies of phytoalexins and glucosinolates in UV irradiated turnip tissue. *Zeitschrift fur naturforschung section C biosciences*, **46** (3–4) 189-93.

Mullin, W.J. and Sahasrabudhe, M.R. (1977) Glucosinolate content of cruciferous vegetable crops. *Canadian Journal of Plant Science*, **57** 1227-30.

Ohtsuru, M. and Hata, T. (1973) General characteristics of the intracellular myrosinase from *A. niger*. *Agricultural and Biological Chemistry*, **37** 2543-48.

Olsen, O. and Sørensen, H. (1979) Isolation of glucosinolates and the identification of O-(α-L-rhamnopyranosyloxy)benzylglucosinolate from *Reseda odorata*. *Phytochemistry*, **18** 1547-52.

Paik, I.K., Robblee, A.R. and Clandinin, D.R. (1980) Products of the hydrolysis of rapeseed glucosinolates. *Canadian Journal of Animal Science*, **60** 481-93.

Quinsac, A., Ribaillier, D., Rollin, P. and Dreux, M. (1992) Analysis of 5-vinyl-1,3-oxazolidine-2-thione by liquid chromatography. *Journal of the American Official Analytical Chemists*, **75** 529-36.

Quinsac, A., Charrier, A. and Ribaillier, D. (1994) Glucosinolates in etiolated sprouts of sea-kale (*Crambe maritima* L.). *Journal of the Science of Food and Agriculture*, **65** 201-207.

Rosa, E.A.S., Heaney, R.K., Fenwick, G.R. and Portas, C.A.M. (1997) Glucosinolates in crop plants. *Horticultural Reviews*, **19** 99-215.

Sang, J.P. and Salisbury, P.A. (1988) Glucosinolate profiles of international rapeseed lines. *Journal of the Science of Food and Agriculture*, **45** 255-61.

Schnug, E. (1987) Eine methode zur schnellen und einfachen bestimmung des gesamtglucosinolatgehaltes in grünmasse und samen von kruziferen durch die quantitative analyse enzymatisch freisetzharen sulfates. *Fat Science Technology*, **89** 438-42.

Smith, T.K., Musk, S.R.R. and Johnson, I.T. (1996) Allyl isothiocyanate selectively kills undifferentiated HT 29 cells *in vitro* and suppresses aberrant crypt foci in the colonic mucosa of rats.

*Biochemical Society Transactions*, **24** (3) s381.

Sones, K., Heaney, R.K. and Fenwick, G.R. (1984a). The glucosinolate content of UK vegetables: cabbages, swede and turnip. *Food Additives and Contaminants*, **1** 289-96.

Sones, K., Heaney, R.K. and Fenwick, G.R. (1984b) Glucosinolates in brassica vegetables: analysis of 27 cauliflower cultivars. *Journal of the Science of Food and Agriculture*, **35** 762-66.

Sones, K., Heaney, R.K. and Fenwick, G.R. (1984c) An estimate of the mean daily intake of glucosinolates from cruciferous vegetables in the UK. *Journal of the Science of Food and Agriculture*, **35** 712-20.

Sørensen, H. (1990) Glucosinolates: structure–properties function, in *Canola and Rapeseed* (ed. F. Shahdi), Van Nostrand, New York, pp. 149-72.

Steinmetz, K.A. and Potter, J.D. (1991) Vegetables, fruit and cancer. I. Epidemiology. *Cancer Causes and Control*, **2** 325-57.

Talalay, P. and Zhang, Y. (1996) Chemoprotection against cancer by isothiocyanates and glucosinolates. *Biochemical Society Transactions*, **24** 806-10.

Thies, W. (1976) *Fette Seifen Anstrichm.*, **78** 231-34.

Tiedink, H.G.M., Hissink, A.M., Lodema, S.M., van Broekhoven, L.W. and Jongen, W.M.F. (1990) Several known indole compounds are not important precursors of direct mutagenic N-nitroso compounds in green cabbage. *Mutation Research*, **232** 199-207.

Tiedink, H.G.M., Malingre, C.E., van Broekhoven, L.W., Jongen, W.M.F., Lewis, J. and Fenwick, G.R. (1991) The role of glucosinolates in the formation of N-nitroso compounds. *Journal of Agricultural Food Chemistry*, **39** 922-26.

Tookey, H.L., VanEtten, C.H. and Daxenbichler, M.E. (1980) Glucosinolates, in *Toxic Constituents of Plant Foodstuffs* (ed. I.E. Liener), Academic Press, New York, pp. 103-42.

Truscott, R.J.W., Burke, D.G. and Minchinton, I.R. (1982) *Biochemical and Biophysical Research Communications*, **107** 1258-64.

Underhill, E.W. and Kirkland, D.F. (1971) *Journal of Chromatography*, **57** 47-54.

Underhill, E.W., Chisholm, M.D. and Wetter, L.R. (1962) Biosynthesis of mustard oil glucosides. *Canadian Journal of Biochemistry and Physiology*, **40** 1505-14.

Underhill, E.W., Wetter, L.R. and Chisholm, M.D. (1973) Biosynthesis of glucosinolates. *Biochemistry Society Symposium*, **38** 303-26.

Van Doorn, H.E., Van Holst, G.J., De Nijs, J., Broer, K., Postma, E., Van Der Kruk, G.C., Raaijmakers-Ruijs, N.C.M.E. and Jongen, W.M.F. (1997) The taste preference for Brussels sprouts is determined by the glucosinolates Sinigrin and Progoitrin (submitted).

VanEtten, C.H. (1969) Goitrogens, in *Toxic Constituents of Plant Foodstuffs* (ed. I.E. Liener), Academic Press, New York, pp. 103-42.

VanEtten, C.H. and Tookey, H.L. (1979) Chemistry and biology effects of glucosinolates, in *Herbivores: their Interaction with Secondary Plant Metabolites* (eds. G.A. Rozenthal and D.H. Janzen), Academic Press, New York, pp. 471-500.

VanEtten, C.H., Daxenbichler, M.E., Williams, P.H. and Kwolek, F. (1976) Glucosinolates and derived products in cruciferous vegetables: analysis of the edible part from 22 varieties of cabbage. *Journal of Agricultural Food Chemistry*, **27** 648-50.

VanEtten, C.H., Daxenbichler, M.E., Tookey, H.L., Kwolek, W.F., Williams, P.H. and Yoder, O.C. (1980) Glucosinolates: potential toxicants in cabbage cultivars. *Journal of the American Society for Horticultural Science*, **105** 710-14.

Verkerk, R., Van Der Gaag, M.S., Dekker, M. and Jongen, W.M.F. (1997a) Effects of processing conditions on glucosinolates in cruciferous vegetables. *Cancer Letters*, **114** 193-94.

Verkerk, R., Krebbers, B., Dekker, M. and Jongen, W.M.F. (1997b) Glucosinolates as contributing factors in the quality of brassica vegetables: stress-induced increase of indole glucosinolates, in *Proceedings of Crop Protection and Food Quality* (in press).

Wattenberg, L.W. (1983) Inhibition of neoplasia by minor dietary constituents. *Cancer Research*, **43** 2448s-2453s.

Wattenberg, L.W. (1985) Chemoprevention of cancer. *Cancer Research*, **45** 1-8.

Wattenberg, L.W. (1992) Inhibition of carcinogenesis by minor dietary constituents. *Cancer Research*, **52** 2085s-2091s.

Zhang, Y., Talalay, P., Cho, C.-G. and Posner, G.H. (1992a) A major inducer of anticarcinogenic protective enzymes from broccoli: isolation and elucidation of structure. *Proceedings of the National Academy of Sciences of the USA*, **89** 2399-2403.

Zhang, Y., Cho, C.-G., Posner, G.H. and Talalay, P. (1992b) Spectroscopic quantitation of organic isothiocyanates by cyclocondensation with vicinal dithiols. *Analytical Biochemistry*, **205** 100-107.

# 4 Natural oestrogenic compounds

Daphne Aldridge and Caroline Tahourdin

## 4.1 Introduction

Research on plant oestrogens is a fast-moving field and this chapter provides a brief overview of representative literature. The overview includes the reasons for interest in these compounds, their occurrence, dietary sources, measurement and reported effects in humans and animals. It does not cover highly specialized areas (e.g. food processing) in detail; for these readers are directed to other, more extensive, reviews (e.g. Verdeal and Ryan, 1979; Price and Fenwick, 1985; Setchell and Adlercreutz, 1988; Adlercreutz, 1995). The present review focuses on the phytoestrogens (plant oestrogens) but very brief reference is made to endogenous animal/mammalian oestrogens in animals. Limited data on the oestrogenic mycotoxin (mycoestrogen), zearalenone, are also provided. Information on environmental oestrogens (exogenous organic chemicals), which may be present in food as contaminants, is not included.

## 4.2 Background

Oestrogens are steroid compounds produced in the mammalian body that serve to maintain female sexual characteristics, the main human oestrogen being 17β-oestradiol (Figure 4.1). Phytoestrogens (plant oestrogens) are a group of non-steroidal compounds produced by a range of plants that, although lacking the classic steroid ring structure (Figure 4.1), have properties similar to 17β-oestradiol. In some plant-derived foods, phytoestrogen concentrations are high and thus their mode of action and possible implications to human health are of interest. Isoflavones are one group of phytoestrogens that has been studied extensively. Other groups include the coumestans, lignans and mycoestrogens such as zearalenone. Zearalenone is a resorcyclic acid lactone produced by various species of *Fusarium* moulds (de Nijs *et al.*, 1996) found in food and fodder plants. Thus zearalenone and its metabolites may also find their way into the human food chain.

The majority of phytoestrogens found in food are isoflavones, therefore these substances have been better characterized than other phytoestrogens such as the coumestans. The basic structures of the four main isoflavones genistein, daidzein, formonetin and biochanin A, together with glycitein (also found in soya), and genistin, daidzin and glycitin (the glucosides of genistein, daidzein and glycitein), are shown schematically in Figure 4.2.

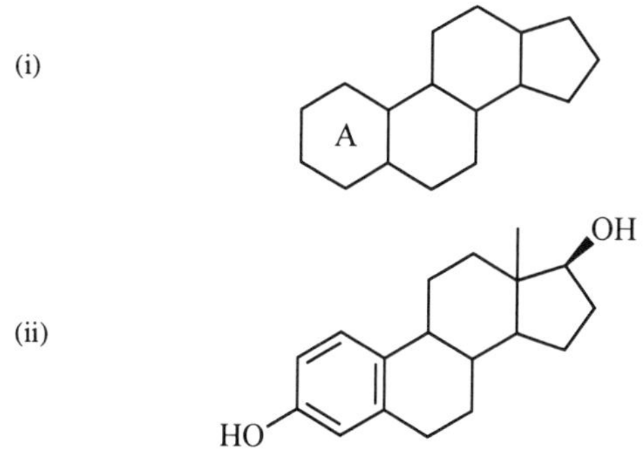

(i)

(ii)

**Figure 4.1**   i) Steroid skeleton and ii) 17β-oestradiol

(NB glycitein and glycitin found in soya, see, for example, Wang and Murphy [1994a], are not reported to be oestrogenic). Figure 4.3 gives the structures of coumestrol and 4'-methoxycoumestrol, the main coumestans. Figure 4.4 shows the structures of the plant lignans, secoisolariciresinol and matairesinol, the mammalian lignans enterolactone and enterodiol (metabolites of secoisolariciresinol and matairesinol), and of equol, a metabolite of a number of the phytoestrogens (e.g. daidzein and formonetin). In plants the isoflavones are usually linked to a sugar molecule at the OH position (as shown on ring A in Figure 4.2 [iii]) forming O-glycosides, which usually occur as malonyl or acetyl esters. The glycosides may undergo hydrolysis to form aglycones. This may be during food processing, for example in the preparation of fermented foods such as soy sauce and miso, or in the human body, probably during transit through the gastrointestinal tract.

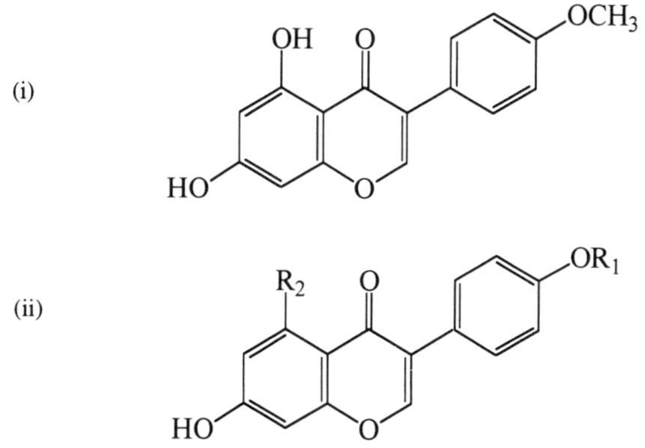

(i)

(ii)

(iii)

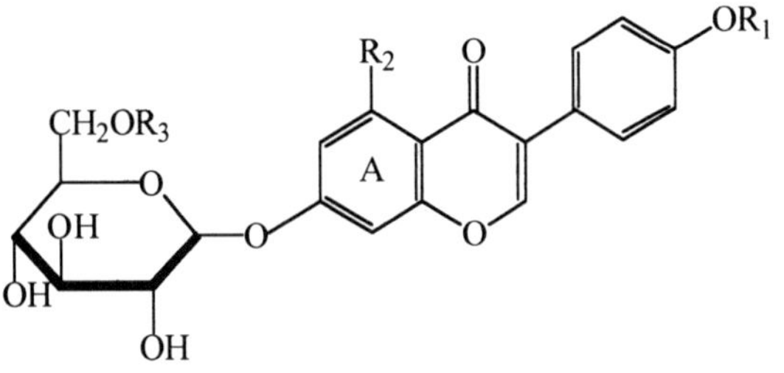

(iv)

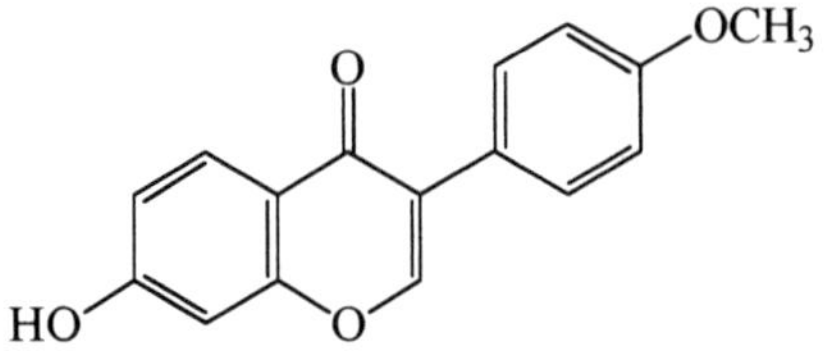

**Figure 4.2**    Structures of daidzein, genistein, glycitein, formonetin, biochanin A and the glucosides of daidzein and genistein and glycitein: (i) biochanin A; (ii) genestein/daidzein/
glycitein:- daidzein: $R_1$ and $R_2$ = H; genistein: $R_1$ = H, $R_2$ = OH; glycitein: $R_1$ =
$OCH_3$, $R_2$ = H; (iii) glucosides:- daidzin: $R_1$, $R_2$ and $R_3$ = H; genistin: $R_1$ = H; $R_2$ =
OH, $R_3$ = H; glycitin: $R_1$ = $OCH_3$, $R_2$ and $R_3$ = H; 6"-$O$-acetyl compound: $R_3$ =
$COCH_3$; 6"-$O$-malonyl compound: $R_3$ = $COCH_2COOH$; (iv) formonetin.

(i)

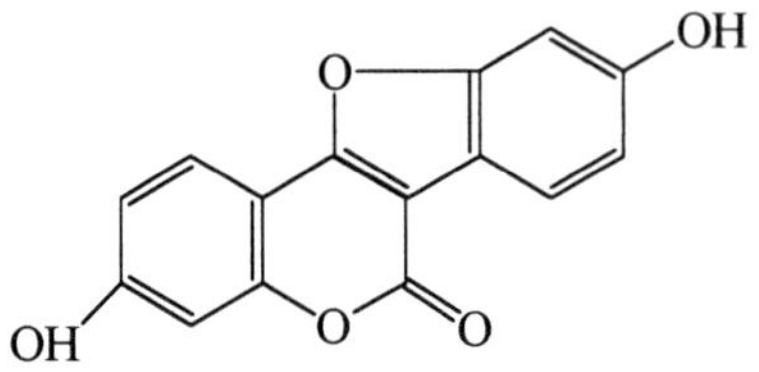

(ii)

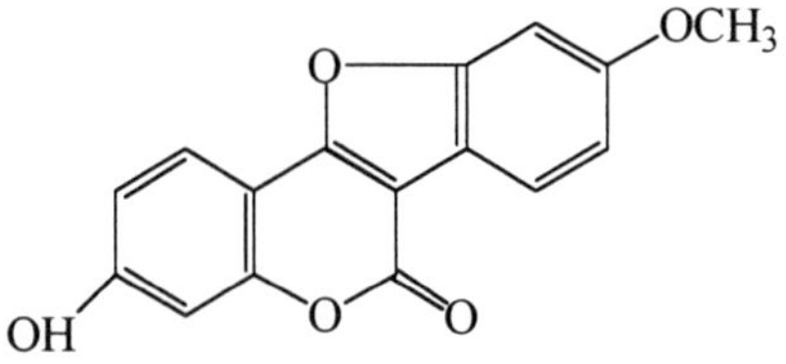

**Figure 4.3**    Structures of coumestrol and 4'-methoxycoumestrol: (i) coumestrol;
(ii) 4'-methoxycoumestrol.

(i)

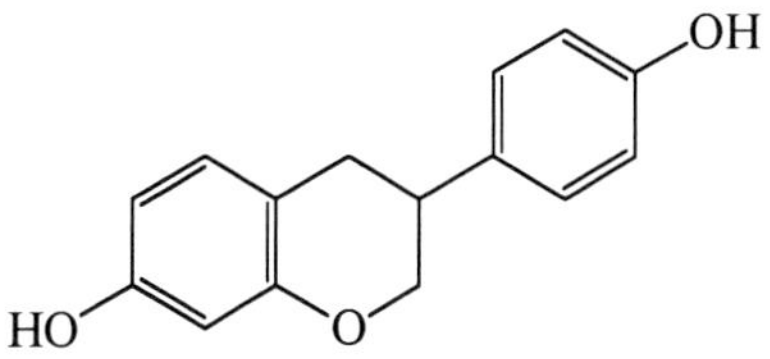


(ii)

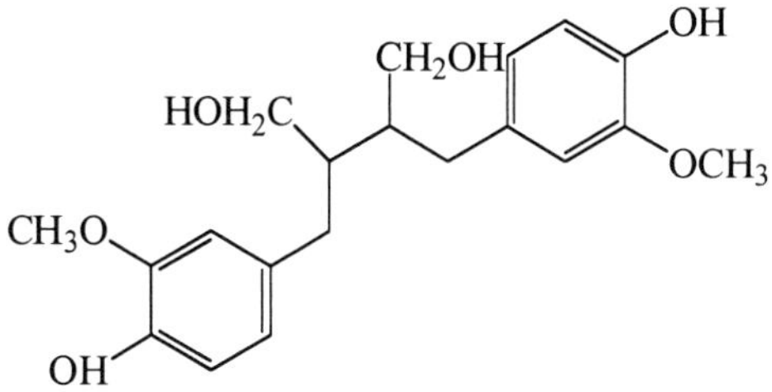


(iii)

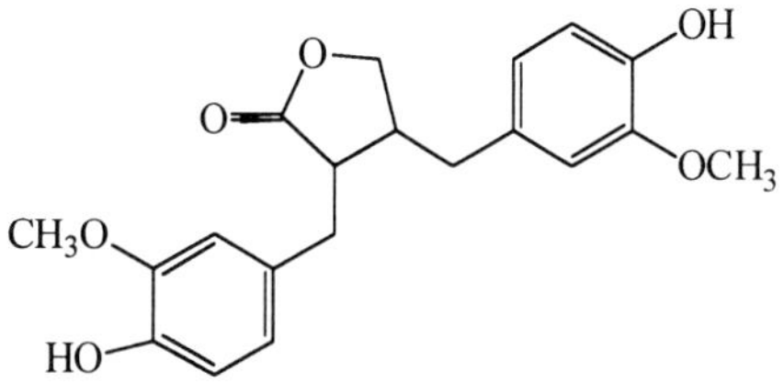


(iv)

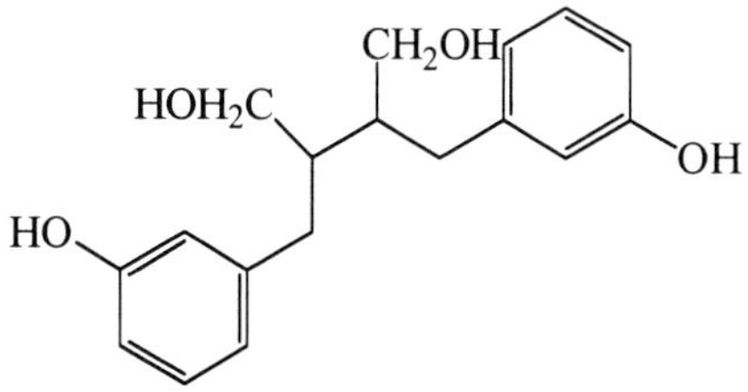


(v)

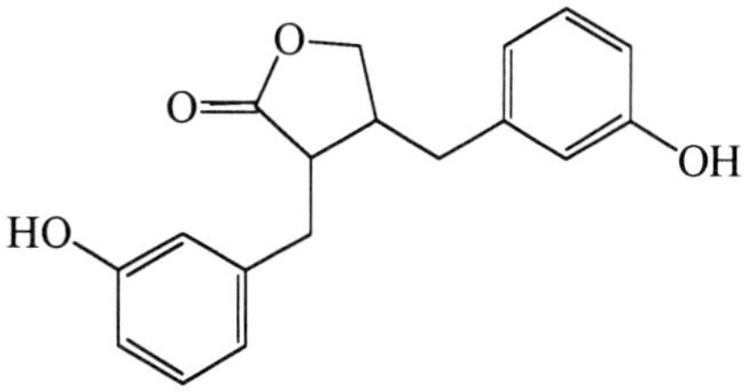


**Figure 4.4** Structures of equol, of the plant lignans secoisolariciresinol and matairesinol, and of the mammalian lignans enterolactone and enterodiol: (i) equol; (ii) secoisolarciresinol; (iii) matairesinol; (iv) enterodiol; (v) enterolactone.

The existence of plants with oestrogenic activity has been known since the 1940s when fertility problems were found in Australian sheep that fed on a diet rich in subterranean clover (*Trifolium subterraneum* L.) (Bennetts *et al.*, 1946). This problem was later identified as being due to the clover's high phytoestrogen content. The actual phytoestrogen content varied widely depending on the cultivar used. Cox (1977) collated figures which show that phytoestrogen content can range from 0.06 to 1.5% dry weight of formonetin, 0.9 to 2.8% genistein and 0.01 to 2% biochanin A. Subsequently it was shown that the oestrogenic effect may not be directly due to any of these compounds but to equol, a metabolite of certain phytoestrogens notably formonetin and daidzein (reviewed in Shutt, 1976). Similar effects have been noted in cattle fed a diet rich in alfalfa (Bickoff *et al.*, 1957; Lookhart, 1980), which can contain high concentrations of coumestrol (a more potent phytoestrogen), and have also been reported in cattle in Finland (Kallela *et al.*, 1984) fed an isoflavone-rich diet.

More recently, there have been reports of a reduction in human sperm count as well as other reports of the feminization of fish and reproductive effects in other wildlife. It has been suggested that these findings may have resulted from exposure to environmental chemicals with oestrogenic or oestrogen-like activity (MRC Institute for Environment and Health, 1995, also reviewed by Kavelock *et al.* [1996] and Colborn *et al.* [1996]). Compounds with such effects are referred to as oestrogen disrupters or, more generally, are classified within the wider category of endocrine disrupters (EDs). Endocrine disrupters were recently defined as 'exogenous substances that cause adverse health effects in an intact organism, or its progeny, consequent to changes in endocrine function' (European Commission, 1997). However, this area is subject to much debate. Despite this, there are many publications on environmental chemicals with oestrogen-disrupting activities such as certain pesticides (mainly organochlorine insecticides), polychlorinated biphenyls (PCBs), dioxins and alkylphenolethoxylates, as well as on the methodology used for assessing oestrogenic potential. There has also been renewed interest in phytoestrogens, which, although not persistent, are ingested in quantities that are orders of magnitude greater than most environmental contaminant EDs.

## 4.3   Occurrence of phytoestrogens

The main source of phytoestrogens in the human diet is usually soya, either in the form of soya foods (e.g. soya milk) or when it is used as an ingredient in numerous processed foods such as bread, snack foods, puddings, pies, etc. However, soya oil was not found to contain phytoestrogens (Eldridge and Kwolek, 1983). The distribution of phytoestrogens varies among plant species. For instance, soya beans are a rich source of isoflavones whereas

**Table 4.1** Some phytoestrogen-containing plants

| Food/plant | Compound(s) identified | Representative references |
|---|---|---|
| Soya beans | Genistein, daidzein, genistin, daidzin, glycitein and glycitin plus acetyl and malonyl esters of the glucosides | Numerous, e.g. Wang and Murphy, 1994a, provides a detailed breakdown |
| Soya sprouts | Daidzein, genistein and their glucosides | Wang et al. (1990) |
| Subterranean clover (*Rifolium subterranneum*) | Coumestrol and formonetin | Various, see text |
| Alfalfa | Coumestrol, formonetin | Knuckles et al. (1976); Lookhart (1980); Saloniemi et al. (1995) |
| Clover sprouts | Coumestrol, formonetin and biochanin A | Franke et al. (1995) |
| Split peas | Daidzein | Franke et al. (1995) |
| Broad beans | Genistein and formonetin | Franke et al. (1995) |
| Flaxseed | Secoisolaricresinol | Obermeyer et al. (1995) |
| Red clover (*Trifolium pratense*) | Formonetin, biochanin A, a small amount of genistein and trace amounts of daidzein | Saloniemi et al. (1995) |
| White clover (*Trifolium repens*) | Coumestrol plus traces of isoflavones | Saloniemi et al. (1995) |

alfalfa, mung beans and certain clovers are rich sources of the coumestans. Table 4.1 lists some major sources of phytoestrogens.

There is an extensive literature on the concentrations of phytoestrogens in a wide variety of plants. The concentrations reported are very variable, not only between species but between different samples of the same species. Data for a given species may vary as a result of the part of the plant investigated, growth, location, temperature, humidity and degree of environmental 'stress', among other factors. Eldridge and Kwolek (1983) showed that the isoflavone content of soya beans varied with season, location and variety, and that for two varieties the highest concentration occurred in the hypocotyl, which represents 2% of soya bean (17565 and 14052 mg/kg), followed by the cotyledon which represents 90% of the soya bean (1585 and 3192 mg/kg), and then the hull, which represents 8% of the soya bean (between 106 and 200 mg/kg for both varieties). Wang and Murphy (1994a) carried out a similar study measuring the effect of harvesting season and location on the isoflavone content (including concentrations of malonylated and acetylated compounds) of eight US and three Japanese varieties of soya beans. These workers demonstrated differences between the isoflavone content and distribution in different varieties, and also that there were differences in the distribution of individual compounds between the US and the Japanese varieties. The Japanese varieties had a higher ratio of 6"-O-malonyl genistin and 6"-O-malonyl daidzin to genistin and daidzin, and a higher concentration of 6"-O-malonyl glycitin than the US varieties. Crop year, and to a much lesser extent location, also influenced isoflavone profiles. These differences are further highlighted in a study by Tsukamoto et al. (1995) who examined the effects of variety, temperature during seed development, seeding and month of harvesting, ambient temperature and geographical location on the isoflavone content of soya beans. They used seven varieties of soya cultivars (four with low and three with normal isoflavone content) planted at two different sites three degrees of latitude apart. Results showed that whereas at the more southerly site the total isoflavone content of whole seeds collected from plants sowed in late June or mid July was found to be consistently higher than for soya planted in April or May, there was no consistent picture at the more northerly site, which was cooler and drier. Further analysis of these data led to the conclusion that the determining factor was the temperature of the seed during development. This hypothesis, that the higher the temperature the lower the isoflavone level, was confirmed by analyzing seeds grown in temperature-controlled cabinets, although the authors noted that other external factors also have an influence on isoflavone content.

Historical data on the concentrations of phytoestrogens should be viewed with a certain degree of caution, since different laboratories used, and still do use, different analytical methodologies. The importance of standardizing analytical methodology has become increasingly apparent and it would be unwise to consider data without reference to the method of analysis used. In an attempt to provide comparative values Reinli and Block (1996) reviewed 22 studies providing data on the phytoestrogen concentrations in foods and normalized the data on a wet weight basis. However, in compiling these data the authors highlighted that data from different laboratories often may not be considered directly comparable because of the different methodologies used. Given these caveats, Table 4.2 presents literature values for the phytoestrogen contents of a range of plant foods, together with the methods of analysis and references. In soya beans most of the isoflavones are present as glycosides, but in processed and especially fermented foods and food products they may be present mainly or completely in the aglycone form.

## 4.4    Measurement of phytoestrogens

In 1978 Kallela and Saastamoinen described the use of high performance liquid chromatography (HPLC) for measuring phytoestrogens in fodder. Although this had the advantage of being relatively quick and enabled both aglycones and glucosides to be identified in the same analytical run, it was superseded by the use of gas chromatography/mass spectrometry (GC/MS) and to a lesser extent liquid chromatography/mass spectrometry (LC/MS). However, with improvements in HPLC methodology this technique is regaining favour. The major disadvantage of using GC/MS is that plant samples that exist as glucosides must be hydrolyzed and then derivatized before they can be measured. Table 4.3 lists the main methods of analysis and their benefits and drawbacks.

## 4.5    Mycoestrogens

Zearalenone is a non-steroidal fungal toxin produced by species of the fungus *Fusarium* and in particular *F. graminearum* and *F. culmorum* (de Nijs *et al.*, 1996; Chapter 7). It has been implicated as the cause of fertility problems in farm animals, including poultry (Chi *et al.*, 1980a), an effect that is highly species-specific. White leghorn chickens and turkeys are highly tolerant (Chi *et al.*, 1980b; Allen *et al.*, 1981). Pigs are particularly susceptible (Chang *et al.* 1979; Young *et al.*, 1982; Sydenham *et al.*, 1988). Effects have also been reported in cows (Kallela and Ettala, 1984). Figure 4.5 shows the structure of zearalenone, the structures of one of its metabolites (α-zearalenol) and zeranol (α-zearalanol), a synthetic analogue used as a growth promoter which has been banned in the European Union since 1988 but sometimes found as a natural zearalenone metabolite. The relative concentrations of the various metabolites are species-specific, for example pigs and man produce more α-zearalenol (a more oestrogenic metabolite) than rodents. This aspect of metabolism has been reviewed by Kuiper-Goodman *et al.* (1987).

Table 4.2 Phytoestrogen concentrations in a selection of human and animal food sources collated from the literature.

| Plant foods[a] | Levels of phytoestrogens[a] (total isoflavones in mg/kg unless specified) | Comments and additional information | Reference and method of analysis |
|---|---|---|---|
| *Sources other than soya* | | | |
| Alfalfa (*Medicago sativa*) (d) | 34 coumestrol | Bud stage | Saloniemi *et al.* (1995) (HPLC) |
| | 65 coumestrol | Early blossom | Franke *et al.* (1995) (HPLC) |
| Alfalfa sprouts (w) | 47 coumestrol | | Saloniemi *et al.* (1995) (HPLC) |
| Clover: White clover (*Trifolium repens*) (d) | 100–600 isoflavones, <1–5.8 coumestrol | Pasture stage (mean of four varieties, four locations) | Saloniemi *et al.* (1995) (HPLC) |
| Clover—Red clover (*Trifolium pratense*) (d) | 400–900 genistein, 6600–10500 formonetin, 3900–14600 biochanin-A | Pasture stage (mean of three varieties, two locations). Samples hydrolyzed before analysis and measured as aglycones | Saloniemi *et al.* (1995) (HPLC) |
| Clover sprouts (w) | 3.5 genistein, 281 coumestrol, 23 formonetin, 4.4 biochanin A[b] | Organically grown in Hawaii Samples hydrolyzed before analysis and measured as aglycones | Franke *et al.* (1995) (HPLC) |
| Flaxseed | 817 secoisolariciresinol | Assumed to be dry weight | Obermeyer *et al.* (1995) (HPLC and LC-MS) |
| Large Lima beans (dry raw) | 15 coumestrol | | Franke *et al.* (1995) (HPLC) |
| *Soya foods: processed products* | | | |
| Cheddar cheese (w) | 34 and 109 | Two sources | Wang and Murphy (1994b) (HPLC) |
| Miso | 1379 (d) 920 (w) | 92% as aglycone for genistein, 91% for daidzein | Coward *et al.* (1993) (HPLC) |
| Miso (w) | 294 | | Wang and Murphy (1994b) (HPLC) |
| Soy milk | 252 (w) 3256 (d) | 5% as aglycone for genistein, 10% for daidzein | Coward *et al.* (1993) (HPLC) |
| Soy milk (d) | 130 daidzein, 92 genistein | Samples hydrolyzed before analysis | Wang *et. al.* (1990) (HPLC) |
| Soya hot dog (w) | 150 | | Wang and Murphy (1994b) (HPLC) |

**Table 4.2** (continued)

| Plant foods[a] | Levels of phytoestrogens[a] (total isoflavones in mg/kg unless specified) | Comments and additional information | Reference and method of analysis |
|---|---|---|---|
| Soya sauce | 90 (d) 23 (w) | 100% as aglycone | Coward et al. (1993) (HPLC) |
| Soyabean paste | 1168 (d) 570 (w) | 76% as aglycone for genistein 82% for daidzein | Coward et al. (1993) (HPLC) |
| Tempeh | 1130 (d) 430 (w) | 59% as aglycone for genistein 74% for daidzein | Coward et al. (1993) (HPLC) |
| Tempeh (w) | 625 | | Wang and Murphy (1994b) (HPLC) |
| Tofu (w) | total as aglycones[b]: 113 daidzein, 166 genistein | Samples hydrolyzed before analysis | Franke et al. (1995) (HPLC) |
| (freeze dried: 13.5% water) | 840 daidzein, 1233 genistein | Calculated values for dry weight:- daidzein 971 (d), genistein 1425 (d) | |
| Tofu (w) | 417 (2031, d); 494 (3827, d) | Two types (i) 11% genistein and 12% daidzein as aglycones (ii) 50% genistein and 7% daidzein as aglycones | Coward et al. (1993) (HPLC) |
| Tofu (w) | 337 | | Wang and Murphy (1994b) (HPLC) |
| Tofu (d) | total as aglycones[a]: 168 to 794 daidzein, 288 to 1321 genistein | Three types: hard soft and dry spiced Samples hydrolyzed before analysis | Wang et. al. (1990) (HPLC) |
| Tofu (w) | Brand 1: 73 to 98 daidzein and 187 to 216 genistein 0.3 mg/kg Biochanin A and 0.8 mg/kg coumestrol found in one brand | Four brands analysed; means for at least two lots of each sample given Samples hydrolyzed before analysis | Dwyer et al. (1994) (GC-MS) |

**Table 4.2** (continued)

| Plant foods[a] | Levels of phytoestrogens[a] (total isoflavones in mg/kg unless specified) | Comments and additional information | Reference and method of analysis |
|---|---|---|---|
| *Soyabeans, soya flour, soya isolate and soya concentrate* | | | |
| Roasted soyabeans (as is) | 1625 | | Wang and Murphy (1994b) (HPLC) |
| Soya bean seeds(d) | total as aglycones[b]: 676 to 1007 daidzein; 940 to 1382 genistein. | Samples hydrolyzed before analysis Three samples grown in US (one organic), one grown in Japan. Further values provided in this reference | Franke et al. (1995) (HPLC) |
| Soya beans (d) | 470 to 3093 depending on variety (four measured) and site. | Measured different varieties grown in the same and different locations | Eldridge and Kwoloek (1983) (LC) |
| Soya beans (original weight) | 5 genistein, 201 genistin | Genistein/genistin only measured[c] | Fugatake et al. (1996) (HPLC) |
| Soya beans (d) 995 | 1636 | | |
| Vinton 81 911 variety | Vinton 81 90H variety Wang and Murphy, 1994b (HPLC) | | |
| Soya beans (d) | Total aglycones: 331 and 507 daidzein, 462 and 680 genistein | Two different sources samples hydrolyzed before analysis | Wang et. al. (1990) (HPLC) |
| Soya beans (d), seven varieties | 200–2137 total at location 1 790–3510 total at location 2 | Diadzin, genistin, glycitin and their malonyl esters, no aglycones or acetyl forms measured. Planting dates between April and July for location 1, and May and July at location 2 | Tsukamoto et al. (1995) (HPLC) |
| Soy concentrate (d) | 2656 | Water extracted: 2% of total as aglycones for genistein, 3% for daidzein | Coward et al. (1993) |

Table 4.2 (continued)

| Plant foods[a] | Levels of phytoestrogens)[a] (total isoflavones in mg/kg unless specified | Comments and additional information | Reference and method of analysis |
|---|---|---|---|
| | 159 | Alcohol extracted 1: 4% total as genistein, 6% total as daidzein | |
| | 443 | Alcohol extracted 2: 23% of total as genistein, 31% as daidzein | |
| Soya flour Asian-style (d) | 1338 | 2% of total as aglycone for genistein/tin and 0% daidzein/zin | Coward et al. (1993) (HPLC) |
| Soya flour (d) | Total as aglycones[a]: 655 daidzein; 1123 genistein | Samples hydrolyzed before analysis | Franke et al. (1995) (HPLC) |
| Soya flour (d) | 1124[d] | 2–3% total as aglycone | Wang and Murphy (1994b) (HPLC) |
| Soy isolate (d) | 466–615 different sources | | Wang and Murphy (1994b) (HPLC) |
| Soy isolate (d) two samples | 848 1158 | 20% and 24% of total as aglycones for genistein, 24% and 27% for daidzein | Coward et al. (1993) (HPLC) |

[a] d = dry weight; w = wet weight; where details are not given it is assumed that the data are for products as sold.

[b] samples hydrolysed before analysis, total agycone (i.e. genistein+ genistin, daidzein + genistin).

[c] NB Wang and Murphy (1994a, b) give values of between 58 and 65 % total isoflavones as genistein/istin.

[d] normalized for molecular weight.

**Table** 4.3 Main methods that may be used to measure phytoestrogens concentrations

|  | HPLC | GC/MS | LC/MS |
|---|---|---|---|
| Advantages | Cheap, quick, can handle multiple samples, no derivatization needed Recent improvements in methodology have increased the applicability of this technique for phytoestrogen analysis | Greater sensitivity and resolution | Good for liquid samples, requires less sample preparation and thus minimal sample loss Selectivity may be increased by using MS/MS Able to measure conjugates (e.g. of phytoestrogens) directly |
| Disadvantages | Less sensitive than the other methods | Requires extensive work-up and derivatization of sample Suitable 2H and 13C standards difficult to obtain Specialist operator desirable | Initial cost of equipment Specialist operator desirable |
| Selected references | Franke and Custer (1996), Jones et al. (1989) | Adlercreutz et al. (1991a, 1995a); Mazur et al. (1996); Wudy et al. (1995) | Coward et al. (1996) |

Zearalenone can be produced by fungi both in the field and during storage, the latter probably being the main site for toxin production (Mirocha et al., 1977; Shotwell, 1977; Pathre and Mirocha, 1980). Optimum growth conditions fall within well-defined limits for temperature and humidity. For instance, it has been reported that optimum conditions for F. moniliforme were a week at 25°C followed by four weeks at 14°C (Martins et al., 1993). However, others have reported that for F. graminearum and F. oxysporum, four weeks at 25°C enhanced zearalenone synthesis but that growth was partially or totally inhibited at 12° to 14°C. (Milano and Lopez, 1991).

Zearalenone can be measured in a variety of ways. The most common methods are HPLC, enzyme-linked immunosorbent assay (ELISA), radio-immunoassay (RIA), thin layer chromatography (TLC) and, less often and less reliably, GC/MS (these methods are reviewed in Leitao et al., 1992).

Zearalenone concentrations in some cereal and other samples (shown to have tested positive for zearalenone contamination) are listed in Table 4.4. More extensive lists are to be found elsewhere, for example in Kuiper-Goodman et al. (1987) or IARC (1993).

(i)

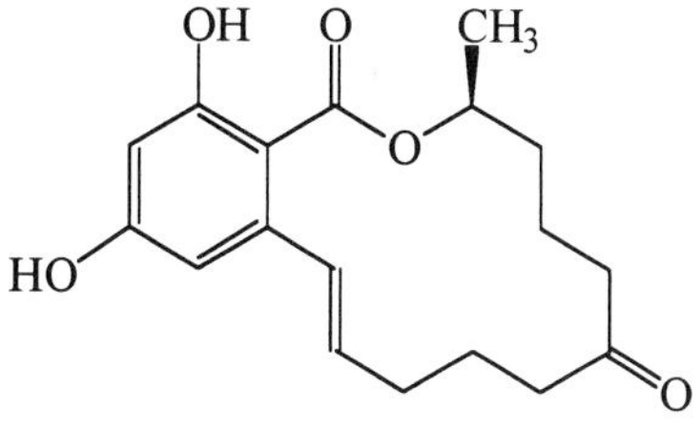

(ii)

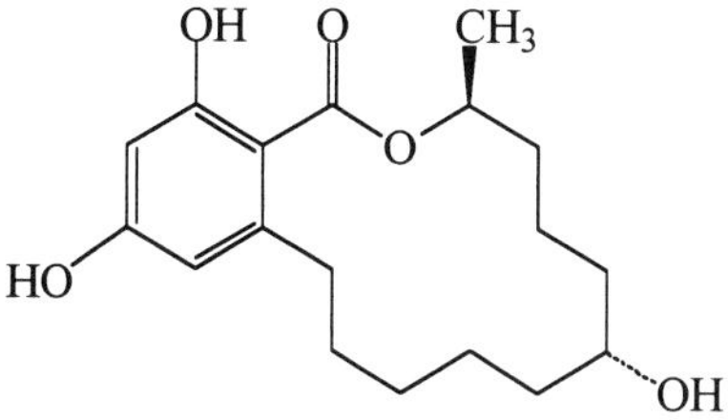

(iii)

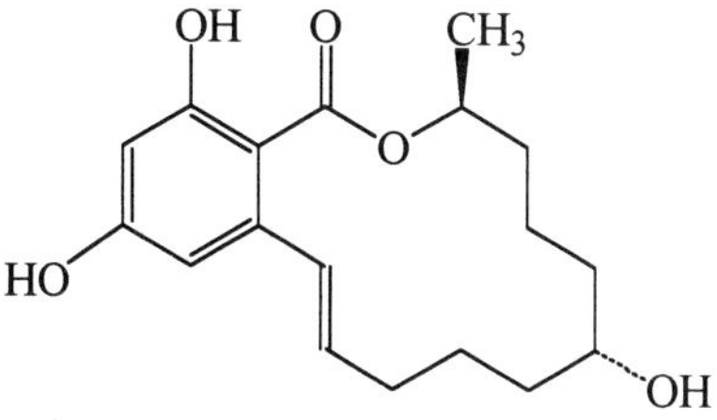

**Figure 4.5**    Structures of zearalenone, one of its metabolites, α-zearalenol, and the synthetic analogue, α-zearalanol (zeranol): (i) zearalenone; (ii) α-zearalanol (zeranol); (iii) α-
zearalenol.

**Table 4.4** Zearalenone concentrations in selected cereals and other samples

| Sample | Concentration (μg/kg) | Number and/or percentage of positive samples (where specified) | Reference and comments |
|---|---|---|---|
| Barley | Maximum 16 | 2/45 (4%) | Scudamore et al. (1997); HPLC |
| Maize | Maximum 510 (five samples at 99 μg/kg or greater) | 13/50 (26%) | Samples from 186 UK animal feed mills sampled in 1992 None found in dried peas and beans, cottonseed, sunflower, palm products or soya |
| Rice bran | 44 | 1/40 (2.5%) | Kim et al. (1993); HPLC |
| Barley | 40–1416 (average 287) | 51% | Tanaka and Ueno (1989); HPLC |
| Cereals from 21 countries | 46 | 45% | Majority of contaminated samples were barley (74%), corn (59%) and oats (50%) |
| Cereals and cereal products | ND–41 | | Patel et al. (1996); HPLC UK survey of ethnic products |
| Herbs and spices | ND–15 | | |
| Pickles and pastes | ND–7 | | |
| Maize | 5–35 | 6% | Ranft et al. (1990); HPLC |
| Maize (field samples) | 300–2200 | | |
| Maize (harvest samples) | 0–1600 | | |
| Maize (stored samples destined for animal feed) | 40–100 | 75% overall | Hussein et al. (1989); TLC |
| Maize (stored samples destined for human consumption) | 40–800 | | |
| Maize kernels | 175–3600 | 100% | Pathre and Mirocha (1980)[a] |
| Maize meal | 40–400 | 12.5% | Doko et al. (1996); TLC |

**Table 4.4** (continued)

| Sample | Concentration (µg/kg) | Number and/or percentage of positive samples (where specified) | Reference and comments |
|---|---|---|---|
| Mixed feed | 4–56 | 20% | Ranft et al. (1990); HPLC |
| Mixed feeds | 850–1250 | 100% | Sydenham et al. (1988) 61–69% sorghum, refused by swine |
| Rye and oats | 7–11 | 2% | Ranft et al. (1990); HPLC |
| Wheat | 22 | 5% | Hietanemi and Kumpulaineu (1991); GC/MS |
| Oats | 63 | 14% | Finnish crops intended for human consumption |
| Wheat | 1–8036 (means ranging from 3.2 ± 1.7[b] to 178 ± 994[c]) | up to 80% | Müller et al. (1997); HPLC |
| Wheat | 4–64 | 7% | Ranft et al. (1990); HPLC |

[a] Submitted for analysis because of possible toxicosis.
[b] In the best year.
[c] For worst year.
ND = not detected.

## 4.6    Other possible sources of plant oestrogens

There are a few reports of other sources of oestrogenic compounds in plants. For instance, Mellanen *et al.* (1996) reported that wood-derived chemicals (possibly β-sitosterol [Figure 4.6] and, to a lesser extent, abietic acid), which can occur in pulp mill effluents, are oestrogenic in fish and in T-47-D cells (a breast cancer cell line that is responsive to oestrogen). However, results from *in vitro* studies using another breast cancer cell line (MCF-7) suggest that the reported oestrogenic activity was not due to β-sitosterol, but to one of its metabolites. Such wood-derived compounds have been linked to the feminization of fish in the vicinity of pulp mill effluents and it has been postulated that the active compound may be a metabolite of β-sitosterol.

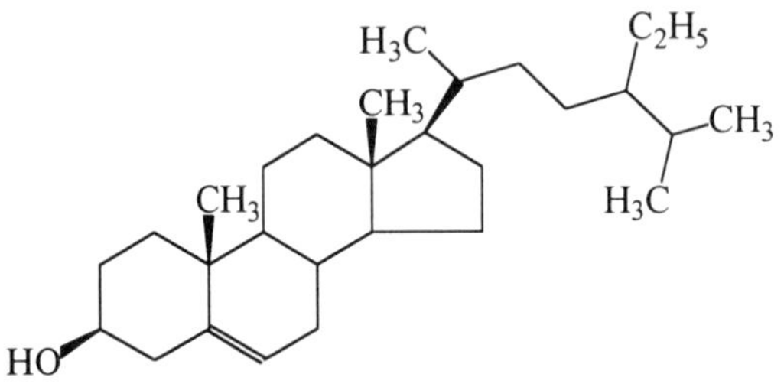

**Figure 4.6**    Structure of β-sitosterol.

There are also reports of steroidal oestrogens in a variety of plants (reviewed in Hewitt *et al.*, 1980). For instance, Young *et al.* (1977) reported the isolation of oestradiol from the French bean (*Phaseolus vulgaris*). Likewise weak oestrogenic properties have been attributed to coffee extracts (Kitts, 1987). However, these reports may need re-evaluation with the introduction and availability of more sophisticated analytical techniques.

## 4.7    Endogenous mammalian oestrogens in meat

All mammals produce a range of oestrogenic compounds throughout their lifetimes. These compounds circulate in the body, where they are mainly bound to protein. The levels of free and bound hormones are regulated by intricate homeostatic mechanisms. This makes quantitative measurements difficult to interpret and therefore comparing the contribution of endogenous oestrogens from animal products in the diet to that from plant oestrogens is extremely difficult. Mammalian hormone concentrations are subject to seasonal, cyclical and intra-individual variations, and no agreed method exists for estimating the relative potency of these compounds (see section 4.8.2).

Much of the analytical work on oestradiol in meat and serum is undertaken as part of veterinary surveillance for drug residues. A recent review by

Lone (1997) quotes muscle oestradiol concentrations for untreated animals of between 7 and 33 ng/kg and oestrone concentrations of 2 to 208 ng/kg in cattle, depending on the sex and, in females, whether pregnant and, if so, the stage of pregnancy. Values for steers were given as 14 ng/kg for oestradiol and 2 ng/kg for oestrone. Surveillance carried out in the UK (Veterinary Medicines Directorate, 1996) for concentrations of oestradiol in the serum of male bovines, of two years or less, showed that none of the 161 animals examined had serum concentrations above an action level of 0.04 µg/kg; 14 animals contained between 0.01 and 0.04 µg/kg oestradiol. However, the proportion of this oestradiol that would be bioavailable to consumers via their food is unknown.

## 4.8    Effects of phytoestrogens in man and animals

### 4.8.1  Exposure

The isoflavones are the most extensively studied of the phytoestrogens. This is probably due to the fact that soya, commonly used in many foodstuffs, is a rich source of these compounds. Exposure of infants to phytoestrogens can occur via ingestion of soya-based infant formulae and via breast milk from mothers who habitually ingest high levels of soya, e.g. vegetarians and some ethnic groups. The reported concentrations of isoflavones in infant formulae vary (Irvine et al., 1995; Setchell et al., 1997; Committee on the Toxicity, Mutagenicity and Carcinogenicity of Chemicals in Food, Consumer Products and the Environment, in press) but it seems likely that infants during their first four months of life may be exposed to intakes of about 4 mg/kg bodyweight per day or more. The concentration of isoflavones in breast milk of mothers fed soya has also been reported (Franke and Custer, 1996). Soya bean challenge led to an isoflavone dose-dependent response in human milk with the maximum concentration observed approximately 12 hours after dosing. The concentrations observed were around 30 to 70 nmol/l, a similar concentration to that observed in the breast milk of Chinese women consuming a normal Asian diet.

Exposure to mammalian oestrogen can also arise from the ingestion of bovine milk. The concentration of oestrogens in bovine milk varies throughout the oestrous cycle and pregnancy, and ranges from 28 to 58 pg/ml (Monk et al., 1975). The oestradiol content of human colostrum and milk has also been estimated to be in the region of 70 pg/ml (Wolford and Argoudelis, 1979). By the third or fourth month post partum, oestradiol is below the level of detection (reviewed by Grosvenor et al., 1992). Earlier reports concerning the concentration of ethinyl oestradiol in the plasma and milk of lactating women administered oral contraceptives (50 µg ethinyl estradiol and 4 mg of megestrol acetate) demonstrated that the ratio of ethinyl oestradiol concentration in plasma to that in milk was 4:1 (Nilsson et al., 1978). Breast enlargement has been observed in breast-fed male and female infants of women taking oral contraceptives. Following discontinuation of breast feeding, breast enlargement subsided (Curtis, 1964, Madhavapeddi and Ramachandran, 1985).

Another study has estimated human exposure to oestrogenic chemicals in terms of oestrogenic equivalents—a function of potency and concentration (Safe, 1995). For phytoestrogens, dietary intake of oestrogenic equivalents by adults was estimated to be 102 µg/day whereas the intakes from hormone replacement therapy (HRT), oestrogen contraceptives and the morning-after pill were 3.35, 16.7 and 333 mg/day respectively. Intake from environmental oestrogens (organic contaminants) was 2.5 pg/day—considerably lower than the intake from plant sources.

Information on exposure can also be gained from measurements of phytoestrogens in plasma and urine. Adlercreutz and co-workers (1993) reported plasma concentrations in Japanese men who habitually ate a diet high in soya and hence phytoestrogens, and Finnish men who consumed a mixed diet. Total plasma isoflavone concentrations in the Japanese men were over 30 times higher than in the Finnish men. Consumption of soya products in Asian cultures is typically 50 to 100 mg isoflavones per day (Barnes *et al.*, 1990; Adlercreutz *et al.*, 1991b; Coward *et al.*, 1993) while in Britain the dietary intake of isoflavones determined from total diet study samples was estimated to be 1 mg per day[1] (Jones *et al.*, 1989). Adding soya to the typical western diet increases urinary isoflavone levels by as much as 1000-fold (Messina *et al.*, 1994). It is interesting to note that only around 30% of individuals are capable of the metabolism of daidzein to equol, a more oestrogenically potent metabolite (Kelly *et al.*, 1995). Other studies have shown that supplementation of the diet with linseed increased plasma lignan concentration by up to 50-fold (Morton *et al.*, 1994), again with wide individual variation. Recently Morton *et al.* (1997) reported the levels of lignans and isoflavones in prostatic fluid. Levels of the plant-derived chemicals were higher in men from Asia than from their European counterparts.

### 4.8.2 *Potency, oestrogen binding and other related cellular effects*

Estimates of the potency of phytoestrogens vary according to the test and species used but, in general, these compounds have a lower potency than 17β-oestradiol. For instance, in a human cancer cell line (Ishikawa Var I line) the relative potencies, based on enhancement of alkaline phosphatase activity with the value for 17β-oestradiol taken as 100, were 0.202 for coumesterol, 0.0984 for genistein, 0.061 for equol, 0.013 for daidzein, <0.006 for biochanin A and <0.0006 for formononetin (Markiewicz *et al.*, 1993). Other *in vitro* studies have measured cell proliferation or protein-

---

[1]However, these figures are not directly comparable since the total diet samples (TDSs) are composite samples of different food groups (for details of TDS see Peattie *et al.*, 1983).

induction response in MCF-7 cells, an oestrogen-responsive breast cancer cell line (Welshons *et al.*, 1990; Mayr *et al.*, 1992; Soto *et al.*, 1992).

The most commonly used *in vivo* test for potency measures relative uterine weight in ovarectomized rodents. This is probably more relevant than the *in vitro* tests noted above. Overall, the potency of isoflavones varies but is low in comparison with 17β-oestradiol. The major isoflavones have been reported to have around 1/500 to 1/10000th of the oestrogenicity of 17β-oestradiol (for a review see Messina *et al.*, 1994). Isoflavones also have low affinity for binding to uterine cytosol. Thus, the relative binding of genistein is 1% (17β-oestradiol is 100%) whereas the binding of daidzein and the other isoflavones tends to be less (for a review see Price and Fenwick, 1985). Coumesterol and zearalenone are approximately two to five times more potent than genistein, with coumesterol apparently being the most potent phytoestrogen.

The action of 17β-oestradiol in the body is strictly controlled by limiting the amount of free hormone. This is achieved by the presence of a sex hormone binding globulin (SHBG) that, as its name suggests, specifically binds 17β-oestradiol and renders it unavailable for action. Results from some studies have shown that phytoestrogens may bind to SHBG (Martin *et al.*, 1978; Arnold *et al.*, 1996). However, such binding is weak in comparison with that of 17β-oestradiol where approximately 90% or more of oestradiol may be bound (Martin *et al.*, 1996).

*In vivo* studies in mammals are generally considered to be more relevant than *in vitro* tests since the results from the former can be more readily extrapolated to exposure of phytoestrogens to humans in everyday life.

Genistein, the most extensively studied of the isoflavones, has been shown to have other intracellular actions. It is an inhibitor of the enzyme protein tyrosine kinase (Akiyama *et al.*, 1987). Protein tyrosine kinase activity is associated with cellular receptors for epidermal growth factor, insulin and insulin-like growth factor, platelet-derived growth factor and mononuclear phagocyte factor, suggesting that the enzyme plays an important role in cell proliferation and transformation (Adlercreutz, 1990; Messina *et al.*, 1994). Genistein also inhibits DNA topoisomerase (Okura *et al.*, 1988) and ribosome S6 kinase (Linassier *et al.*, 1990). It has also been reported to modulate cell cycle phases (Tragonos *et al.*, 1992; Matsukawa *et al.*, 1993) and inhibit differentiation of cancer cell lines (Constantinou *et al.*, 1990). Isoflavones also have antioxidant properties and inhibit superoxide anion, hydrogen peroxide and free radical formation (Wei *et al.*, 1993). Daidzein has also been reported to have similar antioxidant activity (Wei *et al.*, 1995).

### 4.8.3 Effects on reproductive function

Infertility in sheep, as mentioned earlier, was demonstrated to be caused by the sheep grazing on plants with a high isoflavone content after it was first reported in 1946 (Bennetts *et al.*, 1946). Infertility has also been reported in the captive cheetah and this has been linked to a diet high in soya (Setchell *et al.*, 1987). The cheetahs consumed up to 50 mg isoflavones per day. The breeding habits of quails have also been affected by the ingestion of phytoestrogens in their diet (Leopold *et al.*, 1976).

In laboratory animals anovulatory responses and delays in sexual maturity have been observed in young female rats exposed to phytoestrogens during critical periods of development (Whitten and Naftolin, 1992; Whitten *et al.*, 1993, 1995). Besides affecting physiological responses, changes in hormone concentration in neonates can affect areas of the brain, which in turn may affect the development of male and female characteristics (Gorski, 1986; Beyer and Feder, 1987; McEwan, 1987). For example, exposure of young female animals to androgens and oestrogens has been reported to result in enlargement of the sexually dimorphic nucleus of the pre-optic area (SDN-POA) to the size normally associated with young males (Walsh *et al.*, 1982; Tartellin and Gorski, 1988). It has also been reported that neonatal exposure to genistein can result in enlargement of this same area, as well as an alteration in the secretion of luteinizing hormone (LH) from the pituitary (Faber and Hughes, 1991, 1993; Register *et al.*, 1995). Although the development of rodents and humans is not strictly comparable, such experiments raise concerns regarding infants ingesting high quantities of soya soon after birth. However, there is no evidence of developmental problems or infertility in populations that consume large quantities of phytoestrogens, although there is evidence that resistance to the effects of phytoestrogens develops over successive generations in sheep (Croker *et al.*, 1989). In animals, feminization of males has been reported following ingestion of phytoestrogens at critical periods of development (Kaldas and Hughes, 1989; Clarkson *et al.*, 1995; Whitten *et al.*, 1995). Recent work has shown that consumption of modest amounts of soya by premenopausal women who normally consume a western diet resulted in changes to the menstrual cycle and their cyclical surges of LH and follicle stimulating hormone (FSH) (Cassidy *et al.*, 1994, 1995). Reproductive abnormalities in the male may be related to increased oestrogen concentration *in utero* or oestrogen exposure at other critical periods of development. Abnormalities include testicular cancer, cryptorchidism (undescended testes), hypospadias (malformation of the penis) and low sperm count; the reader is directed to a review by Sharpe and Skakkebaek (1993). However, as far as the authors are aware, there is no evidence linking such abnormalities to high phytoestrogen ingestion or exposure to environmental endocrine disrupters.

### 4.8.4 *Other effects of phytoestrogens*
Many people have believed for a number of years that phytoestrogens may protect against coronary heart disease since it is established that endogenous

oestrogens protect premenopausal women from this disease. At menopause and beyond the risk of coronary heart disease for these women increases (Clarkson *et al.*, 1995). A number of experiments in animals and humans have shown that phytoestrogens can reduce total plasma cholesterol (Terpestra *et al.*, 1984; Cruz *et al.*, 1994; Potter, 1995). A recent review of the literature has concluded that three servings of soya products per day would reduce total cholesterol, low density lipoprotein (LDL), cholesterol and triglyceride levels (Anderson *et al.*, 1995).

Observational data from adult populations that habitually ingest high quantities of soya suggest that these individuals have a lower incidence of some types of cancer, such as cancer of the breast, prostate or colon (Adlercreutz *et al.*, 1982; Setchell and Adlercreutz, 1988; Lee *et al.*, 1991; Adlercreutz *et al.*, 1992a, 1995b; Messina *et al.*, 1994). While this theory of a causal link is attractive, it is difficult to separate the effects of phytoestrogens from other differences in diet between the two groups (high soya consumers and others), such as intake of fibre, vitamins, fruit, vegetables, red meat, saturated fat and fish.

There is experimental evidence in laboratory animals that the administration of very high doses of genistein to rats over the neonatal period may reduce mammary tumours induced by dimethyl-benzanthracene, a potent chemical carcinogen (Lamartiniere *et al.*, 1995; Murrill *et al.*, 1996). On the other hand, oestrogens can induce hormone-specific cancers (Sheehan, 1995). For women taking the combined oral contraceptive pill, there is a small increased risk of breast cancer (British National Formulary, 1997). However, the UK's Committee on the Safety of Medicines has advised that this small increased risk is more than counterbalanced by the protective effect against ovarian and endometrial cancer. One recent study has reported that in premenopausal women consumption of soy protein isolate had a stimulatory effect on the female breast, as shown by hyperplastic epithelial changes and elevated plasma oestradiol (Petrakis *et al.*, 1996).

Others have suggested that phytoestrogens play a role in protecting against prostate cancer. Again much of the evidence comes from comparisons of different populations, Asian and western, making it difficult to separate dietary and other factors (Hirayama, 1986; Severson *et al.*, 1989; Shimizu *et al.*, 1991; Adlercreutz *et al.*, 1992a; Messina *et al.*, 1994).

In postmenopausal women it has been reported that ingestion of phytoestrogens may help reduce osteoporosis and flushing (Wilcox *et al.*, 1990; Adlercreutz *et al.*, 1992b; Anderson *et al.*, 1995; Murkies *et al.*, 1995; Baird *et al.*, 1995). There is some evidence that modest ingestion of soya by such women may help reduce flushing but further work is required. With regard to oesteoporosis there have been a number of reports concerning the use of ipriflavone, a synthetic isoflavone used to treat osteoporosis (Agnusdei *et al.*, 1989; Petrilli *et al.*, 1995). Administration of ipriflavone has been shown to maintain bone density. It is tempting to speculate that phytoestrogens have similar effects but, again, further work is needed to verify this issue.

## 4.9 Conclusions

Phytoestrogens, chemicals with oestrogenic and other properties, are present in many different plant foods. In certain groups, such as ethnic populations and vegetarians, intakes can be high while in omnivorous populations intakes are generally low. Phytoestrogens from many different chemical classes (lignans, isoflavones, mycoestrogens and coumestans) have all been shown to have properties similar to, but much weaker than, the endogenous human oestrogen 17β-oestradiol. Nevertheless, because of the high intake of phytoestrogens intracellular concentrations can be high. Effects on fertility and other reproductive functions are well documented in the literature with regard to animals. Because of this there are concerns with regard to the action of these chemicals when consumed by human infants. Thus, much work is going on to elucidate the mechanism of action of phytoestrogens (in particular the isoflavones) and to elucidate their effects, if any, on fertility and reproductive development in humans. However, in populations that ingest large quantities of phytoestrogens there is no evidence of adverse reproductive effects.

Others have ascribed beneficial effects to phytoestrogens, based largely on observed differences in chronic disease between Asian and western populations. Apart from the beneficial effect on plasma cholesterol concentration and possibly coronary heart disease, other benefits appear less well documented. Thus further research is required before definite conclusions can be drawn about the beneficial effects of these compounds. A more critical appraisal of the literature, paying particular regard to the properties of all dietary variables, would probably be a profitable exercise. Researchers should also consider the relevance of *in vitro* experiments in comparison with real life situations before embarking on their research. It is important to understand the mechanism of action of a particular chemical, but the relevance of the dose used, the expected intracellular concentration *in vivo* and other metabolic factors must be considered in designing experiments. Thus *in vitro* experiments and their results cannot be considered in isolation.

## References

Adlercreutz, C.H.T, Goldin, B.R., Gorbach, S.L., Höckerstedt, K.A.V., Watanabe, S., Hämäläinen, E.K., Markkannen, M.K., Mäkelä, T.H., Wähälä, K.T., Hasae, T.A. and Fotis, T. (1995b) Soybean phytoestrogen intake and cancer risk. *Journal of Nutrition*, **125** 757S-770S.
Adlercreutz, H. (1990) Western diet and western diseases—some hormonal and biochemical mechanisms and associations. *Clinical and Laboratory Investigations*, **50** 3-23.

Adlercreutz, H. (1995) Phytoestrogens and cancer. *Environmental Health Perspectives*, **103** (suppl 7) 103-12.

Adlercreutz, H., Fotsis, T., Heinkkinen, R., Dwyer, J.T., Woods, M., Goldin, B.R. and Gorbach, S.L. (1982) Excretion of the lignans enterolactone and enterodiol and of equol in omnivorous and vegetarian postmenopausal women and in women with breast cancer. *Lancet*, **2** 1295-97.

Adlercreutz, H., Fotis, T., Bannwart, C., Wähelä, K., Brunow, G. and Hase, T. (1991a) Isotope dilution gas chromatographic–mass spectrometric method for the determination of lignans and isoflavonoids in human urine, including identification of genistein. *Clin. Chim. Acta*, **199** 263-78.

Adlercreutz, H., Hojo, H., Higashi, A., Fotsis, T., Hämäläinen, E., Hasegawa, T. and Okada, H. (1991b) Urinary excretion of lignans and isoflavinoid phytoestrogens in Japanese men and women consuming a traditional Japanese diet. *American Journal of Clinical Nutrition*, **54** 1093-1100.

Adlercreutz, H., Monsani, Y., Cleoh, J., Höckerstedt, K., Hämäläinen, E.,Wähelä, K., Mäkelä, T. and Haze, T. (1992a) Dietary phytoestrogens and *in vitro* and *in vivo* studies. *Biochemical and Molecular Biology*, **41**, 331-37.

Adlercreutz, H., Hämäläinen, E., Gorbach, S. and Goldin, B. (1992b) Dietary phytoestrogens and the menopause in Japan. *Lancet*, **339** 1233.

Adlercreutz, H., Markkanen, H. and Watanabe, S. (1993) Plasma concentrations of phytoestrogens in Japanese men. *Lancet*, **342** 1209-10.

Adlercreutz, H., van der Wildt, J., Kinzel, J., Attalla, H., Wähalä, K., Mäkelä, T., Hase, T. and Fotis, T. (1995a) Lignan and isoflavinoid conjugates in human urine. *Journal of Steroid Biochemistry*, **52** 97-103.

Agnusdei, D., Zacekei, F., Bigazzi, S., Cepollaro, C., Nard, P., Montagnau, M. and Gennai, C. (1989) Metabolic effects of ipriflavone in postmenopausal osteoporosis. *Drug Exp. Clin. Res.*, **XV** 97-104.

Akiyama, T., Ishida, J., Nakagawa, S., Ogaware, H., Watanabe, S., Itoh, N.M., Shibaya, M. and Fukami, Y. (1987) Genistein, a specific inhibitor of tyrosine-specific protein kinase. *Journal of Biological Chemistry*, **262** 5592-95.

Allen, N.K., Mirocha, C.J., Weaver, G., Aakhus-Allen, S. and Bates, F. (1981) Effects of dietary zearalenone on finishing broiler chickens and young turkey poults. *Poultry Science*, **60** 1165-74.

Anderson, W.J., Johnstone, M.B. and Cooke-Newell, E.M. (1995) Meta-analysis of the effects of soy protein intake on serum lipids. *Medicine*, **333** 276-82.

Arnold, S.F., Robinson, M.K., Notides, A.C., Guillette, L.J. and McLachlan, J.A. (1996) A yeast oestrogen screen for examining the relative exposure of cells to natural and xenoestrogens. *Environmental Health Perspectives*, **104** 544-48.

Baird, D.D., Umbach, D.M., Lansdell, L., Hughes, C.I., Setchell, K.D.R., Weinberg, C.R., Hanley, A.F., Wilcox, A.J. and McLachlan, J.A. (1995) Dietary intervention study to assess estrogenicity of dietary soy among postmenopausal women. *Journal of Clinical Endocrinology and Metabolism*, **80** 1685-90.

Barnes, S., Grubbs, C., Setchell, K.D.R. and Carlson, J. (1990) Soybeans inhibit mammary tumours in models of breast cancer, in *Mutagens and carcinogens in the Diet* (ed. M. Pariza) Wiley-Liss, New York, pp. 239-53.

Bennetts, H.W., Underwood, E.J. and Shier, F.L. (1946) A specific breeding problem of sheep on subterranean clover pastures in Western Australia. *Australian Veterinary Journal*, **22** 2-12.

Beyer, C. and Feder, H.H. (1987) Sex steroids and afferent input, their roles in brain sexual differentiation. *Annual Reviews in Physiology*, **49** 349-64.

Bickoff, E.M., Booth, A.N., Lyman, R.L., Livingston, A.L., Thompson, C.R. and DeEds, F. (1957) Coumestrol, a new estrogen isolated from forage crops. *Science*, **126** 969-70.

British National Formulary (1997) Publication No. 33. The British Medical Association and the Royal Pharmaceutical Society, London.

Cassidy, A., Bingham, S. and Setchell, K. (1994) Biological effects of a diet of soy protein rich in isoflavones on the menstrual cycle of premenopausal women. *American Journal of Clinical Nutrition*, **60** 333-40.

Cassidy, A., Bingham, S. and Setchell, K. (1995) Biological effects of isoflavones in young women: importance of the chemical composition of soyabean products. *British Journal of Nutrition*, **74** 587-601.

Chang, K., Kurtz, H.J. and Mirocha, C.J. (1979) Effects of the mycotoxin zearalenone on swine reproduction. *American Journal of Veterinary Research*, **40** 1260-67.

Chi, M.S., Mirocha C.J., Kurtz, H.J., Weaver, G.A., Bates, F., Robison, T. and Shmoda, W.L. (1980a) Effect of dietary zearalenone on growing broiler chicks. *Poultry Science*, **59** 531-36.

Chi, M.S., Mirocha, C.J., Weaver, G.A. and Kurtz, H.J. (1980b) Effect of zearalenone on female white leghorn chickens. *Applied and Environmental Microbiology*, **39** 1026-30.

Clarkson, T.B., Anthony, M.S. and Hughes, C.L. (1995) Estrogenic soybean isoflavones and chronic disease. *Trends in Endocrinological Metabolism*, **6** 11-16.

Colborn, T., Myers, J.P. and Dumanoski, D. (1996) *Our Stolen Future: how Man-made Chemicals are Threatening our Fertility, Intelligence and Survival*, Little Brown, London.

Committee on the Toxicity, Mutagenicity and Carcinogenicity of Chemicals in Food, Consumer Products and the Environment *1996 Annual Report*, HMSO, London.

Constantinou, A., Kigucki, K. and Huberman, E. (1990) Induction of differentiation and DNA strand breakage in human HL-60 and K-562 leukemia cells by genistein. *Cancer Research*, **50** 2618-24.

Coward, L., Barnes, N.C., Setchell, K.D.R. and Barnes, S. (1993) Genistein, daidzein and their β-glycoside conjugates: antitumor isoflavones in soybean foods from American and Asian diets. *Journal of Agricultural and Food Chemistry*, **41** 1961-67.

Coward, L., Kirk, M., Albin, N. and Barnes, S. (1996) Analysis of plasma isoflavones by reversed phase HPLC–multiple reaction ion monitoring mass spectrometry. *Clin. Chim. Acta*, **247** 121-42.

Cox, R.I. (1977) Plant estrogens affecting livestock in Australia, in *Proceedings of the Joint US–Australian Symposium on Poisonous Plants* (eds. R.F. Keeler, K.R. Van Kampen and L.F. James), Academic Press, Australia.

Croker, K.P., Lightfoot, R.J., Johnson, T.J., Adams, N.R. and Carrick, M.J. (1989) The effects of selection for resistance to clover infertility on the reproductive performances of Merino ewes grazed on oestrogenic pastures. *Australian Journal of Agricultural Research*, **40** 165-76.

Cruz, M.L.A., Wong, W.W., Mimouni, F., Hachey, D.L., Setchell, K.D.R., Klein, P.D. and Tsang, R.C. (1994) Effects of infant nutrition on cholesterol synthesis rates. *Pediatric Research*, **35** 135-40.

Curtis, E.M. (1964) Oral contraceptive feminization of a normal male infant. *Obstetrics and Gynaecology*, **23** 295-96.

Doko, M.B., Canet, C., Brown, N., Sydenham, E.W., Mpuchane, S. and Siame, B.A. (1996) Natural co-occurrence of fumonisins and zearalenone in cereals and cereal-based foods from Eastern and Southern Africa. *Journal of Agricultural and Food Chemistry*, **44** 3240-43.

Dwyer, J.T., Goldin, B.R., Saul, N., Gualtieri, L., Barakat, S. and Adlercreutz, H. (1994) Tofu and soy drinks contain phytoestrogens. *Journal of the American Dietary Association*, **94** 739-43.

Eldridge, A.C. and Kwolek, W.F. (1983) Soybean isoflavones: effect of environment and variety on composition. *Journal of Agricultural Food Chemistry*, **31** 394-96.

European Commission (1997) *Report of the European Workshop on the Impact of Endocrine Disrupters on Health and Human Wildlife* Report EUR 17549, European Commission DGXII, Brussels, p. 5.

Faber, K.A. and Hughes, C.L. (1991) The effect of neonatal exposure to DES, genistein and zearalenone on pituitary responsiveness and sexually dimorphic nucleus volume in the castrated adult rat. *Biology of Reproduction*, **45** 649-53.

Faber, K.A. and Hughes, C.L. (1993) Dose reponse characteristics of neonatal exposure to genistein on pituitary responsiveness to gonadotrophin-releasing hormone and volume of the SDN-POA in post-pubertal castrated female rats. *Reproductive Toxicology*, **7** 35-39.

Franke, A.A. and Custer, L.J. (1996) Daidzein and genistein concentrations in human milk after soy consumption. *Clinical Chemistry* **42**, 955-64.

Franke, A.A., Custer, L.J., Carmencita, M.C. and Narala, K. (1995) Rapid HPLC analysis of dietary phytoestrogens from legumes and from human urine. *Proc. Soc. Exp. Biol. Med.*, **208** 18-26.

Fugatake, M., Takahasi, M., Ishida, K., Kawamura, H., Skugimura, T. and Wakabayashi, K. (1996) Quantification of genistein and genistin in soybeans and soybean products. *Food Chemistry and Toxicology*, **34** 457-61.

Gorski, R.A. (1986) Sexual differentiation of the brain: a model for drug-induced alterations of the reproductive system. *Environmental Health Perspectives*, **70** 163-75.

Grosvenor, C.E., Picciano, M.F. and Baumrucker, C.R. (1992) Hormones and growth factors in milk. *Endocrine Reviews*, **14** 710-28.

Hewitt, S., Hillman, J.R. and Knights, B.A. (1980) Steroidal oestrogens and plant growth and development. *New Phytology*, **85** 329-50.

Hietanemi, V. and Kumpulaineu, J. (1991) Contents of *Fusarium* toxins in Finnish and imported feeds. *Food Additives and Contaminants*, **8** 171-82.

Hirayama, T. (1986) A large-scale cohort study on cancer risk by diet—with special reference to the risk-reducing effects of green yellow vegetable composition. *Diet Nutr. Cancer*, **3** 42-53.

Hussein, H.M., Franich, R.A., Baxter, M. and Andrew, I.G. (1989) Naturally occurring *Fusarium* toxins in New Zealand maize. *Food Additives and Contaminants*, **6** 49-58.

IARC (1993) Toxins derived from *Fusarium graminearum, F. culmorum* and *F. crookwellense*: zearlenone, deoxynivalenol, nivalenol and fusarenone X, in *IARC Monographs on the Evaluation of Carcinogenic Risks to Humans, Vol. 56: Some Naturally Occurring Substances, Food Items and Constituents, Heterocyclic Aromatic Amines and Mycotoxins*, WHO, Geneva, pp. 397-444.

Irvine, C., Fitzpatrick, M., Robertson, I. and Woodhams, D. (1995) The potential adverse effects of soybean phytoestrogens in infant feeding. *New Zealand Medical Journal*, **108** 208-209.

Jones, A.E., Price, K.R. and Fenwick, G.R. (1989) Development of a high performance liquid chromatographic method for the analysis of phytoestrogens. *Journal of Science and Food Agriculture*, **46** 357-64.

Kaldas, R.S. and Hughes, C.L. (1989) Reproductive and general metabolic effects of phytoestrogens in mammals. *Reproductive Toxicology*, **3** 81-89.

Kallela, K. and Ettala, E. (1984) The oestrogenic *Fusarium toxin* (zearalenone) in hay as a cause of early abortions in the cow. *Nordisk Veteriner. Medicin*, **36** 305-309.

Kallela, K. and Saastamoinen, I. (1978) Analysis of plant estrogens in fodder by liquid chromatography. *Kemia Kem.*, **12** 622-23.

Kallela, K., Heinonen, R. and Saloniemi, H. (1984) Plant oestrogens: the cause of decreased fertility in cows—a case report. *Nordisk Veteriner. Medicin*, **36** 124-29.

Kavelock, R.J., Daston, G.P., DeRosa, C., Fenner-Crisp, P., Gray, L., Kaattari, S., Lucier, G., Luster, M., Mac, M.J., Maczka, C., Miller, R., Moore, J., Rolland, R., Scott, G., Sheehan, D.M., Sinks, T. and Tilson, H.A. (1996) Research needs for the risk assessment of health and environmental effects of endocrine disruptors: a report of the US EPA-sponsored workshop. *Environmental Health Perspectives*, **104** (suppl. 4) 715-40.

Kelly, G.E., Joannou, G.E., Reeder, A.Y., Nelson, C. and Waring, M.A. (1995) The variable metabolic response to dietary isoflavones in humans. *Proc. Soc. Exp. Biol. Med.*, **210** 40-43.

Kim, J.-C., Kang, H.-J., Lee, D.-H., Lee, Y.W. and Yoshizawe, T. (1993) Natural occurrence of *Fusarium* mycotoxins (trichothecenes and zearalenone) in barley and corn in Korea. *Applied Environmental Microbiology*, **59** 3798-802.

Kitts, D.D. (1987) Studies on the oestrogenic activity of coffee extract. *Journal of Toxicology and Environmental Health*, **20** 37-49.

Knuckles, B.E., de Fremery, D. and Kohler, G.O. (1976) Coumestrol content of fractions obtained during wet processing of alfalfa. *Journal of Agricultural and Food Chemistry*, **24** 1177-80.

Kuiper-Goodman, T., Scott, P.M. and Watanabe, H. (1987) Risk assessment of the mycotoxin zearalenone. *Reg. Toxicology and Pharmacology*, **7** 253-306.

Lamartiniere, C.A., Moore, J., Holland, M. and Barnes, S. (1995) Neonatal genistein chemoprevents mammary cancer. *Proc. Soc. Expl. Biol. Med.*, **208** 120-23.

Lee, H.P., Gourley, L., Duffy, S.W., Esteve, J., Lee, J. and Day, N.E. (1991) Dietary effects on breast cancer risk in Singapore. *Lancet*, **337** 1197-200.

Leitao, J., Bailly, J.-R. and de Saint Blanquat, G. (1992) Determination of mycotoxins in grains and related products. *Food Science and Technology*, **52** 387-419.

Leopold, A.S., Erwin, M.O.J. and Browning, B. (1976) Phytoestrogens: adverse effects on reproduction in Californian quail. *Science*, **191** 98-99.

Linassier, C.M., Pierre, M., Pecq, J.B.L. and Pierre, J. (1990) Mechanism of action in NIH 3T3 cells of genistein, an inhibitor of EGF receptor tyrosine kinase actvity. *Biochemical Pharmacology*, **39** 187-93.

Lone, K.P. (1997) Natural sex steroids and their xenobiotic analogs in animal production: growth, carcass quality, pharmacokinetics, metabolism, mode of action, residues, methods and epidemiology. *Critical Reviews in Food Science and Nutrition*, **37** 93-209.

Lookhart, G.L. (1980) Analysis of coumestrol, a plant estrogen, in animal feeds by high-performance liquid chromatography. *Journal of Agricultural and Food Chemistry*, **28** 666-67.

Madhavapeddi, R., and Ramachandran, P. (1985) Side effects of oral contraceptive use in lactating women—enlargement of breast in a breast-fed child. *Contraception*, **32** 437-43.

Markiewicz, L., Garey, J., Adlercreutz, C.H.T. and Gurpide, E. (1993) *In vitro* bioassays of nonsteroidal phytoestrogens. *Journal of Steroid Biochemistry and Molecular Biology*, **45** 399-405.

Martin, M.E., Haourigui, M., Pelissero, C., Benassazgay, C. and Nunez, E.A. (1996) Interaction between phytoestrogens and human sex binding protein. *Life Science*, **58** 429-34.

Martin, P.M., Horwitz, K.B., Ryan, D.S. and McGuire, W.L. (1978) Phytoestrogen interaction with estrogen receptors in human breast cancer cells. *Endocrinology*, **103** 1860-67.

Martins, M.L., Peito, M.A.P., Cruz, M.C., Martins, H.M. and Tavora, C.M.A.D. (1993) *In vitro* zearalenone production from *Fusarium* strains, isolated from animal feed. *Revista Portuguesa de Ciencias Veterinarias*, **88** 169-90.

Matsukawa, Y., Marui, N., Sakai, T., Satomi, Y., Yoshida, M., Matsumoto, K., Hishinio, H. and Aoike, A. (1993) Genistein arrests cell cycle progression at G2-M *Cancer Research*, **53** 1328-31.

Mayr, U., Butsch, A. and Schneider, S. (1992) Validation of two *in vitro* test systems for estrogenic activities with zearalenone, phytoestrogens and cereal extracts. *Toxicology*, **74** 135-49.

Mazur, W., Fotis, T., Wähälä, K., Ojala, S., Salakka, A. and Adlercreutz, H. (1996) Isotope dilution gas chromatographic–mass spectrometric method for the determination of isoflavonoids, coumestrol and lignans in food samples. *Analytical Biochemistry*, **233** 169-80.

McEwan, B.S. (1987) Steroid hormones and brain development. Some guidelines for standing action of pseudo hormones and other toxic agents. *Environmental Health Perspectives*, **74**, 177-84.

Mellanen, P., Petä, T., Lehtimäki, J., Mäkëla, S., Bylund, G., Holmbom, B., Mannila, E., Oikari, A. and Santi, R. (1996) Wood-derived estrogens: studies *in vitro* with breast cancer cell lines and *in vivo* with trout. *Toxicology and Applied Pharmacology*, **136** 381-88.

Messina, M.J., Persky, V., Setchell, K.D.R. and Barnes, S. (1994) Soy intake and cancer risk: a review of the *in vitro* and *in vivo* data. *Nutr. Cancer*, **21** 113-31.

Milano, G.D. and Lopez, T.A. (1991) Influence of temperature on zearalenone production by regional strains. *Journal of Food Microbiology*, **13** 329-33.

Mirocha, C.J., Pathre, S.V. and Christensen, C.M. (1977) Zearalenone, in *Mycotoxins in Human and Animal Health* (eds. J.V. Rodricks, C.W. Hesseltine and M.A. Mehlman), Pathotox Publishers, Park Forest South, Illinois, pp. 345-64.

Monk, E.L., Ern, R.E. and Mollett, T.A. (1975) Relationships between immunoreactive estrone and estradiol in milk, blood and urine in dairy cows. *Journal of Dairy Science*, **58** 34-40.

Morton, M.S., Wilcox, G., Wahlqvist, M.L. and Griffiths, K. (1994) Determination of lignans and isoflavinoids in human female plasma following dietary supplementation. *Journal of Endocrinology*, **142** 251-59.

Morton, M.S., Matos-Ferreira, A., Abranches-Monteiro, L., Correia, R., Blacklock, N., Chan, P.F.S., Cheng, C., Lloyd, S., Chieh-ping Wu and Griffiths, K (1997) Measurement and metabolism of isoflavonoids and lignans in the human male. *Cancer Letters*, **114** 145-51.

MRC Institute for Environment and Health (1995) *Environmental Oestrogens: Consequences to*

*Human Health and Wildlife*, MRC IEH, Leicester.

Müller, H.M., Reimann, J., Schumacher, U. and Schwadorf, K. (1997) *Fusarium* toxins in wheat harvested during six years in an area of southwest Germany. *Natural Toxins*, **5** 23-30.

Murkies, A.L., Lombard, C., Strauss, B.J.G., Wilcox, G., Burger, H.G. and Martin, M.A. (1995) Dietary flour supplements decrease post-menopausal hot flushes—effect of soy. *Maturitias*, **21** 189-95.

Murrill, W.B., Brown, N.M., Zhang, J.X., Manzolillo, P.A., Barnes, S. and Lamartiniere, C.A. (1966) Prepubertal genistein exposure suppresses mammary cancer and enhances gland differentiation in rats. *Carcinogenesis*, **17** 1451-57.

de Nijs, M., Rombouts, F. and Notermans, S. (1996) *Fusarium* moulds and their mycotoxins. *Journal of Food Safety*, **16** 15-58.

Nilsson, S., Nygren, K.G. and Johanson, D.B. (1978) Ethynyl estradiol in human milk and plasma after oral administrations. *Contraception*, **17** 131-39.

Obermeyer, W.R., Musser, S.M., Betz, J.M., Casey, R.E., Pohland, A.E. and Page, S.W. (1995) Chemical studies of phytoestrogens and related compounds in dietary supplement: flax and chaparral. *Proc. Soc. Exp. Biol. Med.*, **208** 6-12.

Okura, A., Arakawa, H., Oha, H., Yoshinari, T. and Monden, Y. (1988) Effect of genistein on topoisomerase activity and growth of [VAL12] Ha-*ras*-transformed NIH 3T3 cells. *BBRC*, **157** 183-89.

Patel, S., Hazel, C.M., Winterton, A.G.M. and Mortby, E. (1996) Survey of ethnic foods for mycotoxins. *Food Additives and Contaminants*, **13** 833-41.

Pathre, S.V. and Mirocha, C.J. (1980) Mycotoxins as estrogens, in *Estrogens in the Environment, Symposium* (ed. J.A. McLachlan), Raleigh, North Carolina, pp. 265-78.

Peattie, M.S., Buss, D.H., Lindsay, D.G. and Smart, G.A. (1983) Reorganisation of the British Total Diet Study for monitoring food constituents from 1981. *Food Chemistry and Toxicology*, **21**, 503-507.

Petrakis, N.L., Barnes, S., King, E.B., Lowenstein, J., Wiencke, J., Lee, M.M., Milke, R., Kirk, M. and Coward, L. (1996) Stimulatory influence of soy protein isolate on breast secretion in pre- and postmenopausal women. *Cancer Epidemiology Biomarkers Prev.*, **5** 785-94.

Petrelli, M., Fiorelli, G., Benvenuti, S., Frediani,V., Gori, F. and Brandi, M.L. (1995) Interactions between ipriflavone and the estrogen receptor. *Calcified Tissue International*, **56** 160-65.

Potter, S.M. (1995) Overview of proposed mechanism for the hypo-cholesterolemic affect of soy. *Journal of Nutrition*, **125** 606s -611s.

Price, K.R. and Fenwick, G.R. (1985) Naturally occurring oestrogens in foods—a review. *Food Additives and Contaminants*, **2** 73-106.

Ranft, K., Gerstl, R. and Mayer, G. (1990) Bestimmung und vorkommen von zearalenon in getreide und mischfuffermitteln. *Z. Lebensm. Unters. Forsch.*, **191** 449-53.

Register, B., Bether, M.A., Thompson, D., Walmer, D., Blohm, P., Ayyash, L. and Hughes, C. (1995) The effect of neonatal exposure to DES, coumestrol and beta-sitosterol on pituitary responsiveness and sexually dimorphic nucleus volume in the castrated adult rat. *Proc. Soc. Exper. Biol. Med.*, **208** 72-77.

Reinli, K. and Block, G. (1996) Phytoestrogen content of foods—a compendium of literature values. *Nutr. Cancer*, **26** 123-48.

Safe, S.H. (1995). Environmental and dietary estrogens and human health: is there a problem? *Environmental Health Perspectives*, **103** 346-51.

Saloniemi, H., Wähälä, K., Nykänen-Kurki, P., Kallela, K. and Saastomoinen, I. (1995) Phytoestrogen content and estrogenic effect of legume fodder. *Proc. Soc. Exp. Biol. Med.*, **208** 13-17.

Scudamore, K.A., Hetmanski, M.T., Chan, H.K. and Collins, S. (1997) Occurrence of mycotoxins in raw ingredients used for animal feeding stuffs in the United Kingdom in 1992. *Food Additives Contaminants*, **14** 157-73.

Setchell, K.D.R. and Adlercreutz, H. (1988) Mammalian lignans and phytoestrogens: recent studies on their formation, metabolism and biological role in health and disease, in *Role of the Gut Flora in Toxicity and Cancer* (ed. I.R. Rowland), Academic Press, London, pp. 317-45.

Setchell, K.D.R., Gosselin, S.J., Welsh, M.B., Johnston, J.O., Balistreri, W.F., Kramer, L.W., Dresser, B.L. and Tarr, M.L. (1987) Dietary estrogens—a probable cause of infertility and liver disease in captive cheetah. *Gastroenterology*, **93** 225-33.

Setchell, K.D.R., Zimmer-Nechemias, M.S., Cai, J. and Heubi, J.E. (1997) Exposure of infants to phytoestrogens from soy-based infant formula. *Lancet*, **350** 23-27.

Severson, K.K., Nomura, Y.M.A., Grove, S.J. and Stemmermann, N.G. (1989) A prospective study of demographics, diet and prostrate cancer among men of Japanese ancestry in Hawaii. *Cancer Research*, **49** 1857-60.

Sharpe, R.M. and Skakkebaek, N.E. (1993) Are oestrogens involved in falling sperm counts and disorders of the male reproductive tract? *Lancet*, **341** 1392-95.

Sheehan, D. (1995) The case for expanded phytoestrogen research. *Proc. Soc. Exp. Biol. Med.*, **208** (1) 3-5.

Shimuzu, H., Ross, K.R., Bernstein, L., Yatani, R., Henderson, E.B. and Mack, M.T. (1991) Cancers of the prostate and breast among Japanese and white immigrants in Los Angeles county. *Br. J. Cancer*, **63** 963-66.

Shotwell, O.L. (1977) Assay methods for zearalenone and its natural occurrence, in *Mycotoxins in Human and Animal Health* (eds. J.V. Rodricks, C.W. Hesseltine and M.A.), Mehlman Pathotox, Park Forest South, Illinois, pp. 403-13.

Shutt, D.A. (1976) The effects of plant oestrogens on animal reproduction. *Endeavour*, **35** 110-13.

Soto, A.M., Lin, T.M., Justicia, H., Silvia, R.M. and Sonnenschein,C. (1992) An 'in culture' bioassay to assess the estrogenicity of xenobiotics (E-screen), in *Chemically Induced Alterations in Sexual and Functional Development: the Wildlife/Human Connection* (eds. T. Colborn and C. Clement), Princeton Scientific, Princeton, NJ, pp. 295-309.

Sydenham, E.W., Thiel, P.G. and Marasas, W.F.O. (1988) Occurrence and chemical determination of zearalenone and alternariol monomethyl ether in sorghum-based mixed feeds associated with an outbreak of suspected hyperestrogenism in swine. *Journal of Agricultural and Food Chemistry*, **36** 621-25.

Tanaka, T. and Ueno, Y. (1989) Worldwide natural occurrence of *Fusarium* mycotoxins, nivalenol, deoxynivalenol and zearalenone, in *Mycotoxins and Phycotoxins 88*, 7th IUPAC Symposium on Mycotoxins and Phycotoxins, Japan, 16–18 August, 1988, Elsevier, Amsterdam.

Tartellin, M.F. and Gorski, R.A. (1988) Postnatal influence of DES on the differentiation of the sexually dimorphic nucleus in rats is as effective as perinatal treatment. *Brain Research*, **456** 271-74.

Terpestra, A.H.M., West, C.E., Fennis, J.T.C.M., Schouter, J.A and Van der Veen, E.A. (1984) Hypocholesteriemic effect of dietary soy protein versus caesin in rhesus monkeys. *American Journal of Clinical Nutrition*, **37** 1-7.

Traganos, F., Ardelt, B., Halko, N., Brkuni, S. and Darzynkeizics, Z. (1992) Effects of genistein on the growth and cell cycle progression of normal human lymphocytes and human leukemia MOLT-4 and HL-60 cells. *Cancer Research*, **20** 6200-208.

Tsukamoto, C., Shimada, S., Igita, K., Kudou, S., Kokubun, M., Okubo, K. and Kitamura, K. (1995) Factors affecting isoflavone content in soybean seeds: changes in isoflavones, saponins and composition of fatty acids at different temperatures during seed development. *Journal of Agricultural and Food Chemistry*, **43** 1184-92.

Verdeal, K. and Ryan, D.S. (1979) Naturally occurring estrogens in plant foodstuffs—a review. *Journal of Food Protection* **42** 577-683.

Veterinary Medicines Directorate (1996) *Annual Report on Surveillance for Veterinary Residues in 1995*, Veterinary Medicines Directorate, Byfleet, Surrey.

Walsh, R.J., Brewer, J.R. and Naftolin, F. (1982) Early postnatal development of the arculate nucleus in normal and sexually reversed male and female rats. *Journal of Anatomy*, **135** 733-44.

Wang, G., Kuan, S.S., Francis, O.J., Ware, G.M. and Carman, A.S. (1990) A simplified HPLC method for the determination of phytoestrogens in soybean and its processed products. *Journal of Agricultural and Food Chemistry*, **38** 185-90.

Wang, H.-J. and Murphy, P. (1994a) Isoflavone composition of American and Japanese soyabeans in Iowa: effects of variety, crop year and location. *Journal of Agricultural and Food Chemistry*, **42** 1674-77.

Wang, H.-J. and Murphy, P. (1994b) Isoflavone content in commercial soybean foods. *Journal of Agricultural and Food Chemistry*, **42** 1666-73.

Wei, H., Wei, L., Frenkel, K., Dowen, R. and Barnes, S. (1993) Inhibition of tumor promoter induced hydrogen peroxide formation *in vitro* and *in vivo* by genistein *Nutr. Cancer*, **20** 1-12.

Wei, H., Bowen, R., Cai, Q., Barnes, S. and Wang, Y. (1995) Antioxidant and antipromotional effects of the soybean isoflavone genistein. *Proc. Soc. Exp. Biol. Med.*, **208** 124-29.

Welshons, W.V., Rottinghaus, G.E., Nonneman, D.J., Dolan-Timpe, M. and Ross, P.F. (1990) A sensitive bioassay for the detection of dietary oestrogens in animal feeds. *J. Vet. Diag. Invest.*, **2** 268-73.

Whitten, P.L. and Naftolin, F. (1992) Effects of phytoestrogen diet on oestrogen-dependent reproductive processes in immature female rats. *Steroids*, **57** 56-61.

Whitten, P.L., Lewis, C. and Naftolin, F. (1993) A phytoestrogen diet induces the premature anovulatory syndrome in lactationally exposed female rats. *Biology of Reproduction*, **49** 1117-21.

Whitten, P.L., Lewis, C., Russel, E. and Naftolin, F. (1995) Phytoestrogen influences on the development of behaviour and gonadotropin function. *Proc. Soc. Exp. Biol. Med.*, **208** 82-86.

Wilcox, G., Wahlqvist, M.L., Burger, H.G. and Medley, G. (1990) Oestrogenic effects of plant foods in postmenopausal women. *British Medical Journal*, **301** 905-906.

Wolford, S.T. and Argoudelis, C.J. (1979) Measurement of estrogens in cow's milk, human milk and dairy products. *Journal of Dairy Science*, **62** 1458-63.

Wudy, S.A., Wachter, U.A., Homoki, J. and Yeller, W.M. (1995) 17 α-hydroxyprogesterone, 4-androstenedione and testosterone profiled by routine stable isotope dilution/gas chromatography-mass spectrometry in plasma of children. *Pediatric Research*, **38** 76-80.

Young, I.J., Knights, B.A. and Hillman, J.R. (1977) Oestradiol and its biosynthesis in *Phaseolus vulgaris* L. *Nature*, **267**, 429.

Young, L.G., King, G.J., McGirr, L. and Sutton, J.C. (1982) Moldy corn in diets of gestating and lactating swine. *Journal of Animal Science*, **54** 976-82.

# 5    Nut allergens

Fiona Angus

## 5.1    Introduction

Awareness of nut allergy has increased dramatically in recent years, largely as a result of extensive media coverage of a number of deaths that have occurred in the UK since 1993 from severe allergic reactions to peanuts and other nuts. Despite its having been recognised as a real clinical problem for many years, there has been relatively little funding devoted to the causes, prevalence or management of nut allergy and there is still much that is not known about this disorder.

A major problem in this area has been defining what is a 'nut' and there seem to be few botanical terms that are used more loosely, with different authors defining the terms in different ways. Menninger (1977) provides the broad definition of 'any hard-shelled fruit or seed of which the kernel is eaten by mankind'. Wickens (1995), however, defines nuts as 'hard-shelled fruits or the edible kernels of fleshy drupes, or berries or seeds that are traditionally referred to as nuts'. This chapter includes nuts or seeds that fall within the latter definition, and have been associated with allergic reactions.

## 5.2    Background to food allergy and intolerance

### 5.2.1    Types of reaction

Food allergy and food intolerance are terms that are frequently used interchangeably, but they are not the same reaction. Food intolerance refers to any kind of reproducible, unpleasant reaction to a specific food. A sub-group of food intolerance is food allergy, but a reaction can only be called allergic if it is caused by an immunological response, often involving immunoglobulin E (IgE) antibodies that bind to the food (Royal College of Physicians and British Nutrition Foundation, 1984; Perkin, 1990; Lessof, 1992). Allergy is thought to account for less than 20% of all adverse food reactions.

Immune reactions are classified into four types: I, II, III and IV. Types I, II and III all involve antibodies, whereas type IV reactions are cell-mediated (Perkin, 1990). It is the type I reactions that involve IgE antibodies and are usually very quick. Types II and III have very little importance in food allergy, being involved, for example, in some types of anaemia and kidney disease. Type IV refers to a slow-developing reaction caused by migrating white blood cells (lymphocytes). Coeliac disease is a type IV reaction in which a slow reaction to wheat gluten damages the lining of the intestine.

### 5.2.2 Symptoms

Food allergy and intolerance are associated with a wide range of symptoms. Most commonly, there will be a skin reaction like eczema or urticaria (hives) followed by a gastro-intestinal response including vomiting and diarrhoea (Perkin, 1990). Immune reactions to food often involve type I allergy and may result in anaphylaxis. Anaphylaxis is described as an exaggerated immune response resulting from re-exposure to an allergen (Matsuda and Nakamura, 1993). Anaphylactic symptoms can vary from mild reactions, including lip swelling, itching and urticaria, to more severe reactions such as wheezing, vomiting, coughing and respiratory stress (Kemp *et al.*, 1982).

The presence of the allergen causes a widespread release of inflammatory mediators such as histamine and prostaglandins. These chemicals cause a chain of reactions leading to swelling of the upper airway, severe asthma and a dramatic fall in blood pressure, leading to circulatory collapse (James and Austen, 1964; Ownby, 1995; Hourihane *et al.*, 1995). In extreme cases there may be a sudden onset of vascular shock, resulting in a dramatic fall in blood pressure, coma and even death. Death is usually caused by obstruction of the larynx and epiglottis, and heart failure (Loza and Brostoff, 1995).

The most common symptom of peanut and nut allergy is 'oral allergy syndrome', which involves oral tingling, metallic taste and the classic urticarial rash (Hourihane *et al.*, 1995), but, in more severe cases, anaphylactic reactions have caused death (Yunginger, 1992; Sampson *et al.*, 1992). The response to the allergen is dose-dependent, so larger intakes of the allergen tend to lead to increasingly severe reactions (Yunginger *et al.*, 1989).

From the time of contact with the allergen, onset of symptoms is rapid, usually in the order of a few minutes. Documented cases give the time of onset of initial symptoms for peanut allergy between 'immediate' and 90 min (Boyd, 1989; Settipane, 1989; Yunginger *et al.*, 1989; Sampson *et al.*, 1992). In an investigation of six fatal and six near-fatal cases of food-induced anaphylaxis, by Sampson *et al.* (1992), the children suffered symptoms within 3 to 30 min after ingestion and severe symptoms within 20 minutes (min) and 2.5 hours (h) later. In the most severe cases, it has been shown that many of the victims were also asthmatic (Assem *et al.*, 1990; Metcalfe *et al.*, 1991; Sampson *et al.*, 1992).

Case studies cite the time from ingestion until death as 20 min to 8 days (Boyd, 1989; Yunginger *et al.*, 1989; Assem *et al.*, 1990; Sampson *et al.*, 1992; Ownby, 1995). In some cases symptoms appear to be improving but, after a period of recovery that may be several hours they worsen.

More unusual symptoms have been reported on rare occasions. For example, a case history describes a woman with an intermittent, painful burning sensation on the edge of her tongue. A double-blind placebo-controlled food challenge (DBPCFC) showed that the symptom was caused by ingestion of peanuts (Whitley *et al.*, 1991).

### 5.2.3  Foods implicated

The range of foods that can cause reactions is extensive. Those most commonly implicated include cows' milk, hens' eggs, wheat, soya, fish, shellfish, nuts and peanuts. Many other foods are reported as causing reactions in some people, however, and these include fruits, vegetables, herbs and seeds, as well as some additives. Most of the foods that provoke an immunological or allergic reaction contain glycoproteins or other proteins, of molecular weights between 10 000 and 70 000 (Whitley *et al.*, 1991; Lessof, 1992).

### 5.2.4  Prevalence

Assessing the true prevalence of food intolerance is difficult because of the lack of available practical diagnostic methods and the large number of people required to produce an accurate estimate.

In a cross-sectional population study involving 7500 households in the Wycombe Health Authority area and 7500 households nationwide, Young *et al.* (1994) found that around 20% of those surveyed believed that they suffered from food intolerance. Of these, only 1.4 to 1.8% (depending on the definition used) tested positive. In a similar study of the perceived prevalence of peanut allergy in the UK, Emmett *et al.* (1996) found that 4% of the population perceived themselves to be suffering from food allergy. This finding was based on interviews with 16 434 households,

In the population study of food intolerance by Young *et al.* (1994), 1.6% of the nationwide respondents perceived that they were intolerant to nuts, although, on food challenge, the perceived prevalence of all allergies was found to be overestimated by a factor of ten. In an omnibus survey of perceived prevalence of peanut allergy in the UK, Emmett *et al.* (1996) found that 0.4% of the population reported themselves as being allergic to peanuts. Peanut allergy was strongly associated with other food allergies, particularly to tree nuts and with asthma, eczema and hay fever. In the same study, 0.38% of adult men and women perceived themselves to be allergic to tree nuts and 0.04% reported that they were allergic to sesame seed.

In a cohort study of 1218 children born in the Isle of Wight between 1989 and 1990, Tariq *et al.* (1996) reported that 15 (1.2%) children were sensitised to peanuts or tree nuts by the age of four years. Six of these children had suffered allergic reactions to peanuts (0.5%), one had reacted to hazelnuts and one to cashew nuts. The other seven children had positive skin-prick tests to peanut, but were asymptomatic.

Ewan (1996) reported on 62 cases of food allergy seen at the allergy clinic at Addenbrookes Hospital between 1993 and 1994. Peanuts were the most common cause of allergy, affecting 47 subjects, followed by Brazil nut with 18 subjects affected, almond with 14 subjects and hazelnut with 13 subjects. Early sensitisation (before two years) to peanuts was common, probably because of their introduction into the diet during weaning.

Other studies have suggested estimates of 13 to 15% of children with skin conditions suffering from peanut allergy (Moneret-Vautrin *et al.*, 1993; Hopkins, 1995). Using double-blind food challenges, May and Bock (1978) found that 21% of adolescents aged 3 to 16 years with a history of food-related allergy were allergic to peanuts.

Unlike many other food allergies, peanut allergy is rarely outgrown. Hourihane *et al.* (1995) suggest that if peanut allergy is still present in a child at the age of eight years, in 80% of cases it is likely to remain a life-long problem.

Whitley *et al.* (1991) suggest that, in the US, peanuts are second only to milk and eggs in terms of allergy prevalence. Peanuts do appear to be more allergenic than tree nuts but it has been suggested that this may simply be due to the fact that they are consumed in larger quantities. Peanut allergy is currently thought to be more common in the US than in Europe; however, this is likely to be because the US consumes much larger quantities of peanuts than Europe. This situation is changing, however, as peanuts are currently a cheap source of protein and are becoming increasingly incorporated into processed foods in the European market. It is thought that the incidence of peanut allergy will continue to rise in line with increased consumption (Dutau *et al.*, 1991). Interestingly, it has been suggested that in some north European countries, such as Germany, hazelnut allergy is more common than peanut allergy.

The number of severe reactions caused by food-related anaphylaxis is also not known with any certainty. In the US a prospective survey of the incidence of severe food reactions in Colorado was carried out by Bock (1992). The study involved 73 Colorado emergency departments which identified and recorded emergency cases that were admitted because of severe allergic reactions to food. Bock (1992) identified 25 severe reactions within the two years of the study. Extrapolation of these data to the whole of the US gives an estimate of at least 950 severe food reactions each year. Hide (1993a) related these data to the UK situation and estimated that in the UK there were probably 200 to 250 severe food reactions every year. Of those individuals studied in the prospective survey on the incidence of severe food reactions in Colorado (Bock, 1992), one-third were found to react to peanuts. Relating these data to the UK estimate of approximately 200 to 250 severe food reactions a year gives an estimated incidence of severe reactions to peanuts in the UK of between 65 and 85 per year (Bock, 1992; Hide, 1993a). Peanuts are also the cause of most fatal cases of food-related anaphylaxis.

The number of fatalities from food-related anaphylaxis has not been established. These deaths may be coded under various International Classification of Diseases codes and it is therefore difficult to collect accurate data from death certificates. Again there have been few surveys on the number of fatalities caused by all causes of anaphylaxis, but data extrapolated to the UK from a survey carried out in Canada suggest that there are probably around 20 deaths from all causes of anaphylaxis per year in the UK (this figure includes deaths from bee and wasp stings, and penicillin as well as foods such as peanuts). The number of food-related fatalities is not known, but is generally accepted to be greater than the four to six who die from bee or wasp stings in the UK each year (Hide, 1993a).

### 5.2.5   Family history and other risk factors

Anyone can suffer from peanut or nut allergy but there are certain groups that are thought more likely to be affected. It has been suggested that allergies tend to run in families so that children with allergic parents (not necessarily with allergy to peanuts) would be more likely to develop a peanut allergy (Taylor, 1985; Hourihane et al., 1996), although this is not always the case. The group most at risk appears to be highly atopic children, particularly those with asthma or allergic rhinitis (Settipane, 1989; Zimmerman et al., 1989). Atopic individuals are those that have unusual sensitivity to allergens; this is usually characterised by the amount of IgE in the blood. Atopic children have immune systems that are particularly prone to producing large quantities of IgE in response to foreign proteins. In a study of 141 children, 73 were classified as highly atopic and 82% of the highly atopic patients were found to be sensitive to peanuts, with only 50% of the non-atopic patients being sensitive (Zimmerman et al., 1989).

Reactions to the presence of allergens also tend to be more severe in highly atopic children. In a US study of six fatal and six near-fatal reactions to food in children, Sampson et al. (1992) observed that all the children who had suffered these severe reactions were highly atopic, with current or previous symptoms of asthma, allergic rhinitis or atopic dermatitis. An allergic reaction usually occurs on the second exposure to a particular allergen; the first exposure is referred to as sensitisation and is responsible for the immune system producing IgE specific to the allergen. There are many case studies cited in the literature, however, where an allergic reaction to peanuts (sometimes life-threatening) appears to have occurred on the first exposure to peanuts (Fries, 1982; Asperen et al., 1983; Gerrard and Perelmutter, 1986; DeBolt et al., 1993). For example, of the 30 patients studied by Fries (1982), 14 stated that they had suffered a reaction on their first consumption of peanuts. There is a suggestion that airborne food allergens can sensitise patients (Ownby, 1995).

It has also been suggested that maternal avoidance of a particular food during pregnancy can prevent an infant from developing an allergy. This approach is often recommended when there is a family history of allergy to a particular food. However, maternal avoidance and breast feeding do not guarantee protection against the development of an allergen. While there may be a reduction in the incidence of the allergy in a proportion of infants

(Gerrard and Perelmutter, 1985; Taylor, 1985; Gerrard and Perelmutter, 1986), strict maternal avoidance of peanuts or eggs has still resulted in babies that are sensitised to the food avoided by the mother (Gerrard and Perelmutter, 1986). Some case studies can be cited where the only possible routes of sensitisation are via breast milk (peanut protein has been detected in breast milk) or *in utero* (Gerrard and Perelmutter, 1985; Settipane, 1989; DeBolt *et al.*, 1993). Hourihane *et al.* (1996) suggest that it may be prudent for allergic mothers to avoid peanuts during pregnancy.

It has been proposed that children may be sensitised to peanuts by consumption of peanut oil in infant formula or as a component of vitamin preparations given to the new-born. A study of 40 children found that the incidence of peanut allergy was 5% in those who had been given vitamin preparations not based on peanut oil, 25% in those that had peanut-oil based vitamin preparations monthly and 32% in those that had peanut-oil based vitamin preparations weekly (De Montis *et al.*, 1993).

It has been suggested that the incidence of *in utero* food sensitisation has been underestimated (Hatahet *et al.*, 1994). The area remains controversial, however, with other authors believing *in utero* sensitisation to be relatively unimportant (Loza and Brostoff, 1995).

Studies have shown that individuals suffering fatal or near-fatal anaphylactic reactions nearly always knew that they were allergic to the food consumed. A large percentage of those known to be allergic to peanuts are reported to have inadvertently consumed peanuts over extended periods of study. For example, a study by Bock and Atkins (1989) involved contacting 32 known peanut-sensitive patients between 2 and 14 years after diagnosis. Only eight of these individuals had managed to avoid peanuts completely, 16 had accidentally ingested peanuts in the year before contact, with the other eight accidentally consuming peanuts in a one- to five-year period. Many deaths from peanut anaphylaxis occur in individuals that in the past suffered from only mild reactions to the substance; severe reactions are often associated with individuals that have a history of asthma (Settipane, 1989; Yunginger *et al.*, 1989; Sampson *et al.*, 1992; Ownby, 1995), although there does not appear to be any difference in the severity of the asthma in those patients suffering fatal or near-fatal anaphylactic reactions (Sampson *et al.*, 1992). It has been suggested that asthma may potentiate more severe reactions because of the sensitivity of the lungs to endogenous mediators (Loza and Brostoff, 1995).

A comparison between fatal and near-fatal anaphylactic reactions to foods (the majority caused by peanuts) in the US found that survivors had received an injection of adrenaline soon after ingestion of the allergic substance, often before the onset of severe symptoms. Those suffering fatal anaphylactic reactions delayed the injection of adrenaline, frequently until after the onset of severe symptoms (Settipane, 1989; Sampson *et al.*, 1992).

### 5.3    Peanut allergy

*5.3.1  Botanical aspects*
The peanut (*Arachis hypogaea*) is not related to tree nuts such as hazelnuts
and almonds. Peanuts develop in a seed pod approximately 10 cm below
ground level; hence the alternative name for peanuts, i.e. groundnuts (Fries,
1982; Yunginger and Jones, 1987; Hourihane *et al.*, 1995). Botanically, the
peanut is a member of the legume family, which includes soya beans, peas,
lentils and beans.

   The peanut is harvested as a shelled product with a fruit inside. The fruit
is surrounded by a skin and is formed in two halves (cotyledons) to which
the majority of susceptible individuals are allergic. The skin and germ tissue
have been found to be allergenic in some individuals (Bush *et al.*, 1989).

   There are three types of peanut grown commercially around the world:
Spanish, Runner and Virginia. Peanuts imported into the UK are mainly
American Runners (40 to 60%) and almost all are imported whole and
processed in the UK (Fries, 1982; Yunginger and Jones, 1987; Metcalfe *et
al.*, 1991; Hourihane *et al.*, 1995).

*5.3.2  Major allergens*
Peanut proteins constitute 25 to 28% of the weight of the cotyledons and the
protein is usually separated into two fractions: water-soluble albumins and
saline-soluble globulins. The globulins have been divided into arachin (precipitated in 20% ammonium sulphate) and conarachin. Other peanut proteins have been identified, such as lectins and agglutinins, but these have
less importance than arachin and conarachin. Arachin has been further
divided into seven sub-units with molecular weights ranging from 10 000 to
71 000 (the number of sub-units found may exceed seven depending on the
actual chemical processes used). Conarachin consists of two main components, conarachin I and conarachin II. Conarachin II contains seven sub-
units of molecular weight 18 000 to 62 000 (Hourihane *et al.*, 1995).

   The first reported case of peanut allergy was in 1920 (Blackfan, 1920)
but it is only in the last 15 years or so that work has been done to characterise the allergenic fractions of the peanut (Loza and Brostoff, 1995).
Peanuts are thought to contain a large number of allergenic fractions, many
as yet uncharacterised and unidentified (Hourihane *et al.*, 1995).

   Initial work on the allergens of peanuts identified a fraction called
Peanut I (Sachs *et al.*, 1981); the allergenic material did not, however,
account for all the allergenicity in peanuts. Barnett *et al.* (1983) examined
the allergenicity of μ-arachin, conarachin I, concanavalin A-reactive glyco-
protein, peanut agglutinin and phospholipase D. All the sera collected from
peanut-allergic patients were found to contain IgE antibodies to μ-arachin

and conarachin I; reactions to peanut agglutinin and phospholipase D were less common (Barnett *et al.*, 1983). The main allergens in peanuts have since been identified as *Arachis hypogaea* antigens I and II, usually referred to as Ara h I and Ara h II, and agglutinin. These fractions have respective molecular weights of 63 000, 17 000 and 31 000. The isoelectric points of Ara h I and Ara h II are 4.55 and 5.2, respectively (Burks *et al.*, 1994). Ara h I and II are classified as major allergens since they bind IgE in the blood of those with peanut allergy in *in vitro* tests. Agglutinin, however, is classified as a minor peanut allergen since it binds IgE in the blood of less than half of peanut-allergic patients (Hourihane *et al.*, 1995). It would appear that the allergenic fractions are found in all varieties of peanut (Keating *et al.*, 1990; Burks *et al.*, 1994).

Roasting and heat treatment of peanuts do not seem to reduce the allergic response. Dutau *et al.* (1991) and Yunginger and Jones (1987) have even suggested that the allergenicity of peanuts in some patients is actually increased. Peanuts are unusual in this respect since most allergenic proteins can be made either less allergenic or non-allergenic by heat treatment (Barnett *et al.*, 1983; Matsuda and Nakamura, 1993; Wal, 1993). Chemical denaturation has also been shown to affect the allergenicity of peanut proteins *in vitro* only slightly (Burks *et al.*, 1992).

Historically, those diagnosed as suffering from peanut allergy were advised to avoid all members of the legume family. In more recent years, several research groups have examined the prevalence of cross-reactivity in the legume family. Bernhisel-Broadbent and Sampson (1989) evaluated 69 patients with positive skin prick tests to one or more members of the legume family. The oral food challenges used showed that cross-reactivity in children was very rare (only 5% of those challenged). A similar study by Bock and Atkins (1989) examined 32 children aged 2 to 14 years who reacted to peanuts. Skin prick tests were positive for peas in 15 patients, soya in 17 patients and both in 10 patients. However, only two patients reacted to a test with the suspect food (one to pea and one to soya). Some of these patients reported previous reactions to tree nuts but during the study none of them reacted to challenge with any tree nut. Peanut-allergic subjects do not necessarily therefore cross-react either to other members of the legume family (Boyd, 1989) or to tree nuts (Bock and Atkins, 1989). In some cases, however, cross-reactions to other foods such as tree nuts do occur (Goetz *et al.*, 1991; Loza and Brostoff, 1995). Latex and grass pollen have been shown to cross-react with peanuts (De Martino *et al.*, 1988; Doyle, 1994; Hovanec-Burnes *et al.*, 1995). David (1993) reported the case of a 14-year-old boy who normally developed angiodoema following ingestion of peanuts, but who suffered a life-threatening anaphylactic reaction after eating peanuts five minutes after taking an aspirin. It is reported that the aspirin increased the permeability of the gut mucosa and hence the allergic response. Alcohol also seems to increase the severity of the allergic response to peanuts (Assem *et al.*, 1990).

The amount of peanuts required to elicit an allergic reaction has not been extensively studied but there are many anecdotal case studies. Metcalfe *et al.* (1991) reported that 50 to 100 mg of peanut protein had elicited allergic responses in some children but the most sensitive children at risk of anaphylaxis were not challenged. Settipane (1989) describes peanut as an 'exquisite allergen'. In one study, a wheal-and-flare reaction was induced by the injection of the equivalent of 1/44 000 of a peanut kernel. Case studies report reactions to extremely small quantities of peanuts; for example, children have been reported to suffer symptoms after contact with a table that had been wiped clean of all visible peanut butter. Symptoms have also been induced by kissing or sharing a drink with someone who had recently eaten peanuts and a patient has been described who suffered wheezing and urticaria when a jar of peanut butter was opened in front of him (Fries, 1982; Sampson, 1990; Hopkins, 1995).

## 5.4    Tree nut allergy

### 5.4.1  Botanical aspects
Tree nuts are defined as the edible kernels of the seeds of trees (Woodroof, 1979).

### 5.4.2  Allergenicity

*5.4.2.1  Almonds.* There are two species of almonds (*Amygdalus communis* or *Prunus amygdalus*): sweet almonds and bitter almonds (Woodroof, 1979). Sweet almonds are grown for their edible nuts, while bitter almonds are grown to produce oil or bitter almond (Wickens, 1995). There are two types of sweet almonds, hard- and soft-shell varieties, but most commercial almond cultivars are soft shell.

Almonds are eaten dry or oil-roasted as a dessert nut and find application in confectionery, baking, dairy and snack formulations. In the early 1980s, almond butter was developed and this is used in a number of manufactured products (Wickens, 1995).

Almonds contain 22% protein, 57.7% fat and 15% carbohydrate (Wickens, 1995). Almonds have been associated with severe allergic reactions. In 1995, the UK press reported the death of a 27-year-old woman who died at a Christmas party after allegedly eating Brussels sprouts that had been topped with slivers of almond (Anon, 1996).

Bargman *et al.* (1992) tested the allergenicity of different types and varieties of almonds using immunoblots of almond extracts with sera from almond-allergic individuals. Two major allergens in almonds were identified: one was a heat-stable protein of molecular weight 45 000 to 50 000 and the other was a heat-labile protein of molecular weight 70 000. There were, however, multiple IgE binding proteins in almonds with molecular weights ranging from 38 000 to 70 000.

*5.4.2.2 Brazil nuts.* Brazil nuts are the seed of the *Bertholletia excelsa* or *Bertholletia myrtaceae*. The tree is found principally in the Amazon region and Brazil nuts are a major export from this region. The fruit of the Brazil nut tree is a woody shelled capsule containing a hard pod. Each pod contains 12 to 20 nuts (Woodroof, 1979).

The Brazil nut contains 14% protein, 67% fat and 11% carbohydrate (Wickens, 1995). It has been shown to be a potent allergen. Hide (1983b) highlights four cases of young atopic children who experienced various symptoms including urticaria, swelling of the tongue and lips, and facial oedema after ingestion of, and in some cases touching, a Brazil nut. Sampson (1990) cites the case of a 12-year-old girl with asthma who had a severe life-threatening anaphylactic reaction to Brazil nuts after eating a cookie. Her previous reaction to Brazil nuts was just two weeks before.

Arshad *et al.* (1991) discusses 12 patients aged between 3 and 39 years with Brazil nut allergy in the Isle of Wight. Their symptoms varied from itching around the mouth and swelling through to anaphylaxis, with all the patients reacting within three minutes of ingesting the nut. Five of the patients were followed up over an eight year period and none of them lost their sensitivity to Brazil nuts in this period. Immunoblotting showed that there were several different allergenic fractions in Brazil nuts with molecular weights ranging from less than 5000 to 50 000.

The major allergenic protein in Brazil nuts is reported to be *Ber e* 1, which is a methionine-rich protein made up of two units, 9000 and 3000 in molecular weight (Bush and Hefle, 1996). In recent years, work has been undertaken to improve the methionine content of the soya bean by introducing the gene for this protein from Brazil nuts. However, the allergenicity of the protein was also transferred (Nordlee *et al.*, 1996) and plans to market this transgenic soya bean are reported to have been dropped (Nestle, 1996).

*5.4.2.3 Cashews.* The cashew nut (*Anarcadium occidentale* L.) is a member of the Anacardiaceae family, which includes mango, gingko, poison ivy and oak. The cashew shrub or tree bears kidney-shaped fruit with thick cotyledons (Wickens, 1995). Around 60% of cashews are sold as salted nuts but they are also used in confectionery, bakery products and ethnic foods.

Cashews contain 12.8% protein, 46.7% fat and 18% carbohydrate (Wickens, 1995). Ingestion of cashew nuts has been reported to cause allergy problems and all members of the Anacardiaceae family cause contact dermatitis (Marks *et al.*, 1984). Sampson *et al.* (1992) reported on two fatalities that occurred in the US as a result of severe anaphylactic reactions to cashew nuts. Both were teenage girls who suffered from severe asthma, and both died as a result of eating candy products containing cashew nuts. Marks *et al.* (1984) describe cases of poison-ivy-like dermatitis in 54 people after eating cashew nuts. The reactions were attributed to the presence of urushiol and cardol in the cashew nut shell oil, with which the nuts were found to have been contaminated.

*5.4.2.4  Hazelnuts.* The terms hazelnuts and filberts are used interchangeably to describe plants in the genus *Corylus* (*Corylus avellana* and *C. maxima*). In the UK, a distinction is made between filberts, which have long husks, and cobnuts, which have short husks (Woodroof, 1979). The use of hazelnuts dates back to ancient times, with records from around 5000 years ago. Hazelnuts contain 16.3% protein, 61.2% fat and 11.5% carbohydrate (Wickens, 1995).

Hazelnut allergy has been found to be common among sufferers of tree pollen allergy (Bush and Hefle, 1996). Sampson *et al.* (1992) describe cases of near-fatal anaphylactic reactions to filberts as a result of eating cakes containing them. The subjects, aged 9 and 15 years, were asthmatic.

*5.4.2.5 Macadamia nuts.* Macadamia nuts (*Macadamia intefrifolia*) originate from the rainforests in Queensland and New South Wales, and so are also sometimes referred to as Queensland or Australian nuts (Woodroof, 1979). They belong to the Proteaceae family. The kernels contain 78% fat, the remainder being protein and a small amount of sugar (Wickens, 1995).

As a member of the tree nut family, macadamia nuts could conceivably cause allergy problems. However, no references to these have been found in the literature.

*5.4.2.6  Pecans.* Pecans (*Carya illinoinensis*) belong to the Junlanaceae family (Wickens, 1995). They are cultivated in many parts of the world including the US, Mexico, Australia, South Africa and Israel. The pecan nut contains 70% fat, 10% protein and 13.3% carbohydrate (Wickens, 1995).

Pecans have been reported to cause serious allergic reactions, including fatalities. Yunginger *et al.* (1988) describe the case of a 16-year-old severely asthmatic boy with allergies to peanut and pecan nuts who died following ingestion of pecans in a cheesecake base. Malanin *et al.* (1995) report on the case of a girl who developed IgE antibodies to heated pecans but not to fresh pecans. The allergenic proteins in pecans have a molecular weight of around 15 000.

*5.4.2.7  Pine nuts.* Pine nuts are obtained from the pinon pine (*Pinus edulis*), which is a small tree found in South America. The nuts are obtained from the pine cones, with each cone providing around 100 seeds (Fine, 1987). Pine nuts are also known as pinon nuts, pinoccios, pignoles and pignolas. They have been eaten for centuries but have found increasing use in recent years in pesto sauces, meat dishes, pastries, salads, cakes and biscuits (Koepke *et al.*, 1990).

Pine nuts have been reported as being responsible for recurrent urticaria (Falliers, 1989) and severe anaphylactic reactions (Fine, 1987; Falliers, 1989; Koepke *et al.*, 1990; Nielsen, 1990). Koepke *et al.* (1990) reported on the case of a 21-year-old male who suffered a severe anaphylactic reaction after eating a cookie containing pine nuts. Electrophoresis of pine nut extract showed three protein bands in the molecular weight range 66 000 to 68 000 bound IgE from the subject's serum.

*5.4.2.8 Pistachios.* The pistachio tree (*Pistacia vera* L.) is one of 11 species in the genus *Pistacia* in the family Anacardiaceae, of which cashew and mango are also members. The edible portion of the pistachio is the seed. The size of seeds varies widely in different species of *Pistacia*, but *P. vera* is the only tree capable of producing nuts of a sufficient size for consumption. Pistachio nuts contain 21.4% protein, 50% fat (Wickens, 1995) and carbohydrate, especially sucrose.

Pistachios have been reported as causing allergic reactions. Goldbert *et al.* (1969) reported on a case of pistachio-induced anaphylaxis. Parra *et al.* (1993) have isolated various allergenic proteins in pistachio. The major pistachio IgE-binding protein has a molecular weigh of 34 000; other allergenic proteins are present in the molecular weight range 41 000 to 60 000.

*5.4.2.9 Walnuts.* Walnuts are from the genus *Juglans*, which includes about 15 species and is a member of the Juglandaceae family. The Persian walnut (*Juglans regia*) is most important in terms of world production. Walnuts contain 17% protein, 65% fat and 16.5% carbohydrate.

There is very little published information on walnut allergy. Sampson *et al.* (1992), however, cite the case of a 17-year-old girl with asthma who suffered a near-fatal anaphylactic reaction to walnuts in a cookie.

## 5.5 Other allergenic nuts and seeds

### 5.5.1 Coconuts

The coconut (*Cocos nucifera* L.) belongs to the family Palmae. In strict botanical terms the coconut palm is not a tree but is a monocotyledonous plant that is closely related to bamboo and grasses. Two types of coconut palm exist: tall and dwarf (Ohler, 1984).

Coconut seems to cause allergic reaction only very rarely, but allergic reaction to coconut has been noted in the literature (Bernstein *et al.*, 1982).

### 5.5.2  Sesame

Sesame seed is one of the oldest crops grown for food use, dating back as far as 2350 BC. Its main application nowadays is as a topping for bread, cakes, etc., but sesame seed paste tahini and Turkish halva are becoming increasingly popular. The family Pedialaceae includes 18 species, of which *Sesam indicum* is the most important (Kägi and Wüthrich, 1993).

Both the seeds and the oil have been associated with anaphylaxis, with references in the literature dating back to the 1950s (Rubenstein, 1950; Uvisky, 1956; Tornsey, 1964; Chiu and Haydik, 1991; Kägi and Wüthrich, 1993). Malish *et al.* (1981) describe nine allergens present in sesame seeds with molecular weights ranging from 8000 to 84 000. Kägi and Wüthrich (1993) have suggested that the allergens in sesame may be inactivated by heat. This hypothesis has not been denied or supported in the literature and warrants further investigation.

### 5.5.3  Sunflower seed

The sunflower seed (*Helianthus annuus* L.) is a member of the largest plant family, the Compositae, which includes artichoke, chicory and lettuce (Noyes *et al.*, 1979).

Noyes *et al.* (1979) reported the case histories of three subjects who suffered severe anaphylactic reactions after ingesting sunflower seeds. Allergic contact dermatitis from sunflower seeds has also been reported (Noyes *et al.*, 1979). More recently, Axelsson *et al.* (1994) reported on anaphylactic reactions to sunflower seed that occurred in four patients. It was suggested that sensitisation resulted from the ingestion of airborne sunflower-seed allergens originating in the food of caged birds.

## 5.6    Allergenicity of 'nut' oils

The issue of whether nut oils are allergenic is of great importance. The avoidance of nuts *per se* is relatively straightforward, whereas the avoidance of nut oils as well, which are often labelled simply as 'vegetable oil', is much more difficult.

Until the early 1990s, it had been accepted that refined peanut oils were not allergenic. This theory was based principally on one study carried out by Taylor *et al.* (1981) in the US. Ten patients with well documented reactions to ingestion of peanuts, and who had high levels of IgE antibodies to peanut, were examined. Peanut oil did not cause a wheal-and-flare reaction in skin puncture tests with any of the patients. Oral challenge with quantities of peanut oil exceeding that ever likely to be ingested in one meal caused no immediate or delayed reactions. The conclusion drawn from this study was that peanut oils were not allergenic and did not therefore need to be avoided by peanut-allergic individuals but this study used only one type of peanut oil and studied only ten patients. According to Metcalfe *et al.* (1991), in order to be 95% certain that 95% of those allergic to peanuts will not react to peanut oil, 58 peanut-allergic patients need to be studied and all have to be found to have no reaction to the oil.

There are some anecdotal reports of allergy to peanut oil in the literature. However, close examination of these cases has frequently found that there is another explanation for the allergic reaction. For example, a woman who was known to be peanut-allergic suffered a fatal allergic reaction to a piece of cake (Evans *et al.*, 1988). The cake was known to contain peanut oil but also had almond marzipan icing and hazelnuts on the top. The reaction was initially attributed to the peanut oil but it was later found that the almond paste used to make the icing contained groundnut paste and was the cause of the reaction.

Work by Moneret-Vautrin *et al.* in France (1991, 1994) questioned the relevance of the Taylor *et al.* (1981) study for Europe. Moneret-Vautrin *et al.* (1994) reported four case studies where dermatitis in children was thought to be caused by the peanut oil in commercial infant formula. All infants had positive skin-prick tests to peanuts and subsequent labial and oral challenges with commercial peanut oil caused skin reactions (and swelling of the lip area in one infant). It is reported that peanut-oil-containing formula was removed from the diet of one of the children, resulting in a reduction in the dermatitis. Reintroduction of the formula caused exacerbation of the dermatitis within 36 hours. In the first of these cases, the mothers did not consume peanuts and therefore breast milk sensitisation was unlikely; however, sensitisation *in utero* could not be ruled out (Moneret-Vautrin *et al.*, 1991; Morrow-Brown, 1991; Moneret-Vautrin *et al.*, 1994). As a result of these case studies, a number of infant formula manufacturers in France voluntarily withdrew peanut oil from their formulae.

It is not known how peanut oil elicits allergic reactions but it has been suggested that it may be owing to trace quantities of peanut protein remaining in the processed oil. Some studies have shown that there is no detectable protein in refined peanut oil (Tattrie and Yaguchi, 1973). However, others have suggested levels of protein of up to 500 µg/kg of oil (Klurfeld and Kritchevsky, 1987). Guéant *et al.* (1994) suggested that there is protein in peanut oil, but it is not detected by the usual analytical techniques. They have shown that it is possible to create micelles of oil and protein, and propose that these micelles could be responsible for concealing the protein from analysis (Guéant *et al.*, 1994).

In a recent study undertaken to clarify the position with regard to the allergenicity of peanut oil, however, Hourihane *et al.* (1997) challenged 60 people, with a proven allergy to peanut, to crude and fully refined and deodorised oils from two sources. Six subjects (10%) reacted to the crude oil but none of the subjects reacted to the refined peanut oils. It was concluded that the refined oil was safe for most people suffering from peanut allergy, provided the oil was used properly.

There has been very little work undertaken on the potential allergenicity of other 'nut' oils. The effect of sesame oil in subjects with sesame allergy has been investigated to some extent. It is reported that the oil does contain sesamolin, sesamin and sesamol, which can cause contact dermatitis (Hayakawa *et al.*, 1987). Chiu and Haydik (1991) describe a case of anaphylactic reaction to sesame-seed oil in a patient who was highly sensitive to sesame. Interestingly, in this patient, the oil seemed to provoke more severe reactions than those experienced after exposure to other sesame-seed products.

The safety of sunflower oil in sunflower-seed allergy patients is controversial. Halsey *et al.* (1986) tested the allergenicity of two patients to refined and cold-pressed sunflower oil. The researchers did not detect specific IgE to either of the oils and patients did not react to either oil on challenge. Kanny *et al.* (1994), however, report an allergy to mugwort pollen in a female patient who also suffered anaphylactic reactions as a result of eating sunflower margarine or oil. It is suggested that mugwort pollen allergy cross-reacts with sunflower oil. Frying oil could become a hazard if it becomes contaminated with peanut or nut protein. This can occur, for example, if the oil is used to fry peanut protein-containing products and is then reused (Bush *et al.*, 1989; Hoffman and Collins-Williams, 1994).

It should be remembered that cold-pressed peanut oils are not subjected to the same extremes of processing as fully refined and deodorised oils, and that peanut protein has been found in cold-pressed oils (Hoffman and Collins-Williams, 1994). As with soya, peanut-allergic patients have been advised to avoid cold-pressed oils such as those found in health-food shops.

## 5.7   Implications of nut allergy for the food industry

Peanut-based ingredients are increasingly used by the food industry because of their versatility and competitive price. Unfortunately for the peanut-allergic, these ingredients are not always required to be included on the ingredients listing (Géurin and Géurin, 1995). For example, Häberle *et al.* (1988) cite the case of an allergic reaction to chocolate. The chocolate contained peanut paste, a product often added to cocoa products in Germany to enrich the taste; under current German law, the peanut paste is not required to be declared on the label.

The very small quantities of peanut and nut protein required to cause an allergic reaction that may be fatal is obviously of great concern to the food industry. Traces of peanuts and other nuts have been detected in manufactured foods that should not contain nuts. This is likely to have been caused by cross-contamination in factories that do not use dedicated lines or by the use of nut-containing rework. There are some documented case studies illustrating this point, plus many more anecdotal reports. One case cited in the literature concerns a girl known to be peanut-allergic who suffered an allergic reaction after eating sunflower butter, a product similar to peanut butter but made from sunflower seeds (Yunginger et al., 1983). During the investigation of this reaction, it was found that the manufacturing factory produced peanut butter on the same line as the sunflower butter. Examination of eight samples of sunflower butter identified peanut traces in six of the samples; a radioimmunoassay quantified the contamination as 0.3 to 3.3% peanut butter. The factory thoroughly cleaned the plant each day and had good quality control measures, but this case illustrates the point that it may be necessary to use dedicated lines to prevent accidental contamination. A similar case history reports that 10% of almond butters surveyed contained traces of peanut protein. Again, this was due to peanut butter being manufactured on the same production line (Settipane, 1989).

The food industry is becoming more aware of the special attention required when manufacturing nut-containing and other foods in the same factory. A large number of food manufacturers have altered their production processes to reduce the risk of cross-contamination. This can include scheduling runs of products containing peanuts or other nuts last in the day, adding the nuts at end of the production process and using dedicated production lines for manufacturing nut-containing foods (Gorski, 1997). Others have instigated more detailed labelling, including declaring where nut traces may be accidentally found in a non-nut-containing food and declaring the presence of nuts even when there is not a legal requirement to do so.

Problems have also occurred where peanuts or other nuts have been used in a product in which they would not normally be expected. A well-documented death occurred in a Debenhams restaurant in 1993, caused by a peanut-allergic girl eating a lemon meringue pie that had been topped with ground peanuts (Anon, 1993a,b). Catering outlets have therefore had to make sure that they can identify which of their foods contain or may contain peanuts or nuts. Some restaurants now have a book listing the ingredients in all dishes.

It is now possible to detect peanut proteins in compound foods with the use of immunoassays (Yunginger et al., 1988; Keating et al., 1990; Hefle et al., 1994) and this may be one route that food manufacturers can take to check that their food products do not contain peanut protein. In 1996, ProLab Diagnostics and Cortecs Diagnostics launched enzyme immunoassay kits to detect peanut protein in manufactured foods. The kits have specific antibodies to conarachin A and a sensitivity to around 0.2 ppm.

Most cases of fatal, peanut-induced anaphylaxis have occurred in catering establishments, usually as a result of inadvertent consumption of peanuts (Yunginger et al., 1988; Bock and Atkins, 1989; Sampson et al., 1992). An example in the literature is of a peanut-allergic woman who ordered a beef-burger but was instead supplied with a vegetable burger. The woman suffered an allergic reaction to the peanuts in the burger (Donovan and Peters, 1990).

## 5.8 Conclusions

Allergies to nuts are still rare but numbers are increasing, particularly among children. All nuts and seeds can invoke allergic reactions in susceptible individuals but peanut allergy does appear to be a more common cause of allergic reactions than the other nuts. In addition, it is one of the most potent of the 'nut' allergens, with most of the deaths that have been associated with nuts having been related to exposure to peanuts.

Work is ongoing to characterise the different allergens in nuts but only a small number of the proteins known to be allergenic have been identified. Most work has been on peanuts.

Trace amounts of nut allergens can invoke an allergic response in a sensitive individual and this therefore has enormous consequences for the food and catering industries, particularly in controlling cross-contamination within factory and restaurant environments, and alerting customers to the presence or absence of nuts in prepared food products.

## References

Anon. (1993a) Allergy girl killed by peanuts in a pie. *Daily Telegraph*, 22 December, 5.

Anon. (1993b) Slice of lemon pie kills allergy girl. *Daily Star*, 22 December, 11.

Anon. (1996) Nut allergy kills woman at party. *Daily Telegraph*, 12 December, 9.

Arshad, S.H., Malamberg, E., Krapf, K. and Hide, D.W. (1991) Clinical and immunological characteristics of Brazil nut allergy. *Clinical and Experimental Allergy*, **21** 373-76.

Asperen, P.P., Kemp, A.S. and Mellis, C.M. (1983) Immediate food hypersensitivity reactions on the known first exposure to the food. *Archives of Disease in Childhood*, **58** 253-56.

Assem, E.S.K., Gelder, C.M., Spiro, S.G. and Baderman, H. (1990) Anaphylaxis induced by peanuts. *British Medical Journal*, **300** 1377-78.

Axelsson, I.G.K., Ihre, E. and Zetterstrom, O. (1994) Anaphylactic reactions to sunflower seed. *Allergy: European Journal of Allergy and Clinical Immunology*, **49** (7) 517-20.

Bargman T.J., Rupnow, J.H. and Taylor, S.L. (1992) IgE-binding proteins in almonds (*Prunus amygdalus*) identification by immunoblotting with sera from almond-allergic adults. *Journal of Food Science*, **57** (3) 717-20.

Barnett, D., Baldo, B.A. and Howden, M.E.H. (1983) Multiplicity of allergens in peanuts. *Journal of Allergy and Clinical Immunology*, **72** 61-68.

Bernhisel-Broadbent, J. and Sampson, H.A. (1989) Cross-allergenicity in the legume botanical family in children with food hypersensitivity. *Journal of Allergy and Clinical Immunology*, **83** (2) 435-40.

Bernstein M., Day, J.H. and Welsh, A. (1982) Double-blind food challenge in the diagnosis of food sensitivity in the adult. *Journal of Allergy and Clinical Immunology*, **70** 205-10.

Blackfan, K.D. (1920) *American Journal of Medical Science*, **160** 341-50.

Bock, S.A. (1992) The incidence of severe adverse reactions to food in Colorado. *Journal of Allergy and Clinical Immunology*, **90** (4) 683-85.

Bock, S.A. and Atkins, F.M. (1989) The natural history of peanut allergy. *Journal of Allergy and Clinical Immunology*, **83** (5) 900-904.

Boyd, G.K. (1989) Fatal nut anaphylaxis in a 16-year-old male: case report. *Allergy Proceedings*, **10** (4) 255-57.

Burks, W.A., Williams, L.W., Thresher, W., Connaughton, C., Cockrell, G. and Helm, R.M. (1992) Allergenicity of peanut and soybean extracts altered by chemical or thermal denaturation in patients with atopic dermatitis and positive food challenges. *Journal of Allergy and Clinical Immunology*, **90** (6) Part 1 889-97.

Burks, W.A., Cockrell, G., Connaughton, C. and Helm, R.M. (1994) Allergens, IgE, mediators, inflammatory mechanisms. Epitope specificity and immunoaffinity purification of the major peanut allergen, Ara h I. *Journal of Allergy and Clinical Immunology*, **93** (4) 743-50.

Bush, R.K. and Hefle, S.L. (1996) Food allergens. *Critical Reviews in Food Science and Nutrition*, **36S** S119-63.

Bush, R.K., Steve, M.D., Taylor, S.L. and Nordlee, J.A. (1989) Peanut sensitivity. *Allergy Proceedings*, **10** (4) 261-64.

Chiu, J.T. and Haydik, I.B. (1991) Sesame seed anaphylaxis. *Journal of Allergy and Clinical Immunology*, **88** (3) 414-15.

David, T.J. (1993) *Food and Food Additive Intolerance in Childhood*, Blackwell Scientific Publications, Oxford.

DeBolt, M.F.H., Johansen, K.L. and Yunginger, J.W. (1993) Secretion of peanut allergens in breast milk of nursing mothers. *Journal of Allergy and Clinical Immunology*, January 1993, 342.

De Martino, M., Novembre, E., Cozza, G., De Marco, A., Bonazza, P. and Vierucci, A. (1988) Sensitivity to tomato and peanut allergens in children monosensitized to grass pollen. *Allergy*, **43** 206-13.

De Montis, G., Genfrel, D., Chemillier-Truong, M. and Dupont, C. (1993) Sensitisation to peanut and vitamin D oily preparations. *Lancet*, **341** (8857) 1411.

Donovan, K.L. and Peters, J. (1990) Vegetable burger: all was nut as it appeared. *British Medical Journal*, **300** (6736) 1378.

Doyle, A.J. (1994) Anaphylactic reactions to peanuts. *British Dental Journal*, February 11, 87-88.

Dutau, G., Bremont, F., Moisan, V. and Abbal, M. (1991) L'arachide: allergène d'avenir chez l'enfant at l'adolescent. *Semaine des Hôpitaux de Paris*, **67** (26-27) 1262-65.

Emmett, S., Angus, F., Fry, J. and Lee, P. (1996) Prevalence of peanut allergy in Great Britain and its association with atopic conditions, including other food allergies, and with presence of peanut allergy in other household members (submitted).

Evans, S., Skea, D. and Solovich, J. (1988) Fatal reaction to peanut antigen in almond icing. *Canadian Medical Association Journal*, **139** 231-32.

Ewan, P.W. (1996) Clinical study of peanut and nut allergy in 62 consecutive patients: new features and associations. *British Medical Journal*, **312** 1074-78.

Falliers, C.J. (1989) Pine nut allergy in perspective. *Annals of Allergy*, **62** 186-89.

Fine, A.J. (1987) Hypersensitivity reaction to pine nuts (pinon nuts—Pignolia). *Annals of Allergy*, **59** 183-84.

Fries, J.H. (1982) Peanuts: allergic and other untoward reactions. *Annals of Allergy*, **48** 220-26.

Gerrard, J.W. and Perelmutter, L. (1985) IgE mediated, RAST-positive allergy to peanut, cow's milk and egg: relationship to feeding and maternal diet. *Journal of Allergy and Clinical Immunology*, **75** 178.

Gerrard, J.W. and Perelmutter, L. (1986) IgE-mediated allergy to peanut, cow's milk, and egg in children with special reference to maternal diet. *Annals of Allergy*, **56** 351-54.

Géurin, B. and Géurin, L. (1995) Peanuts: one of the chief sources of food allergens. *Revue Française d'Allergologie et d'Immunologie Clinique*, **35** (1) 39-43.

Goetz, D.W., Lee, C.E., Whisman, B.A. and Goetz, A.D. (1991) Allergenic cross-reactivity among seven tree nuts and peanuts. *Journal of Allergy and Clinical Immunology*, January 1991, 328.

Goldbert, T.M., Patterson, R. and Pruzansky, J.J. (1969) Systemic allergic reactions to ingested antigens. *Journal of Allergy*, **32** 96-107.

Gorski, D. (1997) Reducing allergen risks. *Dairy Foods*, February 1997, 31-34.

Guéant, J.L., Moutété, F., Olszewski, A. and Gastin, I. (1994) Are peanut oils allergenic?, in *Peanut Allergy Seminar, Proceedings of a Conference held at Leatherhead Food Research Association*, 11 March, Leatherhead Food Research Association, Leatherhead, pp. 15-27.

Häberle, M., Baur, X. and Weiss, W. (1988) Erdnußpaste—ein okkultes Allergen in Schokolade. *Allergologie Jahrgang*, **11** (1) 22-26.

Halsey, A.B., Martin, M.E., Ruff, M.E., Jacobs, F.O. and Jacobs, R.L. (1986) Sunflower oil is not allergenic to sunflower seed-sensitive patients. *Allergy*, **49** 561-64.

Hatahet, R., Kirch, F., Kanny, G. and Moneret-Vautrin, D.A. (1994) Sensitisation to peanut allergens in infants aged under four months. Based on 125 cases. *Revue Française d'Allergologie et d'Immunologie Clinique*, **34** (5) 377-81.

Hayakawa, R., Matsunaga, K. and Suzuki, M. (1987) Is sesamol present in sesame oil? *Contact Dermatitis*, **17** 133-35.

Hefle, S.L., Bush, R.K., Yunginger, J.W. and Chu, F.S. (1994) A sandwich enzyme-linked imunosorbent assay (ELISA) for the quantitation of selected peanut proteins in foods. *Journal of Food Protection*, **57** (5) 419-23.

Hide, D. (1993a) Food induced anaphylaxis—death can and must be avoided. *British Journal of Clinical Practice*. **47** (1) 6-7.

Hide, D. (1993b) Clinical curio: allergy to Brazil nut. *British Medical Journal*, **287** 900.

Hoffman, D.R. and Collins-Williams, C. (1994) Cold-pressed peanut oils may contain peanut allergen. *Journal of Allergy and Clinical Immunology*, **93** (4) 801-802.

Hopkins, J. (1995) The very intolerant peanut. *Food Chemical Toxicology*, **33** (1) 81-86.

Hourihane, J., Dean, T.P. and Warner, J.O. (1995) Peanut allergy: an overview. *Chemistry and Industry*, 17 April, 299-302.

Hourihane, J., Dean, T.P. and Warner, J.O. (1996) Peanut allergy in relation to heredity, maternal diet, and other atopic disease: results of a questionnaire survey, skin prick testing and food challenges. *British Medical Journal*, **313** 518-21.

Hourihane, J., Bedwani, S., Dean, T.P and Warner, J.O. (1997) Randomised, double-blind, crossover challenge study of allergenicity of peanut oils in subjects allergic to peanuts. *British Medical Journal*, **314** 1084-88.

Hovanec-Burnes, D., Ordonez, M., Enjamuri, S. and Unver, E. (1995) Identification of another latex-crossreactive food allergen: peanut. *Journal of Allergy and Clinical Immunology*, **95** (1 Part 2) 150.

James, L.P. and Austen, K.F. (1964) Fatal systemic anaphylaxis in man. *The New England Journal of Medicine*, **270** (12) 597-603.

Kägi, M.K. and Wüthrich, B. (1993) Falafel burger anaphylaxis due to sesame seed allergy. *Annals of Allergy*, **71** 127-29.

Kanny, G., Fremont, S., Bicolas, J.P. and Moneret-Vautrin, D.A. (1994) Food allergy to sunflower oil in a patient sentized to mugwort pollen. *Allergy: European Journal of Clinical Nutrition*, **49** (7) 561-64.

Keating, M.U., Jones, R.T., Worley, N.J., Shively, C.A. and Yunginger, J.W. (1990) Immunoassay of peanut allergens in food processing materials and finished foods. *Journal of Allergy and Clinical Immunology*, **86** 41-44.

Kemp, A., Mellis, C., Sharotta, E., Simpson, J. and Barrett, D. (1982) Skin test and clinical reactions to peanut allergens in children. *Australian Paediatric Journal*, **18** (2) 145.

Klurfeld, D.M. and Kritchevsky, D. (1987) Isolation and quantitation of lectins from vegetable oils. *Lipids*, **22** (9) 667-68.

Koepke, J.W., Brock Williams, P., Osa, S.R., Dolen W.K. and Selner, J.C. (1990) Anaphylaxis to pinon nuts. *Annals of Allergy*, **65** 473-76.

Lessof, M.H. (1992) *Food Intolerance*, Chapman & Hall, London.

Loza, C. and Brostoff, J. (1995) Peanut allergy. *Clinical and Experimental Allergy*, **25** 493-502.

Malanin, K., Lundberg, M. and Johnasson, S.G.O. (1995) Anaphylactic reaction caused by neoallergens in heated pecan nut. *Allergy*, **50** 988-91.

Malish, D., Glosky, M.M. and Hofman, D.R. (1981) Anaphylaxis after sesame seed ingestion. *Journal of Allergy and Clinical Immunology*, **67** 35-38.

Marks, J.G., DeMelfi, T., McCarthy, M.A., Witte, E.J., Castagnoli, N., Epstein, W.L. and Aber, R.C. (1984) Dermatitis from cashew nuts. *Journal of the American Academy of Dermatology*, **10** (4) 627-31.

Matsuda, T. and Nakamura, R. (1993) Molecular structure and immunological properties of food allergens. *Trends in Food Science and Technology*, **4** 289-93.

May, C.D. and Bock, S.A. (1978) A modern clinical approach to food hypersensitivity. *Allergy*, **33** 166.

Menninger, E.A. (1977) *Edible Nuts of the World*, Horticultural Books Inc., Stuart, FL.

Metcalfe, D.D., Sampson, H.A. and Simon, R.A. (1991) *Food Allergy: Adverse Reactions to Foods and Food Additives*, Blackwell Scientific Publications, Oxford.

Moneret-Vautrin, D.A., Hatahet, R., Kanny, G. and Ait-Djafer, Z. (1991) Allergenic peanut oil in milk formulas. *Lancet*, **338** (8775) 1149.

Moneret-Vautrin, D.A., Kirch, F. and Fremont, S. (1993) Choc anaphylactique mortel à l'arachide. *Archives Française de Pédiatrie*, **50** 721-26.

Moneret-Vautrin, D.A., Hatahet, R. and Kanny, G. (1994) Risks of milk formulas containing peanut oil contaminated with peanut allergens in infants with atopic dermatitis. *Paediatric Allergy and Immunology*, **5** 184-88.

Morrow-Brown, H. (1991) Allergenic peanut oil in milk formulas. *Lancet*, **338,** 14 December, 1523.

Nestle, M. (1996) Allergies to transgenic foods—questions of policy. *New England Journal of Medicine*, **334** (11) 726-27.

Nielsen, N.H. (1990) Systemic allergic reaction to pine nuts. *Annals of Allergy*, **64** 132-33.

Nordlee, J.A., Taylor, S.L., Townsend, J.A., Thomas, L.A. and Bush, R.K. (1996) Identification of a Brazil nut allergen in trasngenic soybeans. *New England Journal of Medicine*, **334** (11) 688-92.

Noyes, J.H., Boyd, G.K. and Settipane, G.A. (1979) Anaphylaxis to sunflower seed. *Journal of Allergy and Clinical Immunology*, **63** (4), 242-44.

Ohler, J.G. (1984) *Coconut, Tree of Life*, FAO, Rome.

Ownby, D.R. (1995) The whole body. *Allergy*, **50** (suppl. 20) 27-30.

Parra, F.M., Cuevas, M., Lezaun, A., Alonso, M.D., Beristain, A.M. and Losada, E. (1993) Pistachio nut hypersensitivity: identification of pistachio nut allergens. *Clinical and Experimental Allergy*, **23** 996.

Perkin, J.E. (1990) Major food allergens and principles of dietary management, in *Food Allergies and Adverse Reactions*, Aspen Publishers Inc., Gaithersburg, pp. 51-63.

Royal College of Physicians and British Nutrition Foundation (1984) Food intolerance and food adversion. *Journal of the Royal College of Physicians*, **18** (2) 1-5.

Rubenstein, L. (1950) Sensitivity to sesame seed and sesame oil. *New York State Journal of Medicine* **50** 343-44.

Sachs, M.I., Jones, R.T. and Yunginger, J.W. (1981) Isolation and partial purification of a major peanut allergen. *Journal of Allergy and Clinical Immunology*, **67** 27-34.

Sampson, H.A. (1990) Peanut anaphylaxis. *Journal of Allergy and Clinical Immunology*, **86** (1) 1-3.

Sampson, H.A., Medelson, L. and Rosen, J.P. (1992) Fatal and near-fatal anaphylactic reactions to food in children and adolescents. *New England Journal of Medicine*, **327** (6) 380-84.

Settipane, G.A. (1989) Anaphylatic deaths in asthmatic patients. *Allergy Proceedings*, **10** (4) 271-74.

Tariq, S.M., Stevens, M., Matthews, S., Ridout, S., Twiselton, R. and Hide, D.W. (1996) Cohort study of peanut and nut sensitisation by age of 4 years. *British Medical Journal*, **313** 514-17.

Tattrie, N.H. and Yaguchi, M. (1973) Protein content of various processed edible oils. *Canadian Institute of Food Science and Technology Journal*, **6** (4) 289-90.

Taylor, S.L. (1985) Food allergies. *Food Technology*, **39** (2) 98-105.

Taylor, S.L., Busse, W.W., Sachs, M.I., Parker, J.L. and Yunginger, J.W. (1981) Peanut oil is not allergenic to peanut-sensitive individuals. *Journal of Allergy and Clinical Immunology*, **68** 372-75.

Torsney, P.J. (1964) Hypersensitivity to sesame seed. *Journal of Allergy*, **35** 514-19.

Uvisky, I.H. (1956) Sensitivity to sesame seed. *Journal of Allergy*, **22** 377-78.

Wal, J.-M. (1993) Food allergy: proteins as true food allergens or carriers for potentially allergenic xenobiotics, in *Food Ingredients Europe*, Maarsen Expoconsult Publishers, Maarsen, pp.182-90.

Whitley, B.D., Holmes, A.R., Shepherd, M.G. and Ferguson, M.M. (1991) Peanut sensitivity as a cause of burning mouth. *Oral Surgery, Oral Medicine and Oral Pathology*, **72** 671-74.

Wickens, G.E. (1995) *Edible Nuts*, FAO, Rome.

Woodroof, J.G. (1979) *Tree Nuts*, 2nd edn, AVI Publishing Company, Connecticut.

Young, E., Stoneham, M.D., Petruckevitch, A., Barton, J. and Rona, R. (1994) A population study of food intolerance. *Lancet*, **343,** May 7, 1127-30.

Yunginger, J.W. (1992) Anaphylaxis. *Current Problems in Paediatrics*, March 1992, 130-46.

Yunginger, J.W. and Jones, R.T. (1987) *A review of peanut chemistry. Arbeiten aus dem Paul-Ehrlich-Institut, dem Georg-Speyer-Haus und dem Ferdinand-Blum-Institut*, Band 80, Gustav Fisher Verlag, Stuttgart, New York.

Yunginger, J.W., Gauerke, M.B., Jones, R.T., Dahlberg, M.J.E. and Ackerman, S.J. (1983) Use of radioimmunoassay to determine the nature, quantity and source of allergenic contamination of sunflower butter. *Journal of Food Protection*, **46** (7) 625-28.

Yunginger, J.W., Sweeney, K.G., Sturner, W.Q., Giannandrea, L.A., Teigland, J.D., Bray, M., Benson, P.A., York, J.A., Biedrycki, L., Aquillace, D.L. and Helm, R.M. (1988) Fatal food-induced anaphylaxis. *Journal of the American Medical Association*, **260** (10) 1450-52.

Yunginger, J.W., Squillace, D.L., Jones, R.T. and Helm, R.M. (1989) Fatal anaphylactic reactions induced by peanuts. *Allergy Proceedings*, **10** (4) 249-53.

Zimmerman, B., Forsyth, S. and Gold, M. (1989) Highly atopic children: formation of IgE antibody to food protein, especially peanut. *Journal of Allergy and Clinical Immunology*, **83** (4) 764-70.

# 6 Bacterial toxins found in foods

Ian Millar, David Gray and Helen Kay

## 6.1 Introduction

The World Health Organisation (WHO) has defined foodborne disease as 'a disease of an infectious or toxic nature caused by, or thought to be caused by, the consumption of food or water.' The incidence of foodborne disease continues to rise and represents a significant economic cost to developed countries (for example, an estimated $7 billion per annum in the USA), while in developing countries it is a significant cause of mortality among children under five (Adams and Moss, 1995).

The vast majority of reported bacterial foodborne illnesses are the result of infection and subsequent multiplication of bacteria in the gut of a susceptible host following consumption of food contaminated with these organisms. Disease is caused by a number of mechanisms, such as toxin production in the case of *Escherichia coli* O157:H7 (Schmidt, 1995). However, food poisoning can also result from the ingestion of food containing pre-formed toxin, which is produced during the growth and multiplication of bacteria in the food. The ingested toxin is then absorbed into the host via the intestine. The resulting illness is thus caused by an intoxication rather than an infection. The organisms that are most commonly responsible for such outbreaks are *Clostridium botulinum*, *Staphylococcus aureus* and *Bacillus cereus* (Granum *et al.*, 1995). This chapter will be concerned with these organisms and the toxins that they produce.

## 6.2 *Clostridium botulinum*

### 6.2.1 Properties of C. botulinum

*C. botulinum* is a Gram-positive spore-forming rod that is obligately anaerobic. Some of its basic microbiological properties are summarised in Table 6.1. The figures for temperature, pH, etc. show the range over which these bacteria can survive and grow, but these should not be interpreted as absolute values as they can vary according to the particular bacterial strain and with the growth medium used.

Despite their grouping as a single species, strains of *C. botulinum* have widely varying physiological and biochemical characteristics (Adams and Moss, 1995). The single common factor is the production of potent neurotoxins that are the cause of botulism (Hauschild, 1989). Seven serologically distinct toxins are produced, namely types A, B, C, D, E, F and G, with the associated strains being classified on the basis of the type of toxin produced. Generally, only one type of toxin is produced by a particular strain of *C. botulinum*, although in rare instances more than one toxin type can be elaborated with the second toxin type being produced in lesser amounts (Hauschild, 1989). The species is further subdivided into four groups (Table 6.2), mainly according to the degree of proteolytic activity. The main strains of concern in foods are group I proteolytic strains types A, B and F, and group II non-proteolytic strains types B, E and F.

In culture media botulinum toxin is produced during the exponential phase of bacterial growth and is released from the cell into the growth medium; as the cells cease to grow and divide, toxin is also released partly as a result of cell lysis (Siegel and Metzger, 1979).

### 6.2.2  Types and structures of botulinum toxins
Botulinum toxins occur in foods in the form of complexes (Hauschild, 1989) consisting of a botulinum toxin subunit and one or more non-toxic subunits (Hatheway, 1990). The size of the complexes formed depends on the strain of *C. botulinum*, the type of food and the growth conditions.

Purified botulinum toxins are single-chain polypeptides (Simpson, 1986), with a molecular weight of 150 000 Da (Daltons). Proteolytic cleavage, either endogenous or exogenous, is necessary to generate active toxin. The nicked toxin consists of a heavy (100 000 Da) and a light (50 000 Da) chain connected by a disulphide bridge (Hauschild, 1989). Both chains are required for toxin activity (Montecucco and Schiavo, 1995). Further information on toxin structure can be found in reviews by Hatheway (1990), DasGupta (1989) and Montecucco and Schiavo (1995).

### 6.2.3  Toxicity, mode of action and effects of botulinum toxins
Botulinum toxin is one of the most poisonous substances known, with an estimated minimum lethal dose (MLD) in mice of 0.3 ng/kg (Middlebrook, 1989). The lethal dose for type A botulinum toxin in humans is estimated to be 0.1 to 1.0 μg (Schantz and Sugiyama, 1974). Lund (1990) calculated that the lethal dose in humans is 0.005 to 0.1 μg toxin for proteolytic strains, and 0.1 to 0.5 μg toxin for non-proteolytic strains. Studies involving the oral administration of toxin to mice have shown that the lethal dose decreases as the size of the toxin complex increases (Sakaguchi *et al.*, 1981; Sakaguchi *et al.*, 1984). This is probably owing to the greater stability of large complexes at low pH, making them more resistant to the action of digestive enzymes (Sakaguchi *et al.*, 1984).

The toxicity of these toxins is due to their specificities and their mode of action (Montecucco and Schiavo, 1995). Botulinum toxins bind very specifically to receptors at the neuromuscular junction and act enzymically

**Table 6.1** Properties of *C. botulinum*

| Gram stain | Morphology | Spore formation | Metabolism | Growth temperature range (°C) (optimum) | pH range for growth | Inhibitory pH | Inhibitory NaCl concentration (%) | Minimum $a_w$ for growth | Number of toxin types |
|---|---|---|---|---|---|---|---|---|---|
| +ve | Straight or slightly curved rods, 2 to 10μm long, motile by pertrichous flagella | Yes | Obligate anaerobe | Gp I: 10–48 (35–40)<br>Gp II: 3.3–45 (18–25)<br>Gp III: 15 (40)<br>Gp IV: (37) | Gp I: 4.6–9.0<br>Gp II: 5.0–9.0 | Gp I: 4.6<br>Gp II: 5.0 | Gp I: 10<br>Gp II: 5 | Gp I: 0.94<br>Gp II: 0.97 | 7 |

Data taken from: Adams and Moss (1995); Hatheway (1995); Hauschild (1989) and Kim and Foegeding (1992).
$a_w$: water activity

**Table 6.2** Characteristics of *C. botulinum* Groups I–IV

| Characteristic | *C. botulinum* group | | | |
|---|---|---|---|---|
| | I | II | III | IV |
| Toxin type | A, B, F | B, E, F | C, D | G |
| Proteolytic | + | - | +/- | + |
| Associated with human outbreaks | + | + | - | - |
| Optimum growth temperature (°C) | 35–40 | 18–25 | 40 | 37 |
| Minimum growth temperature (°C) | 10 | 3.3 | 15 | ND |
| Heat resistance of spores (°C) | 112 | 80 | 104 | 104 |

Compiled from Hauschild (1989) and Hatheway (1995).
ND: not determined.

as zinc endopeptidases cleaving specific proteins involved in the release of the neurotransmitter acetylcholine. By blocking the release of acetylcholine, neurotransmission between nerve fibres is prevented (Montecucco and Schiavo, 1994). For reviews of the mode of action of botulinum toxin see Montecucco and Schiavo (1993, 1994, 1995).

Initial symptoms can take from two hours to eight days to appear, but are usually apparent between 12 and 48 h after the consumption of food contaminated with toxin. Symptoms include a flaccid paralysis, nausea, vomiting, constipation, urine retention, double vision, difficulty in swallowing, dry mouth and difficulty in speaking. Without treatment, death results from respiratory or heart failure (Adams and Moss, 1995). The mortality rate is high (20 to 50%) but depends on various factors including the toxin type, the amount ingested, the type of food and the speed of application of appropriate medical treatment (Adams and Moss, 1995).

### 6.2.4 Incidence and occurrence of foodborne botulism

Spores of *C. botulinum* are widely found in the environment including soils, aquatic and marine sediments, and they can also be found in the alimentary tracts of birds, mammals and fish (Hauschild, 1989; Adams and Moss, 1995). Owing to their ubiquitous nature there is, therefore, the potential for *C. botulinum* spores to contaminate many different types of foods. If conditions are favourable for spore germination and the growth of vegetative cells, toxin will be produced. Foods and food products associated with food poisoning outbreaks due to botulinum toxin, and food packaging techniques that pose a risk of botulism, are reviewed in sections 6.2.5 and 6.2.6, respectively.

Surveys have also shown geographical variations in the types of spores found, and a possible link with the 'local' form of botulism. *C. botulinum* type A spores, for example, predominate in soil samples from the western USA, Brazil and Argentina, while type B strains predominate in the eastern USA (Dodds and Hauschild, 1989). The pattern in the USA correlates with the incidence of foodborne botulism there. Between 1978 and 1984, west of the Rocky Mountains, 47 outbreaks were due to type A and four to type B; east of the Rocky Mountains, 12 outbreaks were due to type A and 13 to type B (Smith and Sugiyama, 1988). Spores of non-proteolytic type B strains predominate in the UK and Europe (McClure *et al.*, 1994b). In almost all countries where surveys have been made, *C. botulinum* type E predominates in aquatic environments and adjacent soils (Dodds and Hauschild, 1989).

Data illustrating the incidence of foodborne botulism is presented in Table 6.3. Botulism has a high incidence in the USA, with a total of 597 cases of foodborne botulism between 1971 and 1989 (Hauschild, 1992). The former Soviet Union also had a high incidence, mainly linked to preserved fish, meats and vegetables (Smith and Sugiyama, 1988). In Japan, foodborne botulism is mainly associated with preserved fish and other seafoods (Smith and Sugiyama, 1988). Botulism is a major health problem in Iran, with most outbreaks there also being associated with fish and fish products (Hauschild, 1992). Accurate data about the incidence of botulism in Europe is limited but, between 1979 and 1988, 148 outbreaks (comprising more than 225 cases and four deaths) were recorded at the Institut Pasteur, France, and it is estimated that these represent about half the total number of outbreaks (Lund, 1990). The largest number of outbreaks and cases *per capita* world-wide has been reported from Poland, most of the implicated foods being canned (Hauschild, 1992). Germany also has a high incidence of foodborne botulism in comparison to other European countries (Smith and Sugiyama, 1988). The UK has a much lower incidence than the USA or the rest of Europe, with only three outbreaks between 1955 and 1989 (Hauschild, 1992). The largest recorded outbreak in the UK was in 1989, when 27 people were affected (with one death) due to the consumption of contaminated hazelnut yoghurt (O'Mahony *et al.*, 1990). Tropical countries have a very low incidence of foodborne botulism, probably due to the limited use of food preservation (Smith and Sugiyama, 1988).

**Table 6.3** Botulism outbreaks

| Period | Country | No. of outbreaks | No. of cases | Deaths |
|--------|---------|------------------|--------------|--------|
| 1984–87 | Poland | 1301 | 1791 | 46 |
| 1958–83 | China | 986 | 4377 | 548 |
| 1971–89 | USA | 272 | 597 | 63 |
| 1978–89 | France | 175 | 304 | 7 |
| 1983–89 | Germany | 99 | 206 | 4 |
| 1951–87 | Japan | 97 | 479 | 110 |
| 1958–64 | former Soviet Union | 95 | 328 | 95 |
| 1971–89 | Canada | 79 | 202 | 28 |
| 1971–89 | Alaska | 51 | 122 | 8 |
| 1955–89 | UK | 3 | 33 | 3 |

Adapted from Hauschild (1992).

According to Hauschild (1992), type E toxin is the most common cause of botulism in colder regions such as Alaska, Canada, Greenland, Scandinavia, parts of the former Soviet Union, Iran and northern Japan. Types A and B are most frequently implicated in more temperate regions. Type A accounts for the majority of the outbreaks in the western USA, Argentina, Brazil and China whereas type B predominates in European outbreaks (Poland, the former Czechoslovakia, Germany, France, Belgium, Spain, Portugal and Italy).

*6.2.5  Foods and food products associated with botulism outbreaks*
Botulism has been associated with a number of foods (Table 6.4) including
meats (Roblot *et al.*, 1994), fish (Huss, 1981), dairy products (O'Mahony *et
al.*, 1990; Aureli *et al.*, 1996) and vegetables (McClure *et al.*, 1994b; Brent
*et al.*, 1995).

**Table 6.4**  Incidence of botulism outbreaks related to food type

| Food type | Country | % of total outbreaks | Period |
|---|---|---|---|
| Vegetables[a] | USA | 59 | 1971–89 |
| | Spain | 60 | 1969–88 |
| | Italy | 77 | 1979–87 |
| | China | 86 | 1958–83 |
| Fish products | Alaska | 52 | 1971–89 |
| | former Soviet Union | 67 | 1958–64 |
| | Japan | 99 | 1951–87 |
| | Norway | 84 | 1961–90 |
| | Iran | 97 | 1972–74 |
| Meat products[b] | Germany (West) | 78 | 1983–88 |
| | Poland | 83 | 1984–87 |
| | France | 89 | 1978–89 |
| | Denmark | 100 | 1984–89 |
| | former Czechoslovakia | 72 | 1979–84 |
| | Hungary | 89 | 1985–89 |
| | former Yugoslavia | 100 | 1984–89 |
| | Canada | 72 | 1971–89 |

[a] Especially after home preservation by heat treatment or fermentation.
[b] For example, home-cured hams.
Adapted from Hauschild (1992).

*6.2.5.1  Fish.* Fish and fish products account for the majority of cases of
foodborne botulism in Alaska, Japan, Scandinavia, Iran and the former
Soviet Union. Most cases are caused by type E toxin although in Norway
and the former Soviet Union, approximately half are due to type B toxin and
type A toxin, respectively (Hauschild, 1992).

Unprocessed eviscerated fish and fish fillets pose few problems with
regard to *C. botulinum* as spoilage by other bacteria is rapid and occurs
before *C. botulinum* can grow and produce toxin. However, when fish is
subjected to preservation procedures to increase its shelf life, such as smoking, drying, salting, marinating or fermenting, the risk of botulism is
increased. The reason for this is that these processes selectively destroy or
inhibit the spoilage bacteria common to raw fishery products but frequently
have little or no inhibitory effect on *C. botulinum* spores (Eklund, 1992).

*C. botulinum* spores are more frequently found in fish products (1 to
29%) than other types of foods, with the number of spores varying from 1
to 170 per kilogram of food (Hauschild, 1989). In general, the types of fish

products associated with botulism are home-processed, uncooked or lightly cooked (for example, hot smoked), traditionally stored at ambient temperature and then eaten without further cooking. Also, many of the processed fish products are acidic and prepared from fatty fish species which are often ungutted (Huss, 1981).

Three major outbreaks of botulism (21 cases, nine deaths) associated with fish occurred in the USA between 1960 and 1963 owing to commercially prepared smoked fish from the Great Lakes (Osheroff *et al.*, 1964). Many of the outbreaks linked to smoked fish products have been caused by a failure to understand that these products may become hazardous if they are improperly processed or stored without refrigeration (Eklund, 1992). However, botulism in fishery products in the USA (Alaska) and Canada is mainly linked to the preparation and consumption of traditional 'ethnic' fish products, such as fermented salmon and salmon eggs, by native Inuits (Smith and Sugiyama, 1988). Consumption of the fermented fish products izushi and kirikomi accounts for virtually all cases of foodborne botulism in Japan (Hauschild, 1992). During 1992 in Egypt faseikh, an uneviscerated fish product that had been poorly fermented and salted, was responsible for a large outbreak of type E botulism (Weber *et al.*, 1993).

Pickled fish have also been involved in botulism outbreaks, for example pickled herring in Canada (Eklund, 1992). Salted fish, salted and dried fish (such as kapchunka), and salted fish eggs, can also cause botulism (Hauschild, 1992). Kapchunka (also known as ribbetz) caused an outbreak of botulism that affected eight people (one death) in the USA and Israel in 1987. It was concluded that poor packaging and lack of refrigeration allowed toxin production to occur (Slater *et al.*, 1989). Subsequently, at least two other outbreaks have been attributed to kapchunka in the USA (McClure *et al.*, 1994b).

6.2.5.2 *Meats.* The level of contamination of meats with *C. botulinum* is generally low—estimates range from less than 0.1 to 7 spores per kilogram (Lucke and Roberts, 1992). The incidence is lower in North America than in Europe (Dodds, 1992). In continental Europe the single major cause of botulism is home-cured smoked ham, particularly in France, Belgium, Germany and Poland (Hauschild, 1992; Roblot *et al.*, 1994).

Salted pork is apparently the predominant vehicle for meatborne botulism in Belgium, Norway and Spain (Lucke and Roberts, 1992). Pork products cause botulism more frequently than those from beef or lamb, while poultry and poultry products have not to date been associated with botulism (Lucke and Roberts, 1992).

Type B toxin is most commonly responsible for botulism caused by meats (Hauschild, 1992). Type E toxin has been associated with botulism caused by the consumption of raw or parboiled meats from marine mammals such as seals, whales and walruses by the native Inuit population in Canada and Alaska (Hauschild, 1989).

*6.2.5.3 Cheese and other dairy products.* The level of contamination of dairy products with *C. botulinum* is very low (Dodds, 1992) and their involvement in foodborne botulism is rare, accounting for less than 1% of the total number of outbreaks recorded since 1899 (Collins-Thompson and Wood, 1992).

Hazelnut yoghurt was responsible for the largest recorded outbreak of foodborne botulism (type B) in the UK during June 1989, affecting 27 people and resulting in one death. Hazelnut conserve used to flavour the yoghurt had been sweetened with aspartame rather than sugar. This increased the water activity of the product and thus created an environment in which *C. botulinum* could grow. Post-canning treatment of the conserve was insufficient to destroy the *C. botulinum* spores that were present within it (O'Mahony *et al.*, 1990).

The most recent outbreak of botulism (type A) in dairy products involved eight people (one death) in four cities in southern Italy during August and September 1996, and was traced to Mascarpone cheese. Spores from *C. botulinum* type A, which can grow at temperatures as low as 10°C, were found in the cheese. As there were no other control factors to prevent growth of *C. botulinum* (section 6.2.7), it is thought that raised storage temperature of the Mascarpone cheese at some point in the distribution chain allowed *C. botulinum* to grow and produce toxin (Aureli *et al.*, 1996; Simini, 1996).

Other dairy products that have caused outbreaks of botulism include cheese spread, cottage cheese, soft cheese and Brie (Collins-Thompson and Wood, 1992).

*6.2.5.4 Vegetables.* In the USA, Argentina, Spain, Italy and China vegetables were most frequently implicated in outbreaks of foodborne botulism. These were commonly home canned, except in China where they were fermented (Hauschild, 1992). Virtually all outbreaks involving fruit and vegetables have been caused by type A and type B toxins (Notermans, 1992).

The frequent presence of *C. botulinum* spores in raw products is a major factor contributing to the risk of botulism. Soil and organic fertilisers are the major sources of contamination of raw fruit and vegetables (Notermans, 1992). A wide variety of fruits and vegetables have been involved in botulism outbreaks including peanuts, peppers, tomatoes, mushrooms and garlic, and some examples are given below. Frequently, the product responsible was stored for long periods at ambient temperatures under almost anaerobic conditions and was treated inadequately with regard to the inactivation or elimination of spores (Notermans, 1992).

Commercially prepared chopped garlic in soybean oil, which was used to make garlic butter served on sandwiches in a restaurant, was responsible for an outbreak of botulism (type B) that affected 36 people in Canada (St Louis *et al.*, 1988). The chopped garlic in oil had been stored at room temperature for several months.

Inadequately heat-treated canned beetroot was responsible for an outbreak of type B botulism involving 10 people in the former Soviet Union (Podreshetnikova *et al.*, 1970). The US Food and Drug Administration has designated baked or boiled potatoes as potentially hazardous food products for botulinum toxin production and recommends that they are stored at 7°C or less, or above 60°C (Hauschild, 1989). Potato salad has caused at least four outbreaks of botulism in the USA (Seals *et al.*, 1981; Brent *et al.*, 1995). Stuffed aubergines were responsible for the largest recorded outbreak of foodborne botulism (type A, 230 cases, 40% mortality), which occurred in 1933 in Dniepropetrosk in the former Soviet Union (Smith and Sugiyama, 1988).

### 6.2.6 Food packaging techniques and the risk of botulism

One aim of food packaging is to prolong the shelf life of food. Problems can arise when the processing of food is insufficient to destroy contaminating *C. botulinum* spores and cells, where the process is flawed or when packaged foods are subsequently stored incorrectly (temperature abuse). Increasing the shelf life has the disadvantage of increasing the time available for *C. botulinum* to grow and produce toxin, if permissible conditions arise.

*6.2.6.1 Canning.* The safety of canned foods depends on effective sealing and heat treatment. The heat treatment must be sufficient to destroy spores as well as vegetative cells (section 6.2.7.1). After heating, the containers must be cooled and container integrity maintained to avoid recontamination of the can through punctures or leaks. A fatal outbreak of botulism (type E) in the UK in 1978, involving imported canned Alaskan salmon, was suspected to have been caused by contamination with *C. botulinum* spores after heat processing, possibly via a defect in the tin during cooling. A small hole in the tin probably allowed any gas produced to escape and therefore the appearance and smell of the tinned salmon appeared normal to the persons eating it (Ball *et al.*, 1979). Canning poses the greatest risk when carried out in the home environment. For example, home canned vegetables have been implicated in most botulism outbreaks in the USA, Argentina, Spain and China (Hauschild, 1992).

When food is canned aseptically the food and containers are sterilised separately, the food is then cooled to a suitable temperature for filling and the containers are filled and sealed under aseptic conditions. The finished product can then be stored at ambient temperature for prolonged periods

(Shapton and Shapton, 1991). Obviously, there is a greater risk of post-heat treatment contamination with *C. botulinum* spores and so greater care must be taken with technical and quality control. Low-acid, aseptically packaged foods pose a particular risk of botulism and appropriate sterilisation processes must be employed (Shapton and Shapton, 1991).

*6.2.6.2 Vacuum and modified atmosphere packaging.* Vacuum packaging (VP) involves placing the food in a gas impermeable plastic bag and removing air by applying a vacuum, then chilling or freezing the product. Modified atmosphere packaging (MAP) involves placing the food in a plastic tray, overlaying with a gas mixture, sealing and then chilling. VP and MAP have been proposed as means of extending the shelf life and of improving the quality of foods, in particular of perishable chilled foods, which are also known as REPFEDs (refrigerated, processed foods of extended durability). These foods are very varied and include ready meals, salads, soups, fresh pasta and hot-smoked fish products. The food is cooked or processed prior to packaging and receives little or no additional heat treatment prior to consumption (Lund and Notermans, 1992).

Challenge test studies have been carried out involving the inoculation of food with *C. botulinum* spores, followed by incubation at various temperatures and subsequent assessment of toxin production. Such studies have shown a higher rate of toxin production in vacuum-packaged fish compared to non-vacuum-packed fish (Pace and Krumbiegel, 1973). In addition, vacuum-packed hot-smoked trout was responsible for an outbreak of botulism in Germany (Bach *et al.*, 1971).

Of concern has been the finding that the type of atmosphere used in MAP can actually promote the germination of *C. botulinum* spores, resulting in growth and toxin production. For example, depending on the concentration, carbon dioxide may stimulate *C. botulinum* so concentrations of carbon dioxide in MAP must be carefully controlled (Kim and Foegeding, 1992).

*6.2.6.3 Sous vide.* Such foods represent one of the most common types of REPFEDs. The food is packaged in heat-stable, air-impermeable bags under vacuum, the bags are then sealed and the product is cooked (pasteurised), cooled and stored under refrigeration (Lund and Notermans, 1992). The heat treatments used will inactivate vegetative bacteria but any bacterial spores present will often survive these treatments, including those of *C. botulinum* (Simpson *et al.*, 1995). The prepared foods are stored at chill temperatures for up to 30 days (Simpson *et al.*, 1995) prior to reheating and consumption.

There is concern that prolonged refrigeration, combined with low salt levels, high pH and an oxygen-free environment, may allow growth and toxin production by *C. botulinum*, in particular by psychrophilic group II strains but also by group I strains, if temperature abuse occurs (i.e. exposure to temperatures above 10°C) (Simpson *et al.*, 1995). It has been shown that refrigerator and refrigerated food product temperatures can exceed 10°C (Tolstoy, 1991).

Although to the authors' knowledge there have been no documented cases of botulism involving *sous vide* foods, many challenge test studies have shown that it is possible for *C. botulinum* to grow and produce toxin in *sous vide* processed foods, including beef, chicken and salmon (Crandall *et al.*, 1994; Meng and Genigeorgis, 1994; Simpson *et al.*, 1995). Although opinions are divided over whether or not *sous vide* foods pose a risk of botulism (Church and Parsons, 1993), the general consensus is that there is a risk and that appropriate control measures in addition to chill temperatures should be taken (Crandall *et al.*, 1994; Meng and Genigeorgis, 1994).

### 6.2.7 Control measures

There is extensive literature on the control of botulinum toxin formation in foods. Strategies include the destruction of *C. botulinum* spores, inhibition of the germination of spores, inhibition of growth and toxin production by vegetative cells, and the destruction of preformed toxin in foods.

In most studies data on the effects of external factors, e.g. pH and water activity, on the growth of foodborne pathogens such as *C. botulinum* has been obtained by varying only one or two factors, with the others remaining near optimal (Adams and Moss, 1995). However, in foods these factors are usually present at an individually sub-optimal level but collectively are able to affect the ability of microorganisms to grow. This is known as the hurdle effect (Leistner, 1978). This multi-factorial approach for preserving foods has been applied empirically for many years, for example for smoked fish where a combination of factors (salt, smoke and drying) all contribute to the overall preservation and microbial safety of the food (Adams and Moss, 1995). Clearly, the hurdle effect has to be taken into account when assessing the risk of *C. botulinum* toxin production in a food. Conditions that permit *C. botulinum* to grow and produce toxin constitute a greater risk than conditions that permit the germination of *C. botulinum* spores (Sperber, 1982).

### 6.2.7.1 Destruction/inactivation of *C. botulinum spores*. The most effective and widely used method to inactivate spores is heat treatment. This treatment is designed to inactivate very large numbers of spores of *C. botulinum*. The amount of heat required to inactivate *C. botulinum* spores varies widely, depending mainly on the composition of the food. The pH of the foods is particularly important, and 'low-acid' foods with a pH higher than 4.5 require a 'botulinum cook' in the UK (Shapton and Shapton, 1991). The 'botulinum cook' is the minimum sterilisation process required to eliminate *C. botulinum* spores and is also known as the 12 D reduction process

(12 decimal reductions). This is defined as the heat required to inactivate a theoretical contamination by $10^{12}$ C. botulinum spores. For most foods this requires an $F_0$ of three (where one $F_0$ equals one minute at 121°C, assuming instantaneous heating and cooling), therefore an $F_0$ of three is three minutes at 121°C. Meats usually receive an $F_0$ of six.

The Campden guidelines give the heat treatment that is required to reduce the probability of C. botulinum spores surviving in no more than 1 in $10^{12}$ cans. This treatment takes into account the size and volume of the containers, thus giving an extra margin for safety as it requires more lethal heat than the standard 12 D concept.

Spores of proteolytic type A and B strains are more resistant to heat than non-proteolytic strains (Table 6.2). The survival of non-proteolytic strains is, however, of particular concern in REPFEDs because of their ability to grow at refrigeration temperatures (Hauschild, 1989). A recent study on the effect of various heat treatments on non-proteolytic C. botulinum type B, E and F spores demonstrated that they could withstand some heat treatments and subsequently produce toxin. For example, after heating at 85°C for 19 min, followed by storage at 12°C, toxin was detected after 28 days while visible growth was only detected after 42 days. It has been proposed that foods given such heat treatment should be stored below 12°C for no more than 28 days (Peck et al., 1995).

Peck and Fernandez (1995) have shown that the presence of lysozyme in foods can influence the survival of non-proteolytic spores of C. botulinum (types B, E and F) subjected to heat treatment (19.8 minutes at 90°C). Spores heated in the absence of lysozyme and subsequently stored at 8, 12, 16 or 25°C showed no vegetative cell growth or toxin formation but spores heated in the presence of lysozyme did germinate, grow and produce toxin, even when stored at 8°C. It seems likely that lysozyme acts as a substitute for a germination mechanism that has been inactivated by the heat treatment (Gould, 1984). The effect of lysozyme on the germination of heat-damaged spores should be taken into account when assessing the heat treatment necessary to ensure the safety of REPFEDs (Lund and Notermans, 1992).

Ionising radiation can also be used to inactivate spores of C. botulinum, types A and B being the most resistant. Foods tend to have a protective effect, while food additives can act as sensitizers (e.g. sodium chloride) or protectors (Kim and Foegeding, 1992). According to these authors irradiation has been approved by the health and safety authorities in 36 countries for the treatment of more than 49 different foods.

It is not always practical or desirable to inactivate C. botulinum spores as a means of control as the treatments involved are often harsh and may adversely affect the taste, appearance and nutritional value of the food, as well as increasing the processing cost.

*6.2.7.2 Prevention of* C. botulinum *spore germination.* C. botulinum spores can germinate over a wide temperature range (from below 4 to 70°C) with an optimum of 37°C (Kim and Foegeding, 1992). Thus temperature alone is of little use as a control measure. Generally, *C. botulinum* spores cannot germinate and grow in high-moisture acidic foods (pH of less than 4.5) but the spores do remain viable (Lund, 1990).

There has been considerable research into the use of chemical preservatives to inhibit the germination of *C. botulinum* spores. Nitrite can inhibit spore germination in defined media, but not at the levels allowed in foods, and low levels of nitrite can actually stimulate spore germination. Salt can only inhibit *C. botulinum* spore germination at levels that would be unacceptable in food products. Sorbates, EDTA (ethylene diamine tetra-acetic acid) and some spice oils have also been shown to be inhibitory to spore germination (Kim and Foegeding, 1992).

*6.2.7.3 Prevention of* C. botulinum *growth and toxin production.* The control of *C. botulinum* in most foods is achieved by the inhibition of growth and toxin production, and in most foods inhibition is the result of a combination of factors rather than a single factor (Hauschild, 1989).

The temperature limits for the growth of *C. botulinum* are given in Table 6.1. Generally, the major concern is with growth of group II non-proteolytic strains of *C. botulinum* in refrigerated foods. There is particular concern about foods packed under vacuum or modified atmosphere and *sous vide* foods (REPFEDs; Lund and Notermans, 1992) where temperature may be the major controlling factor preventing growth and toxin production. Non-proteolytic strains may have sufficient time to grow in refrigerated foods if the shelf life is extensive, whereas group I proteolytic strains will only grow in these foods if temperature abuse occurs (Kim and Foegeding, 1992). The mild heat treatments associated with VP and MAP foods may select for *C. botulinum* and allow toxin to form in products without any visual indication that this has occurred.

The acid tolerance of *C. botulinum* depends on the strain, food composition, type of acidulant, presence of preservatives and prior heat and/or other treatments. Water activity ($a_w$) and the presence of oxygen also affect acid tolerance (Kim and Foegeding, 1992). It is generally accepted that *C. botulinum* cannot grow and produce toxin in foods with a pH of 4.6 or lower, however this is not the case if large amounts of protein are present. Currently, only canned, pasteurised, acidic or acidified fruits and vegetables are protected by acidity alone because of their relatively low protein content (Kim and Foegeding, 1992). *C. botulinum* can be controlled in high-moisture foods by maintaining a pH of less than 4.5 (Lund, 1990).

Salt is widely used to inhibit the growth of *C. botulinum* in foods, the inhibitory effect being due to the suppression of water activity. The effectiveness of salt depends on its concentration in the aqueous phase, i.e. the brine concentration (Hauschild, 1989). The minimum water activities for growth of *C. botulinum* are given in Table 6.1, with $a_w$ of 0.94 and 0.97 corresponding to salt (brine) concentrations of approximately 10% and 5%, respectively (Hauschild, 1989). The type of solute used to control water activity also affects growth and toxin production. Generally, sodium chloride, potassium chloride, glucose and sucrose have similar effects, while glycerol permits growth at lower water activity values. The absolute water activity limits for growth and toxin production in foods depend on other factors including temperature, pH, redox potential and added food preservatives; the limiting water activity can be raised significantly by adding preservatives or increasing acidity (Kim and Foegeding, 1992).

Since *C. botulinum* is anaerobic, it is commonly assumed that it cannot grow in foods that are exposed to oxygen or in foods with a high redox potential $(E_h)$. In practice, the $E_h$ of most foods exposed to oxygen is generally low enough to permit growth (Sperber, 1982).

The use of preservatives to control growth and toxin production by *C. botulinum* has been comprehensively reviewed by Kim and Foegeding (1992), and except where stated otherwise the following information is from this source. Sodium and potassium salts of nitrite and nitrate have been used for many years to cure meats and fish. Nitrite is the functional constituent and although nitrate has no antibotulinal activity it can be converted to nitrite by other microorganisms present in the food. The effectiveness of nitrite inhibition depends on temperature, pH, sodium chloride concentration, storage time, the number of spores present and the composition of the food (Cook and Pierson, 1983). Nitrite delays the growth of *C. botulinum* and subsequent toxin production but does not prevent it. A major concern with the use of nitrite is the formation of nitrosamines, some of which are known to be carcinogenic and mutagenic.

Sorbic acid and its salts have been examined as possible replacements for nitrite in cured meats. At the appropriate pH, sorbic acid will delay growth and toxin production by inhibiting the growth of vegetative cells. The inhibitory effect of sorbate on the growth of *C. botulinum* increases with decreasing pH (7.0 to 4.9) (Lund *et al.*, 1987).

Nisin is a polypeptide antimicrobial compound produced by some strains of *Streptococcus lactis* which has been used in various foods, mainly cheese and other dairy products, to control *C. botulinum* by inhibiting its growth. It is less effective in meat products.

Polyphosphates are used in foods for the purpose of controlling microbial growth but they also appear to enhance the inhibition of antibotulinal agents such as nitrite and sorbate. Ascorbate (vitamin C) and isoascorbate (erythorbate) are used to accelerate the meat-curing process and have also been found to enhance the inhibitory activity of nitrite, as do EDTA, other chelating agents and cysteine. EDTA is approved for use in a variety of foods including processed meats, seafood and vegetables.

Smoke exerts a preservative effect through a combination of drying and the deposition of chemicals derived from the thermal decomposition of wood. Smoking, in combination with appropriate concentrations of sodium chloride, is effective in preventing growth and toxin production by *C. botulinum* types A and B. However, smoking alone should not be considered an effective substitute for sodium chloride or refrigeration.

Sulphur dioxide (in the form of sodium metabisulphite), mace, bay leaf and nutmeg extracts, garlic and onion oils, spice oils, *n*-monoalkyl maleates and fumarates, and lactate salts have all been shown to have antibotulinal activity.

The addition of lactic acid bacteria to foods can prevent *C. botulinum* growth and toxin production in meat products by acidification. It may, however, be necessary to add a fermentable carbohydrate to ensure that enough acid is produced. The inhibitory efficiency of this approach depends on the initial pH, the type and level of inoculum, the type and level of the carbohydrate, the buffering capacity of the product and the presence of inhibitory compounds (Conner *et al.*, 1989).

There is increasing consumer resistance to the use of preservatives in foods and a desire for 'fresher' more 'natural' foods, but there is increased risk, when traditional preservation techniques are modified or replaced, of situations arising where botulinum toxin can be formed in foods. This was the case with the hazelnut yoghurt outbreak (O'Mahony *et al.*, 1990).

The effect of irradiation on foodborne organisms including *C. botulinum* has been reviewed comprehensively by Monk *et al.* (1995). Vegetative cells are inactivated by low doses of radiation, but the main disadvantage is that such doses have little or no effect on the spores (Eklund, 1992).

*6.2.7.4 Destruction of preformed* C. botulinum *toxin in foods.* Developing processes to inactivate botulinum toxins in foods without destroying the nutritional value or palatability of the food has proved difficult. Botulinum toxin can be inactivated by heat but the stability of the toxin depends on the nature of the heating medium; for example proteins, colloids and high ionic strength have a protective effect (Lund, 1990). Heat treatment at 79°C for 20 min or 85°C for 5 min can be viewed as a guideline for the inactivation of toxin types A, B, E and F (Hauschild, 1989).

The stability of botulinum toxin to the effects of irradiation also depends on the chemical and physical nature of the food (Lund, 1990). Botulinum toxin was found to be more resistant to gamma radiation than *C. botulinum* spores (Siegel, 1992). Substances in foods exert a significant protective effect. For example, a dose of 8 kGy was sufficient to destroy type A toxin in buffer, while in minced beef slurries the same dose reduced the amount of toxin present by only 55%, as determined by immunoassay (Rose *et al.*, 1988). This study also showed, however, that the biological activity of type A was more sensitive to irradiation than its immunological activity. Botulinum toxins cannot be reliably inactivated by radiation doses that do not adversely affect the palatability and nutritional value of the food (Siegel, 1992). Irradiation should only be used in conjunction with good manufacturing practice and other control measures, and should not be relied upon as a sole means of control.

### 6.2.8 HACCP
The hazard analysis critical control point (HACCP) concept encompasses a systematic approach to hazard identification, assessment and control (ICMSF, 1988). It involves identifying critical control points (CCPs) in a process (e.g. the temperature of cans during heat processing) and establishing procedures to monitor and verify that these CCPs are under control by, for example, continuous temperature monitoring of cans. Corrective action is required when a CCP falls outside the designated limits. The HACCP system is now mandatory for the processing of seafoods in the USA (Garrett *et al.*, 1995) and is increasingly being adopted world-wide for the manufacture of other foodstuffs. It is undoubtedly of value in controlling spore survival, growth and toxin production by *C. botulinum* in foods (ICMSF, 1988; Shapton and Shapton, 1991).

### 6.2.9 Predictive modelling of C. botulinum growth and thermal inactivation
Mathematical modelling of microbial growth and toxin production has been proposed as an alternative to the traditional approach of challenge testing (Williams *et al.*, 1992). In the UK, a multi-centre research programme resulted in the creation of mathematical models based on experimental data that allow predictions of the growth, survival and thermal inactivation of foodborne pathogenic bacteria to be made (McClure *et al.*, 1994a). This has led to the production of 'Food MicroModel', a software package that can be used to predict both the growth and thermal inactivation of non-proteolytic *C. botulinum* strains by inputting data on temperature, pH, water activity, etc. Predictive models allow the risk of growth to be quickly assessed, especially if a new food product formulation is being considered, but they do not entirely eliminate the need for challenge testing.

### 6.2.10 Methods for detecting botulinum toxins in foods
At present the most sensitive, reliable and reproducible method for the detection, quantification and typing of botulinum toxins is the mouse bioassay (Andrews and Messer, 1990). The test involves injecting mice intraperitoneally with 0.5 ml of food extracts and observing for typical symptoms of

botulism over a 72 h period. Positive samples are typed by means of neutralisation tests using monovalent antisera for each toxin type (Andrews and Messer, 1990).

Since the test is ethically undesirable, time-consuming (taking up 4 days) and requires expensive and specialised facilities, great efforts have been made to replace it. These have included enzyme-linked immunosorbent assays (ELISAs; Dezfulian *et al.*, 1984; Shone *et al.*, 1985), ELISA–ELCA (enzyme-linked coagulation assay; Doellgast *et al.*, 1993), substrate-based ELISA (Hallis *et al.*, 1996), latex agglutination (Horiguchi *et al.*, 1984) and biosensors (Kumar *et al.*, 1994). While some of these methods have attained similar sensitivities to the mouse bioassay, greater numbers of false positives and negatives are frequently obtained, and none of these methods are able to detect all types of botulinum toxin.

## 6.3   Staphylococcus aureus

Some of the basic microbiological properties of *S. aureus* are summarised in Table 6.5. It is Gram positive, facultatively anaerobic and does not form spores. The cells are cocci and characteristically form clusters, appearing like bunches of grapes under microscopic examination (Baird-Parker, 1990).

**Table 6.5** Properties of *S. aureus*

| Gram stain | Morphology | Spore formation | Metabolism | Growth temperature range (°C) (optimum) | pH range for growth (optimum) | Minimum $a_w$ for growth (optimum) | Number of toxin types |
|---|---|---|---|---|---|---|---|
| +ve | Coccus with spherical to ovoid cells, ≈ 1 μm diameter | No | Facultative anaerobe | 7–48 (35–37) | 4.0–10.0 (6.0–7.0) | 0.83 (0.98) | >7 |

Data taken from Adams and Moss (1995), Bergdoll (1989), Concon (1988) and Baird-Parker (1990).

$a_w$: water activity.

The growth temperature range is 7 to 48°C and the bacterium can grow over a wide pH range, 4 to 10, with a pH of 6 to 7 being optimal (Baird-Parker, 1990). The effect of pH on *S. aureus* growth varies with the strain and is affected by the inoculum level, growth medium, sodium chloride concentration, temperature and redox potential.

An important characteristic of *S. aureus* is that it can tolerate high levels of salt—it can grow in media containing 5 to 7% sodium chloride, with some strains capable of growth in the presence of 20% sodium chloride.

*S. aureus* can also grow over a much wider water activity range than other foodborne pathogens; growth can occur down to an $a_w$ of 0.83 and the optimum is greater than 0.99. The minimum water activity supporting growth by *S. aureus* depends on a number of factors, including type of humectant, pH and redox potential (Bergdoll, 1989).

The growth of *S. aureus* can be significantly affected by the presence of other foodborne bacteria. *S. aureus* is not good at competing with other foodborne bacteria for essential nutrients and they can inhibit its growth by the production of acidic products that lower the pH, and by the production of hydrogen peroxide, volatiles and antibiotics (Genigeorgis, 1989). Factors affecting the inhibitory effect of various foodborne bacteria on *S. aureus* include the proportion of *S. aureus* to competitors, temperature, atmosphere, pH, water activity, redox potential and the ability of other foodborne bacteria to produce inhibitory factors (Genigeorgis, 1989).

### 6.3.1 Types and structures of S. aureus enterotoxins

At least seven serologically different types of *S. aureus* enterotoxins (SEs) are known (A, B, $C_1$, $C_2$, $C_3$, D, E), with others yet to be identified (Bergdoll, 1989). In accordance with the current nomenclature for these toxins, they will be referred to here as SEA to SEE, where SEA is the abbreviation for staphylococcal enterotoxin A.

Strains of *S. aureus* have been found that produce enterotoxin F (SEF; Bergdoll *et al.*, 1981) and enterotoxin H (SEH; Su and Wong, 1995), while Betley *et al.* (1992) isolated a strain of *S. aureus* possessing the gene for enterotoxin G (SEG). So far, SEF and SEG have not been linked with food poisoning; SEF has been implicated in toxic shock syndrome. There is some recent evidence that SEH may be involved in staphylococcal food poisoning. This toxin was implicated in a familial outbreak in Brazil caused by cheese (Pereira *et al.*, 1996), with both an SEH-producing *S. aureus* strain and low levels of SEH being detected in the cheese. Additionally, a study by Su and Wong (1996) using an ELISA method showed that 10 out of a total of 21 strains previously shown to produce enterotoxins of unknown type, produced SEH.

SEs are small single-chain polypeptides with molecular weights ranging between 26 000 and 34 100 Da (Freer and Arbuthnott, 1986). The amino acid compositions of SEA, SED and SEE are similar, as are those of SEB and SEC (Bergdoll, 1989).

SEs are resistant to the digestive enzymes of the human intestinal tract, except to pepsin when the pH is less than 2.0 (Genigeorgis, 1989). SEs are stable over a wide pH range, from 2.0 to 11.0 (Genigeorgis, 1989).

The conditions under which SEs are produced are shown in Table 6.6. The optimum temperature for SE production is higher than that for growth, ranging from 40 to 45°C. The pH range for toxin production is from 4 to 9.6, with an optimum of pH 7 to 8. As is the case with growth, the effect of pH on SE production varies with the strain and is affected by the inoculum level, growth medium, sodium chloride concentration, temperature and redox potential. The optimum $a_w$ is 0.98, with values ranging from 0.85 to greater than 0.99 for aerobic growth, and 0.90 to greater than 0.99 for anaerobic growth (Baird-Parker, 1990). The minimum $a_w$ supporting enterotoxin production by *S. aureus* depends on a number of factors, including type of humectant, pH and redox potential. It is important to note that *S. aureus* can grow in conditions of temperature, pH and water activity that will not support enterotoxin production (Baird-Parker, 1990).

**Table 6.6** Factors affecting *S. aureus* enterotoxin production

| Factor | Aerobic Range | Aerobic Optimum | Anaerobic Range or lower limit |
|---|---|---|---|
| Temperature (°C) | 10–48 | 40–45 | 10–45 |
| pH | 4.0–9.6 | 7.0–8.0 | 5.3 |
| $a_w$ | 0.85–>0.99 | 0.98 | 0.90 |
| NaCl (%) | 0–10 | 0 | ND |
| Oxygen (% DO) | 5–50 | 5–20 | NA |

Data taken from Baird-Parker (1990) and Tranter and Brehm (1990).
$a_w$: water activity.
% DO: dissolved oxygen.
ND: not determined.
NA: not applicable.

SEs (A to E) can be divided into two groups on the basis of their amino acid composition and the way in which they are produced. According to Baird-Parker (1990), the production of SEB and SEC is controlled by plasmids and occurs mainly at the end of the stationary phase of cell growth. The production of SEA, SED and SEE is under chromosomal control and occurs throughout the logarithmic phase. This difference is reflected by differences in the formation of toxins in foods. SEA and SED are produced under a much wider range of pH, water activity and redox potential than SEB or SEC (Bergdoll, 1989). SEA, SED and SEE are produced in relatively small amounts and their production is closely related to the growth of the organism whereas SEB and SEC can be produced in relatively large amounts and their production is more closely related to the incubation conditions (Bergdoll, 1989). It is because of its relatively large enterotoxin yield that most research on toxin production by *S. aureus* has been conducted using SEB-producing strains.

Other species of staphylococci (*S. intermedius* and *S. hyicus*) are also capable of producing enterotoxins (Adesiyun *et al.*, 1984; Hirooka *et al.*, 1988). Their role in staphylococcal food poisoning is as yet unclear.

*6.3.2  Effects, toxicity and mode of action of* S. aureus *enterotoxins*

Staphylococcal food poisoning is characterised by a rapid onset, symptoms appearing within one to six hours of ingesting enterotoxin-containing food. The main symptoms are vomiting and diarrhoea, while others include muscular cramps, abdominal pain, headache, sweating and dehydration. Acute symptoms usually last from one to eight hours but complete recovery can take up to two days. SEs can cause enteritis, fever, leukocytosis and in rare instances can be fatal (Bergdoll, 1989). However, illness is usually mild, normally only lasting for up to 24 h (Freer and Arbuthnott, 1986).

Studies using human volunteers have shown that ingestion of 0.4 µg enterotoxin (SEA, SEB and SEC) per kilogram body weight causes illness, with a minimum dosage of 0.05 µg/kg. These results suggest that less than 1 µg of toxin may cause illness in sensitive individuals (Bergdoll, 1989). In a large outbreak of *S. aureus* enterotoxin A food poisoning, linked to the consumption of chocolate milk, it was estimated that 200 mg or less of SEA can cause illness in sensitive individuals (Evenson *et al.*, 1988).

The precise mode of action of SEs is not known but the vomiting and diarrhoeal response is probably caused via stimulation of local neuroreceptors in the intestinal tract, with transmission of stimuli to the vomiting centre of the brain via the vagus and sympathetic nervous systems (Baird-Parker, 1990).

*6.3.3  Outbreaks of* S. aureus *food poisoning*

Staphylococci are widely distributed and can be found in air, water, milk, sewage, humans and animals, and also in anything that comes into contact with these things. The presence of low numbers of *S. aureus* in foods is therefore not uncommon. However, animals and humans are the main reservoir for these organisms, with 30–50% of humans carrying *S. aureus*, mainly in the nose but also in the throat and on the skin (Bergdoll, 1989). Staphylococcal food poisoning is mainly caused by coagulase-positive *S. aureus* but occasionally coagulase-negative *S. aureus* strains have been implicated in foodborne outbreaks (Gomez-Lucia *et al.*, 1988). The role of the coagulase enzyme, which coagulates human serum, is, however, unclear.

Data relating to the incidence of staphylococcal food poisoning are presented in Table 6.7. Food poisoning due to SEs is one of the four most common types of reported food poisoning world-wide (Genigeorgis, 1989) although as a relatively mild illness of short duration it is more likely than some other types of food poisoning to be under-reported. Most reported cases are linked to food poisoning outbreaks with far fewer sporadic cases being documented. Between 1983 and 1987, 7.8% of reported food poisoning outbreaks in the USA were due to staphylococci, while during the same period in England and Wales the figure was 1.9% (Adams and Moss, 1995). It is significant that of 359 incidents recorded in the UK between 1969 and

**Table  6.7** Foodborne outbreaks due to *S. aureus* and *B. cereus*

| Period | Country | % of food poisoning outbreaks due to *S. aureus* | % of cases of food poisoning due to *S. aureus* | % of food poisoning outbreaks due to *B. cereus* | % of cases of food poisoning due to *B. cereus* |
|---|---|---|---|---|---|
| 1973–82 | Canada | 26.9 | 16.8 | 7.3 | 2.2 |
| 1976–84 | England & Wales | 2.2 | 1.9 | 2.3 | 0.7 |
| 1975–84 | Finland | 39.5 | 15.6 | 11.9 | 17.8 |
| 1960–68 | Hungary | 56.0 | 34.0 | 8.0 | 15.0 |
| 1976–80 | Japan | 30.8 | 20.9 | 0.8 | 0.7 |
| 1977–82 | Netherlands | 17.7 | 10.3 | 22.4 | 11.5 |
| 1973–85 | Scotland | 1.0 | 1.4 | 0.9 | 0.8 |
| 1972–82 | USA | 26.6 | 26.6 | 2.9 | 1.3 |

Data taken from Kramer and Gilbert (1989).

1990, over half occurred in the months of June, July and August each year, with more incidents occurring in years with especially hot summers (Wieneke *et al.*, 1993). This emphasizes the importance of adequate refrigeration and good hygiene in preventing staphylococcal food poisoning.

SEA-producing strains were found in 69% of the reported outbreaks in the USA and UK. Strains producing SED alone or with SEC accounted for 10% while strains producing only SEB were rarely found (Freer and Arbuthnott, 1986). According to Baird-Parker (1990), the predominance of SEA and SED in the causation of staphylococcal food poisoning is a consequence of their production being possible over the wide range of conditions found in foods.

### 6.3.4  Foods and food products associated with S. aureus food poisoning
Most foods associated with staphylococcal food poisoning are cooked, have a high protein content, are contaminated during handling and allowed to remain at room temperature or refrigerated in large masses for several hours, often overnight (Genigeorgis, 1989).

#### 6.3.4.1  Fish and shellfish.
There is concern in the USA over the microbiological safety of cooked ready-to-eat shrimp and crabmeat with regard to contamination with *S. aureus* and subsequent enterotoxin production, especially as these foods are often imported from countries with questionable food hygiene and processing practices. A survey by Ellender *et al.* (1995) showed that cooked ready-to-eat crabmeat was frequently contaminated with *Staphylococcus* species, including *S. aureus*, and that contamination probably occurred during the processing and/or distribution phases. If contamination with vegetative cells has occurred there is a risk of subsequent staphylococcal enterotoxin production should the temperature of the crabmeat rise above 7°C for any significant period of time.

In the USA, the Centres for Disease Control (CDC) reported two seafood-associated outbreaks of staphylococcal food poisoning between 1978 and 1987 involving 12 cases. Nine of these cases were associated with shellfish and the other three with other seafood products. All were due to infected food handlers contaminating the products with *S. aureus* (Ahmed, 1991). In the UK, fish and shellfish accounted for 7% of staphylococcal-associated food poisoning outbreaks (Wieneke *et al.*, 1993).

#### 6.3.4.2  Meats.
Between 1969 and 1990, meat, poultry or their products were the most frequently implicated foods in outbreaks of staphylococcal food poisoning in the UK, being responsible for 75% of incidents (Wieneke *et al.*, 1993). This is also the case in the USA. Salted meats, for example corned beef and hams, are high-risk foods for staphylococcal enterotoxin outbreaks owing to the ability of *S. aureus* to tolerate high levels of salt,

combined with the inhibitory effects of salt on the normal food spoilage flora (Adams and Moss, 1995).

Many outbreaks involving large numbers of people have been linked to baked hams, usually at picnics (Bergdoll, 1989). Ham was also responsible for a notable outbreak that involved 196 of a total of 344 passengers and one steward on a flight from Tokyo to Paris. The ham was found to contain enterotoxin, while one of the cooks who had prepared the ham was found to have lesions on his hand containing enterotoxigenic staphylococci. Only those passengers who ate ham prepared by the cook with lesions fell ill (Eisenberg *et al.*, 1975).

Sausages are rarely implicated in staphylococcal food poisoning, but outbreaks have been caused by fermented sausage products—this subject has been comprehensively reviewed by Nychas and Arkoudelos (1990). Genoa sausage, for example, which is fermented without heating, has caused outbreaks of staphylococcal food poisoning. This has occurred when staphylococci have been able to grow and produce enterotoxin before the bacterial starter cultures, used in the meat fermentation, were able to produce enough acid to inhibit growth.

In 1979, canned corned beef processed in five different countries was linked to staphylococcal food poisoning in four countries (including the UK). It appeared that the source of the problem was faulty seams in the cans, which allowed staphylococci to enter the cans during cooling. SEA-producing staphylococci were found in corned beef from two of the processing countries (Bergdoll, 1989). In the UK, corned beef accounted for nine incidents involving 85 people and SEA-producing *S. aureus* strains were isolated (Wieneke *et al.*, 1993).

In July 1975 in the UK, 71 out of 147 pupils and staff became ill after a school lunch that included cooked chicken. The strain responsible for the outbreak was isolated from the chicken, the affected individuals and one food handler, and was found to produce SEA. The toxin was also detected in the remaining chicken, which had been thawed overnight, roasted the following day and stored at ambient temperature prior to being served cold (Wieneke *et al.*, 1993).

*6.3.4.3 Milk and milk products.* The occurrence of staphylococci in milk and milk products has been comprehensively reviewed by Gilmour and Harvey (1990). Milk and milk products can become contaminated if good hygiene is not practiced on farms, the milk is inadequately pasteurized (or not heat treated) and precautions are not taken to prevent contamination and growth of staphylococci during the manufacturing process and in the finished product (Gilmour and Harvey, 1990). In the UK, this food grouping accounted for 8% of staphylococcal food poisoning incidents between 1969 and 1990 (Wieneke *et al.*, 1993).

Many outbreaks have occurred due to cheese contaminated with staphylococcal enterotoxin but the wider adoption of pasteurised milk for cheese manufacture has reduced its occurrence (Bergdoll, 1989). A particular risk in cheese manufacture is the use of a starter culture with inadequate initial activity (Gilmour and Harvey, 1990). Butter is very rarely associated with staphylococcal food poisoning outbreaks, although in the USA in 1977 over 100 people fell ill after eating whipped butter, the butter being made from cream that was contaminated with *S. aureus* after pasteurisation (Bergdoll, 1989).

In the USA, milk is infrequently implicated in staphylococcal food poisoning. However, one outbreak among school children was linked to chocolate milk (Evenson *et al.*, 1988). The milk was held at a warm temperature for 4 to 5 h prior to pasteurisation, during which time the staphylococci grew and produced enterotoxin. The subsequent pasteurisation process was insufficient to inactivate the SEA present in the milk. In the UK between 1951 and 1960, raw milk was responsible for 20 outbreaks (590 cases) of staphylococcal food poisoning, while cream was responsible for two outbreaks (26 cases) between 1981 and 1984 (Gilmour and Harvey, 1990). Cream-filled bakery goods are often implicated in staphylococcal food poisoning incidents, especially during the warmer summer months; again inadequate refrigeration and poor hygiene are believed to be responsible (Bergdoll, 1989). In the UK and USA ice cream is infrequently associated with staphylococcal food poisoning outbreaks, but in Hungary it is the most common food vehicle (Adams and Moss, 1995).

*6.3.4.4 Other foods.* Vegetables are occasionally linked to staphylococcal food poisoning, mainly in the form of salads, for example potato salad (Bergdoll, 1989). In addition, *S. aureus* can grow and produce enterotoxin in unventilated, overwrapped mushrooms (Martin and Beelman, 1996).

In 1985, an international outbreak of staphylococcal food poisoning involving four countries was traced to dried lasagne pasta sheets produced in Italy, from which *S. aureus* producing SEA was isolated. SEA was detected at a level of 1 to 10 µg per 100 g lasagne, which was apparently contaminated with *S. aureus* due to inadequately pasteurised liquid egg (Woolaway *et al.*, 1986). In Japan, rice balls moulded by hand are the commonest vehicle of staphylococcal food poisoning (Adams and Moss, 1995).

*6.3.5 Canned foods*
Canned foods have rarely been implicated in staphylococcal food poisoning because the organism is readily destroyed by post-canning heat treatments. However, post-processing contamination through faulty seals is possible, with the entry of *S. aureus* cells into an environment both free of microbial competition and conducive to its growth (Hardt-English *et al.*, 1990). Four

outbreaks of staphylococcal food poisoning in the USA in 1989, affecting 102 people, were linked to canned mushrooms from China (Centers for Disease Control, 1989). An investigation by Hardt-English *et al.* (1990) found that the mushrooms were transported over long distances, without refrigeration in sealed plastic bags, to the canning plants, where upon examination prior to canning they appeared unspoiled. The same authors carried out a study recreating these conditions and found that a modified atmosphere (increased carbon dioxide) was created in the plastic bags as a result of the respiration of the mushrooms. This study also showed that *S. aureus* could grow and produce toxins under these conditions within 48 h. The lack of spoilage was most likely due to inhibition of spoilage bacteria by the modified atmosphere. Thermal processing records indicated that the canned mushrooms were subsequently inadequately processed (Centres for Disease Control, 1989) and sufficient levels of enterotoxin survived the canning process to cause illness (Hardt-English *et al.*, 1990). Further studies have also shown that preformed staphylococcal enterotoxin in mushrooms can survive the typical thermal processes given to canned foods, reinforcing the need to prevent contamination by, and growth of, *S. aureus* in foods prior to processing through proper staff and plant hygiene, and adequate refrigeration (Anderson *et al.*, 1996).

### 6.3.6    Control measures

*S. aureus* and other staphylococci are widely distributed in the environment and at least 50% of humans carry these microorganisms in their nasal passages, throat or hands. Any foods subjected to human handling during preparation and processing are therefore at risk. Although not all strains are enterotoxigenic, between 50 and 70% may be (Bergdoll, 1989). In the UK between 1969 and 1990 most contamination of foods by *S. aureus* occurred in the home, followed by restaurants and shops (Wieneke *et al.*, 1993).

Effective control measures to reduce the risk of staphylococcal food poisoning include the minimising of food handling, the employment of proper personal hygiene by food handling and processing personnel, the maintenance of proper plant and process hygiene by food handling and processing personnel, and the storage of foods at adequate refrigeration temperatures before, during and after processing.

*6.3.6.1 Destruction/inactivation of* S. aureus. *S. aureus* is not heat resistant, log-phase cultures in milk having $D$ values of 20 to 65 s at 62°C, and 41 s at 72°C. Heat resistance can vary depending on the growth stage of the microorganism, with $D$ values increasing three-fold with stationary phase cultures (Adams and Moss, 1995). Heating is considered to be the most effective method for inactivating staphylococci in foods (Bergdoll, 1989).

Freezing and thawing have very little effect on the viability of *S. aureus* but storage for prolonged periods does decrease the number of viable

*S. aureus* in meat (Bergdoll, 1989). Drying also lowers the number of recoverable *S. aureus* from beef products, for example corned beef (Bergdoll, 1989). *S. aureus* cells are also easily killed by irradiation (Baird-Parker, 1990).

*6.3.6.2 Prevention of* S. aureus *growth and toxin production.* Increasing the level of the initial inoculum enables staphylococci to grow under more adverse conditions. Highly inhibitory foods require a heavier level of contamination before growth can take place (Genigeorgis, 1989). Many commercially processed foods are excellent substrates for *S. aureus*, allowing both growth and enterotoxin production to occur with as few as 100 cells per gram (Ibrahim *et al.*, 1981; Bennett and Amos, 1982; Mansfield *et al.*, 1983; Kovats *et al.*, 1984). Conditions should therefore, if possible, be optimised to prevent growth and enterotoxin production.

The production of enterotoxin is more sensitive to decreases in the storage temperature of foods than the growth of *S. aureus* and growth can occur at a slightly lower $a_w$ than can enterotoxin production (Table 6.6).

Although *S. aureus* can grow and produce toxin in the presence of high levels of sodium chloride, enterotoxin production is affected. In a study by Baird-Parker (1971), the amount of enterotoxin produced was found to decrease in the presence of 7 to 9% sodium chloride and was undetectable at 10 to 14%, although the growth of the organism was unaffected even at the latter concentration. In high salt conditions, enterotoxin production is influenced by temperature and pH. In general, more enterotoxin is produced at higher temperatures and more alkaline pHs protect against the inhibitory effects of sodium chloride.

The levels of salt, pH and nitrite normally found in typical non-fermented, non-pickled, cured meats that are not extensively dried will not prevent growth and enterotoxin production under aerobic conditions but may be inhibitory under anaerobic conditions (e.g. vacuum packaging). Prevention of growth and enterotoxin production by sorbates is enhanced by decreasing the storage temperature, pH and level of inoculum (Genigeorgis, 1989).

Low pH can be used to inhibit growth and toxin production. As the pH decreases, higher levels of staphylococci are required to initiate growth. The type of acidulant can affect the sensitivity to changes in pH; for example, acetic acid is more inhibitory towards *S. aureus* than lactic acid (Minor and Marth, 1972).

Most of the foodborne bacteria inhibitory to *S. aureus* are from the genera *Streptococcus*, *Lactobacillus* and *Leuconostoc*. The presence and/or growth of other bacteria and their effects on *S. aureus* growth and enterotoxin production are of most importance in milk and other dairy products, and fermented meats (Genigeorgis, 1989).

Vegetative cells of *S. aureus* are sensitive to low doses of irradiation, 0.1 to 0.6 kGy resulting in death (Baird-Parker, 1990). This topic has been reviewed in detail by Monk *et al.* (1995).

*6.3.6.3 Destruction of preformed* S. aureus *enterotoxins in foods.* The heat stability of SEs is well documented (Denny *et al.*, 1966; Tatini *et al.*, 1976). Enterotoxin in food is not easily inactivated by heat, with higher levels of toxin requiring higher levels of heat for inactivation (Bergdoll, 1989). Generally, SEs are more rapidly denatured at higher temperatures and up until recently the temperatures used in conventional canning processes were considered sufficient to inactivate levels of SEs that may be typically present in foods. Levels of 0.5 to 10 µg per 100 g food are usually found in foods associated with staphylococcal enterotoxin outbreaks (Bergdoll, 1989). There is evidence, however, that SEA, SEB, SEC and SED may survive legal heat processing temperatures and times (Tibana *et al.*, 1987; Bennett and Berry, 1987; Anderson *et al.*, 1996). The thermal inactivation of SEs is affected by the purity of the toxin, the serological type of toxin, the amount of toxin present, the heating medium and the pH of the medium (Genigeorgis, 1989).

SEs are very resistant to gamma irradiation (Genigeorgis, 1989), with more than 2.7 rads and 9.7 rads required to give one decimal reduction in SEB in buffer and milk, respectively (Read and Bradshaw, 1967). Rose *et al.* (1988) showed that SEA was more resistant to irradiation than type A botulinum toxin. Again, food was shown to have a protective effect. Up to 26% of SEA remained biologically active after a dosage of 23.7 kGy, which is twice the dose proposed for legal acceptance in the UK.

### 6.3.7 HACCP

As for *C. botulinum* (section 6.2.8), HACCP is undoubtedly of benefit in both assessing and controlling the risk of *S. aureus* contamination, growth and enterotoxin production in food products (ICMSF, 1988).

### 6.3.8 Predictive modelling of S. aureus growth and enterotoxin production

Food MicroModel contains models for the growth of *S. aureus* and can be used to predict the likelihood of growth under a given set of conditions (McClure *et al.*, 1994a). The USDA Pathogen Modelling Programme also contains similar information to that of Food MicroModel. As more experimental data is gathered, existing predictive modelling programmes are updated (Eifert *et al.*, 1996), while new programmes are created, for example to assess the risk of growth and enterotoxin production by *S. aureus* in a cooked meat product (Walls and Scott, 1997). While models can be used to indicate growth rates in foods, they should not be relied on as sole safety measures as in some instances the growth rate can be underestimated, for example in challenge testing of sterile foods with *S. aureus* (Walls *et al.*, 1996).

### 6.3.9 *Methods for detecting* S. aureus *enterotoxins in foods*

A comprehensive review of detection methods for SEs has been published by Su and Wong (1997).

The AOAC approved standard method for detecting SEs in foods is the microslide gel double diffusion test. This is a qualitative method with a sensitivity of 10 to 100 ng/ml of enterotoxin in culture supernatant and concentrated food extracts (Andrews and Messer, 1990). The sensitivity of this method is barely adequate for detecting the small levels of toxin likely to be present in foods (0.5 to 10 mg/100g; Bergdoll, 1989).

Agglutination methods, including reverse passive latex agglutination (RPLA), have been developed for detecting SEs. The RPLA test uses latex particles sensitized with purified anti-staphylococcal-enterotoxin antibodies, which agglutinate in the presence of homologous enterotoxins. Commercial RPLA kits are available that give a sensitivity of 1 to 2 ng/ml (sufficient to detect SEs in most foods associated with outbreaks) but the test is subjective and takes 24 h to complete (Berry *et al.*, 1987; Fujikawa and Igarashi, 1988). Another RPLA method using high-density latex particles has been reported that can detect 0.5 ng/ml of enterotoxin in 3 h (Fujikawa and Igarashi, 1988). RPLA methods also suffer from the problem of non-specific binding and agglutination of food extracts. This problem can be prevented by using larger fluid volumes for food extractions but this reduces the sensitivity of the method to less than that required for determining the safety of foods (Bergdoll, 1989). Another drawback is the cost of commercial RPLA kits, which renders them impractical for the routine screening of large numbers of food samples.

Two commercially available immunoassay kits for SEs (TECRA and RIDASCREEN) have been evaluated by Park *et al.* (1993, 1994, 1996). They found that the TECRA ELISA kit (utilising polyvalent antibodies for SEA to SEE) produced a significant number of false-positive samples when used to detect enterotoxins in seafoods, in particular shellfish, and this could only be prevented by employing various sample treatments prior to assaying (Park *et al.*, 1993, 1996). The RIDASCREEN kit (utilising monovalent antibodies for SEA to SEE) was found to be rapid (three hours per test), specific and sensitive, and had minimum detection limits of 0.20 to 0.30 ng/ml in extracts of ham, salami and mushroom, 0.30 to 0.35 ng/ml in cheese extracts, and 0.50 to 0.75 ng/ml in foods such as noodles, ham, salami, cheese and turkey (Park *et al.*, 1994).

Other ELISA methods have also been developed and proposed for use in detecting SEs in foods. Bhatti *et al.* (1994) developed a fluorogenic enzyme-linked immunosorbent assay (FELISA) that can detect 0.1 fg/ml pure toxin and 10 pg/g enterotoxin in artificially contaminated food (minced beef, cheese). Using an amplified ELISA method, Morissette *et al.* (1991) were able to detect SEB in artificially contaminated cheese at a level of 0.5 to 1.0 ng/ml. The applicability of these methods for the detection of *S. aureus* in foods has yet to be determined.

An automated immunosensor has been developed for the detection of SEB, using anti-SEB antibodies coated on polymethylmethacrylate beads, with a claimed sensitivity of 5 ng/g in samples of spiked cream (Strachan *et al.*, 1997). Several biosensors have been developed for detecting SEs. Tempelman *et al.* (1996) have described a sensor that can detect 0.5 ng/ml SEB in buffer and 10 ng/ml in spiked ham samples, while DeSilva *et al.* (1995) have developed an immunobiosensor that can detect as little as 0.389 ng/ml SEB in buffer. However, the suitability of these systems for routine use in examination of food samples has not been determined.

An assay for the biological activity of SEA has been developed based on the proliferation of human and rat lymphocytes (T-cells). This assay may be applicable to the detection of SEA in food samples (Rasooly *et al.*, 1997). As little as 1 pg/ml SEA stimulated proliferation and using this assay system 1 ng/ml SEA was detected in food samples (Rasooly *et al.*, 1997). This is, therefore, a promising alternative to the current test for SEA biological activity that requires monkeys or kittens (Bergdoll, 1978).

## 6.4   *Bacillus cereus*

### 6.4.1   *Properties of* B. cereus

*B. cereus* is a Gram-positive, facultatively anaerobic spore-forming rod. The genus *Bacillus* can be divided into three groups. Species of group 1 are the main concern in food poisoning (Kramer and Gilbert, 1989).

A summary of the basic microbiological properties of *B. cereus* is shown in Table 6.8. The typical temperature range for growth is 10 to 50°C, with an optimum of 28 to 35°C (Kramer and Gilbert, 1989). Of concern in recent years, however, has been the finding of psychrotrophic variants of *B. cereus* that are capable of growth and toxin production down to 4°C (van Netten *et al.*, 1990).

### 6.4.2   *Types, structures and formation of* B. cereus *toxins*

There are seven different types of toxins produced by *B. cereus* but only emetic (vomit-inducing) toxin and diarrhoeal enterotoxin are involved in food poisoning (Granum, 1994).

*6.4.2.1   Emetic toxin.* Little is known about the structure and function of *B. cereus* emetic toxin except that it is heat stable and can withstand heating at 121°C for 90 min. It is resistant to proteolysis and is stable at pH values between 2 and 11 (Kramer and Gilbert, 1989; Granum, 1994). The optimum temperature for the production of emetic toxin was reported to be 25 to 30°C in rice culture (Melling and Capel, 1978). This toxin is thought to be of low molecular weight (less than 10 000 Da) and has been variously speculated to be a peptide (Kramer and Gilbert, 1989) or a lipid (Shinagawa *et al.*, 1992).

There is conflicting evidence as to whether toxin production occurs at the late exponential phase of growth or during sporulation of vegetative *B. cereus* cells in the stationary phase (Kramer and Gilbert, 1989). Emetic toxin may be formed as a result of the enzymatic modification of the food in which *B. cereus* is growing, but this has yet to be established (Granum, 1994).

*6.4.2.2 Diarrhoeal enterotoxin.* *B. cereus* diarrhoeal enterotoxin is a thermolabile protein inactivated by heating at 56°C for five minutes, and has a molecular weight of approximately 40 000 Da (Granum *et al.*, 1993). It is unstable below pH 4 and above pH 11, and is degraded by digestive enzymes including pepsin, trypsin and chymotrypsin, calling into question the ability of preformed toxin in foods to cause disease (Kramer and Gilbert, 1989). The optimum temperature for toxin production is 32 to 37°C and it is produced towards the end of the exponential growth phase (Kramer and Gilbert, 1989).

There is, however, conflicting evidence as to whether the symptoms caused by *B. cereus* diarrhoeal enterotoxin are due to the presence of preformed enterotoxin in foods or are the result of ingestion of *B. cereus* cells or spores and subsequent enterotoxin production in the small intestine (Kramer and Gilbert, 1989; Granum, 1994). Although Granum (1994) took the view that, on balance, the evidence was weighted towards infection rather than intoxication, preformed *B. cereus* diarrhoeal enterotoxin has been detected in foods in a recent study (Tan *et al.*, 1997). Lund (1990) states that *B. cereus* enterotoxin is both preformed in food and formed by the bacterium in the intestine. Whether or not the preformed toxin is stable enough to cause illness after ingestion is uncertain (Kramer and Gilbert, 1989; Granum, 1994).

*6.4.3 Effects and mode of action of* B. cereus *toxins*

*6.4.3.1 Emetic toxin.* The onset of illness is rapid, within 1 to 5 h of consuming food contaminated with the toxin. The main symptoms are nausea, vomiting and malaise with occasional subsequent diarrhoea. The duration is short, with symptoms usually lasting for less than 24 h (Kramer and Gilbert, 1989; Granum, 1994). The mode of action of this toxin is, to date, unknown.

*6.4.3.2 Enterotoxin.* The onset of illness is usually 8 to 16 h after ingestion of food contaminated with the toxin. It is characterised by abdominal pain and profuse watery diarrhoea, accompanied by rectal spasms and nausea. The symptoms are usually of short duration, lasting for 12 to 24 h (Kramer and Gilbert, 1989; Granum, 1994). The enterotoxin has been found to exert its action by disrupting cell membranes, resulting in cell leakage (Granum *et al.*, 1993).

### 6.4.4 *Occurrence of* B. cereus *food poisoning*

*B. cereus* spores and vegetative cells are widely distributed in the environment in soils, clays, sediments, dust and water and are also found in many different types of foods including cereals, flour, milk and other dairy products, meats, vegetables, dried foods and spices (Goepfert *et al.*,1972; Norris *et al.*, 1981; Kneifel and Berger, 1994). However, milk products and food products of plant origin are the main sources of *B. cereus* food poisoning (Granum, 1994). *B. cereus* is now well established as a significant cause of foodborne illness, accounting for up to 23% of reported outbreaks of known bacterial cause (Kramer and Gilbert, 1989). Data relating to the incidence of *B. cereus*-related food poisoning are given in Table 6.8.

**Table 6.8** Properties of *B. cereus*

| Gram stain | Morphology | Spore formation | Metabolism | Growth temperature range (°C) (optimum) | pH range for growth | Minimum $a_w$ for growth | Number of toxin types |
|---|---|---|---|---|---|---|---|
| +ve | Rod, 1 μm × 3 to 5 μm long, in chains, motile by peritrichous flagella | Yes | Facultative anaerobe | 4–50 (28–35) | 4.35–9.30 | 0.83–0.95 | 7 |

Data taken from Adams and Moss (1995) and Kramer and Gilbert (1989).

*6.4.4.1 Outbreaks due to emetic toxin.* Food poisoning due to *B. cereus* emetic toxin was first identified in the early 1970s in the UK and was associated with consumption of cooked rice from Chinese restaurants and take-away outlets (Lund, 1990). Most reported cases of *B. cereus* food poisoning in the UK have been attributable to the emetic form of toxin (Kramer and Gilbert, 1989). Similar outbreaks have also been reported in Canada, Finland, India, Japan, The Netherlands, Norway and the USA (Turnbull, 1986).

Illness due to *B. cereus* emetic toxin is almost exclusively linked to farinaceous (flour-based) foods, in particular cooked rice (Lund, 1990). The association with Chinese restaurants is due to the practice of cooking rice in bulk, then allowing it to cool and dry at room temperature, with portions being fried quickly with beaten egg when required. The cooked rice is left at room temperature, usually overnight, and sometimes for up to three days. This allows time for heat-resistant spores originally present in the raw rice to germinate and for vegetative cells to grow and produce toxin. Vegetative cell growth is rapid in cooked rice held at ambient temperatures (Kramer and Gilbert, 1989).

Although the vast majority of cases of *B. cereus* emetic toxin food poisoning are due to consumption of Cantonese-style cooked rice, other foods that have been involved include other ethnic rice dishes (curries, risotto and rice salad), vanilla slices, pasteurised cream, milk pudding, chicken supreme, infant milk formulas and cooked pasta (Turnbull, 1986; Kramer and Gilbert, 1989). In most cases it is the holding of foods for too long at improper temperatures, allowing spores to germinate and vegetative cells to grow and produce toxin, that is the most important factor in the causation of the emetic form of *B. cereus* food poisoning.

*6.4.4.2 Diarrhoeal enterotoxin.* As already discussed (section 6.4.2.2), there is considerable controversy as to whether this toxin can cause disease by means of intoxication. Since food poisoning due to this toxin was first described in 1950, following four outbreaks in Norway, a large number of outbreaks due to *B. cereus* diarrhoeal enterotoxin has been recorded in many countries including the UK, USA, Canada, Australia, China, Japan, Brazil, India, Hungary, The Netherlands and Bulgaria (Lund, 1990). Illness due to *B. cereus* diarrhoeal toxin is primarily associated with proteinaceous foods, vegetables, sauces and puddings; other foods that have been implicated include casseroles, other cooked meat and poultry dishes, sausages, meat and vegetable soups and, occasionally, fish, pasta, milk and ice cream (Goepfert *et al.*, 1972; Kramer and Gilbert, 1989). Where *B. cereus* is recovered from suspect food vehicles, it is usually present in large numbers ($5 \times 10^5$ to $9.5 \times 10^8$ colony-forming units per gram; Kramer and Gilbert, 1989).

The emergence of psychrotrophic strains of *B. cereus*, which are capable of growing at temperatures as low as 4°C, is of considerable concern. These enterotoxin-producing strains have been found in pasteurised milk, mousses and cook/chill meals (REPFEDs) (van Netten *et al.*, 1990). Van Netten *et al.* (1990) showed that temperature abuse prior to storage at 7°C resulted in a substantial reduction (two to six days) in the time required for enterotoxin formation, indicating that unless REPFEDs are stored below 4°C throughout, they present a risk of *B. cereus* intoxication.

*6.4.5 Control measures*

Due to the widespread occurrence of *B. cereus* it is impossible to prevent contamination of raw foods. However, the ingestion of low numbers of *B. cereus* is not harmful (Kramer and Gilbert, 1989). Freshly cooked food eaten hot is safe but if the food is maintained at temperatures between 10°C and 60°C, spores that have survived cooking can germinate and the result-ing vegetative bacteria can multiply in the food (Lund, 1990). Effective con-trol measures depend on the prevention of spore germination and the prevention of the growth and toxin production of *B. cereus* cells in cooked, ready-to-eat foods (Kramer and Gilbert, 1989).

To date there has been limited research on control measures to prevent *B. cereus* food poisoning. This may be due, at least in part, to its relatively recent recognition as a foodborne pathogen and to the short duration of the illness that it causes.

As is the case with *C. botulinum*, the hurdle effect (section 6.2.7) should be taken into account when assessing the risk of *B. cereus* toxin production in food. Food MicroModel (section 6.2.9), which includes data on the growth of both mesophilic and psychrotrophic *B. cereus* strains, can be used to assist in this process. HACCP (section 6.2.8) is also undoubtedly of benefit in both assessing and controlling *B. cereus* contamination, growth and toxin production in food products (ICMSF, 1988).

*6.4.5.1 Destruction/inactivation of* B. cereus *spores.* The heat resistance of *B. cereus* spores depends on the type of food in which they are found; the $D100°C$ values for skim milk and low acid foods (above pH 4.5) are 2.7 to 3 min and 5 min, respectively (Concon, 1988). While, on the whole, *B. cereus* spores possess unremarkable heat resistance compared to other spore-forming bacteria in their growth temperature range, it has been shown that a single spore in a total spore population of $10^6$ can show an unusually high resistance to heat (Kramer and Gilbert, 1989). For example, a study by Parry and Gilbert (1980) demonstrated greater thermal resistance among ten strains that caused emetic toxin food poisoning associated with rice ($D95°C$ = 22 to 36 min), as compared to nine routine isolates from raw rice ($D95°C$ =1.5 to 6 min). Steaming under pressure, thorough roasting and grilling are most likely to destroy spores; cooking at or below 100°C will permit the sur-vival of some *Bacillus* spores (Kramer and Gilbert, 1989).

*B. cereus* spores appear to show resistance to irradiation. In challenge test studies using spores of six strains of *B. cereus* (one emetic toxin-pro-ducing and five enterotoxin-producing strains) in various vacuum-packed meats, irradiation at doses between 0 and 4 kGy did not have a significant effect on spore survival (Thayer and Boyd, 1994).

*6.4.5.2 Prevention of* B. cereus *spore germination.* Spore germination may be greatly reduced by unfavourable conditions such as low temperature, low pH (below 4.5) and low water activity (Kramer and Gilbert, 1989). Although spore germination can occur over a broad temperature range (−1°C to 59°C), the optimum temperature is 30°C (Concon, 1988) Thus refrigeration of foods will help to minimise spore germination.

Nisin has been shown to prevent germination of *B. cereus* spores isolated from crumpets (Jenson *et al.*, 1994); nisin is now a permitted additive in crumpets and other high moisture flour based products in Australia (Anon., 1989).

*6.4.5.3 Prevention of* B. cereus *growth and toxin production.* Growth and multiplication of vegetative *B. cereus* cells typically occurs between 10°C and 50°C, with an optimum of 28 to 35°C (Kramer and Gilbert, 1989). For many strains therefore, refrigeration is sufficient to prevent or minimise growth and toxin production. Maintaining the pH of the food below pH 6 is also effective (Benedict *et al.*, 1993). Growth and toxin production of psychrotropic strains (capable of growing at temperatures as low as 4°C) can be prevented by storage below 4°C and maintaining the pH of the food at 6 or below (van Netten *et al.*, 1990).

There is little published data on the effect of water activity. Kramer and Gilbert (1989) suggested that an $a_w$ of approximately 0.9 can be regarded as the lower limit for growth and toxin production. An $a_w$ of 0.94 has been reported as inhibitory for psychrotrophic strains (van Netten *et al.*, 1990).

The use of preservatives for the control of *B. cereus* growth and toxin production has been limited to date. Nisin is effective in preventing growth of *B. cereus* cells in crumpets, although a higher level was required to inhibit vegetative cells compared with spores (Jenson *et al.*, 1994). Sorbic acid, potassium sorbate and garlic extract have also been shown to be inhibitory (Kramer and Gilbert, 1989).

Thayer and Boyd (1994) have shown that irradiation to a maximum dose of 3.0 kGy will significantly reduce the number and viability of *B. cereus* vegetative cells in mechanically deboned chicken meat and they conclude that irradiation of meat or poultry could provide significant consumer protection from vegetative cells of *B. cereus*. Monk *et al.* (1995) have reviewed the effect of irradiation on this organism.

### 6.4.6  Destruction of preformed toxin in foods

As discussed previously (sections 6.4.2.1 and 6.4.2.2), emetic toxin is considered heat stable, whereas the diarrhoeal enterotoxin is heat labile. However, a recent study has shown that the thermostability of the enterotoxin is four times greater in milk than in buffer (Baker and Griffiths, 1995). This suggests that enterotoxin may be more stable than previously thought when preformed in foods.

### 6.4.7  Methods for detecting B. cereus toxins in foods

At present there are no practical tests available for detecting *B. cereus* emetic toxin in foods. Enterotoxin has been detected in foods using a commercial reversed passive latex agglutination kit (Oxoid; van Netten *et al.*,

1990). The manufacturer claims the sensitivity of this kit to be four nanograms of enterotoxin per gram of food macerate. A commercially available ELISA kit has also been used to detect *B. cereus* enterotoxin in food samples (Tan *et al.*, 1997).

### 6.4.8 *Other* Bacillus *species implicated in food poisoning*

A number of other *Bacillus* species have also been implicated in food poisoning, including *B. subtilis*, *B. licheniformis* and *B. pumilis* (Kramer and Gilbert, 1989). However, a causal link between these species of *Bacillus* and food poisoning has not been firmly established. It is not known whether these species are toxigenic and, if so, whether they can produce toxin in foods.

Although considered to be an insect pathogen, *B. thuringiensis* has recently been implicated in a gastro-enteritis outbreak linked to onion powder, and was found to produce an enterotoxin with the same cytotoxic activity as that produced by *B. cereus* (Jackson *et al.*, 1995). Further research is required, however, to determine the role of this organism and its toxin in food poisoning.

## 6.5 Concluding remarks

Foodborne intoxications due to toxin formation in foods by *C. botulinum*, *S. aureus* and *B. cereus* continue to remain a problem world-wide. Individual countries, and even areas or districts of countries, can have problems with specific microbial intoxications, for example type A botulism in the western USA. The increasing globalisation of the food supply is potentially leading to a greater risk of these intoxications being spread outside their normal geographic boundaries. It is also increasingly likely that other toxins produced by these bacteria, and which may also be important in food intoxications, have yet to be identified. At the same time, other species of bacteria are increasingly being suspected of being involved in foodborne intoxications, for example *B. thuringiensis*. Food processors need to be aware of these risks, especially when producing new food products or adopting novel food processing regimes, such as *sous vide*. They must also be aware of the need to adhere to good hygienic practices and HACCP. Consumers also need to be made more aware of the risks of bacterial toxins in foods, primarily through better education in hygiene during food handling and preparation. Both food processors and consumers need to use appropriate storage conditions for foods at all points in the chain of processing, distribution and consumption.

# References

Adams, M.R. and Moss, M.O. (1995) *Food Microbiology*, The Royal Society of Chemistry, Cambridge, 398 pp.

Adesiyun, A.A., Tatini, S.R. and Hoover, D.G. (1984) Production of enterotoxins by *Staphylococcus hyicus*. *Veterinary Medicine*, **9** 487-95.

Ahmed, F.E. (ed.) (1991) *Seafood Safety*, National Academy Press, Washington, DC, 432 pp.

Anderson, J.E., Beelman, R.R. and Doores, S. (1996) Persistence of serological and biological activities of staphylococcal enterotoxin A in canned mushrooms. *Journal of Food Protection*, **59** 1292-99.

Andrews, W.H. and Messer, J. (1990) Microbiological methods, in *Official Methods of Analysis of the Association of Official Analytical Chemists*, 15th edn (ed. K. Helrich), AOAC Inc., Arlington, Virginia, pp. 459-61.

Anon. (1989) *Commonwealth of Australia Gazette*, Australian Government Publishing Service, Canberra, December 15.

Aureli, P., Franciosa, G. and Pourshaban, M. (1996) Foodborne botulism in Italy. *Lancet*, **348** 1594.

Bach, R., Wenzel, S., Muller-Prasuhn, G. and Glasker, H. (1971) Teichforellen als Trager von *Clostridium botulinum* und ursache von botulinus. *Archiv fur Lebensmittelhygiene*, **22** 107-12.

Baird-Parker, A.C. (1971) Factors affecting the production of bacterial food poisoning toxins. *Journal of Bacteriology*, **84** 181-97.

Baird-Parker, A.C. (1990) The staphylococci: an introduction. *Journal of Applied Bacteriology Symposium Supplement*, **69** 1S-8S.

Baker, J.M. and Griffiths, M.W. (1995) Evidence for increased thermostability of *Bacillus cereus* enterotoxin in milk. *Journal of Food Protection*, **58** 443-45.

Ball, A.P., Hopkinson, R.B., Farrell, I.D., Hutchison, J.G.P., Paul, R., Watson, R.D.S., Page, A.J.F., Parker, R.G.F., Edwards, C.W., Snow, M., Scott, D.K., Leone-Ganado, A., Hastings, A., Ghosh, A.C. and Gilbert, R.J. (1979) Human botulism caused by *Clostridium botulinum* type E: the Birmingham outbreak. *Quarterly Journal of Medicine*, **48** 473-91.

Benedict, R.C., Partridge, T., Wells, D. and Buchanan, R.L. (1993) *Bacillus cereus*: aerobic growth kinetics. *Journal of Food Protection*, **56** 211-14.

Bennett, R.W. and Amos, W.T. (1982) *Staphylococcus aureus* growth and toxin production in nitrogen-packed sandwiches. *Journal of Food Protection*, **45** 157-61.

Bennett, R.W. and Berry, M.R. (1987) Serological reactivity and *in vivo* toxicity of *Staphylococcus aureus* enterotoxins A and D in selected canned foods. *Journal of Food Science*, **52** 416-18.

Bergdoll, M.S. (1978) Staphylococcal intoxications, in *Foodborne Infections and Intoxications*, 2nd edn (eds H. Rieman and F.L. Bryan), Academic Press, New York, pp. 444-94.

Bergdoll, M.S. (1989) *Staphylococcus aureus*, in *Foodborne Bacterial Pathogens* (ed. M.P. Doyle), Marcel Dekker, New York, pp. 463-523.

Bergdoll, M.S., Cross, B.A., Reisser, R.F., Robbins, R.N. and Davis, J.P. (1981) A new staphylococcal enterotoxin, enterotoxin F, associated with toxic-shock-syndrome *Staphylococcus aureus* isolates. *Lancet*, **ii** 1017-21.

Berry, P.R., Rodhouse, J.C., Wieneke, A.A. and Gilbert, R.J. (1987) Use of commercial kits for the detection of *Clostridium perfringens* and *Staphylococcus aureus* enterotoxins. *Society for Applied Bacteriology Technical Series*, **24** 245-54.

Betley, M.J., Borst, D.W. and Regassa, L.B. (1992) Staphyloccal enterotoxins, toxic shock syndrome toxin and streptococcal pyrogenic exotoxins: a comparative study of their molecular biology. *Chemical Immunology*, **55** 1-35.

Bhatti, A.R., Siddiqui, Y.M. and Micussan, V.V. (1994) Highly sensitive fluorogenic enzyme-linked immunosorbent assay: detection of staphylococcal enterotoxin B. *Journal of Microbiological Methods*, **19** 179-87.

Brent, J., Gomez, H., Judson, F., Miller, K., Rossi-Davis, A., Shillam, P., Hatheway, C., McCroskey, L., Mintz, E., Kallander, K., McKee, C., Romer, J., Singleton, E., Yager, J. and Sofos, J. (1995) Botulism from potato salad. *Dairy, Food and Environmental Sanitation*, **15** 420-22.

Centres for Disease Control (1989) Multiple outbreaks of staphylococcal food poisoning caused by canned mushrooms. *Morbidity and Mortality Weekly Report*, **38** 417-18.

Church, I.J. and Parsons, A.L. (1993) Review: *sous vide* cook-chill technology. *International Journal of Food Science and Technology*, **28** 563-74.

Collins-Thompson, D.L. and Wood, D.S. (1992) Control in dairy products, in *Clostridium botulinum. Ecology and Control in Foods* (eds A.H.W. Hauschild and K.L. Dodds), Marcel Dekker, New York, pp. 261-77.

Concon, J.M. (1988) Bacterial food contaminants: bacterial toxins, in *Food Toxicology. Part B: Contaminants and Additives*, Marcel Dekker, New York, pp. 771-841.

Conner, D.E., Scott, V.N., Bernard, D.T. and Kautter, D.A. (1989) Potential *Clostridium botulinum* hazards associated with extended shelf-life refrigerated foods: a review. *Journal of Food Safety*, **10** 131.

Cook, F.K. and Pierson, M.D. (1983) Inhibition of bacterial spores by antimicrobials. *Food Technology* **37** (11) 115.

Crandall, A.D., Winkowski, K. and Montville, T.J. (1994) Inability of *Pediococcus pentosaceus* to inhibit *Clostridium botulinum* in *sous vide* beef with gravy at 4 and 10°C. *Journal of Food Protection*, **57** 104-107.

DasGupta, B.R. (1989) The structure of botulinum neurotoxin, in *Botulinum Neurotoxin and Tetanus Toxin* (ed. L.L. Simpson), Academic Press, New York, pp. 53-67.

Denny, C.B., Tan, P.L. and Bohrer, C.W. (1966) Heat inactivation of staphylococcal enterotoxin A. *Journal of Food Science*, **31** 762-67.

DeSilva, M.S., Zhang, Y., Hesketh, P.J., Maclay, G.J., Gendel, S.M. and Stetter, J.R. (1995) Impedance based sensing of the specific binding reaction between *Staphylococcus* enterotoxin B and its antibody on an ultra-thin platinum film. *Biosensors and Bioelectronics*, **10** 675-82.

Dezfulian, M., Hatheway, C.L., Yolken, R.H. and Bartlett, J.G. (1984) Enzyme-linked immunosorbent assay for detection of *Clostridium botulinum* type A and type B toxins in stool samples of infants with botulism. *Journal of Clinical Microbiology*, **20** 379-83.

Dodds, K.L. (1992) *Clostridium botulinum* in foods, in *Clostridium botulinum. Ecology and Control In Foods* (eds A.H.W. Hauschild and K.L. Dodds), Marcel Dekker, New York, pp. 209-32.

Dodds, K.L. and Hauschild, A.H. (1989) Distribution of *Clostridium botulinum* in the environment and its significance in relation to botulism, in *Recent Advances in Microbial Ecology. Proceedings, 5th International Symposium on Microbial Ecology* (eds T. Hattori, Y. Ishida, Y. Maruyama, R.Y. Morita and A. Uchida), Scientific Societies Press, Tokyo, pp. 472-76.

Doellgast, G., Triscott, M.X., Beard, G.A., Bottoms, J.D., Cheng, T., Roh, B.H., Roman, M.G., Hall, P.A. and Brown, J.E. (1993) Sensitive enzyme-linked immunosorbent assay for detection of *C. botulinum* neurotoxins A, B and E using signal amplification via enzyme-linked coagulation assay. *Journal of Clinical Microbiology*, **31** 2402-2409.

Eifert, J.D., Gennings, C., Carter, Jr, W.H., Duncan, S.E. and Hackney, C.R. (1996) Predictive model with improved statistical analysis of interactive factors affecting the growth of *Staphylococcus aureus* 196E. *Journal of Food Protection*, **59** 608-14.

Eisenberg, M.S., Gaarslev, K., Brown, W., Horwitz, M. and Hill, D. (1975) Staphylococcal food poisoning aboard a commercial aircraft. *Lancet*, **2** 595-99.

Eklund, M.W. (1992) Control in fishery products, in *Clostridium botulinum. Ecology and Control In Foods* (eds A.H.W. Hauschild and K.L. Dodds), Marcel Dekker, New York, pp. 209-32.

Ellender, R.D., Huang, L., Sharp, S.L. and Tettleton, R.P. (1995) Isolation, enumeration and identification of gram-positive cocci from frozen crabmeat. *Journal of Food Protection*, **58** 853-57.

Evenson, M.L., Hinds, M.W., Bernstein, R.S. and Bergdoll, M.S. (1988) Estimation of human dose of staphylococcal enterotoxin A from a large outbreak of staphylococcal food poisoning involving chocolate milk. *International Journal of Food Microbiology*, **7** 311-16.

Freer, J.H. and Arbuthnott, J.P. (1986) Toxins of *Staphylococcus aureus*, in *Pharmacology of Bacterial Toxins* (eds F. Dorner and J. Drews), Pergamon Press, Oxford, pp. 581-633.

Fujikawa, H. and Igarashi, H. (1988) Rapid latex agglutination test for detection of SEs A to E that uses high-density latex particles. *Applied and Environmental Microbiology*, **54** 2345-48.

Garrett, E.S., Hudak-Roos, M. and Ward, D.R. (1995) Implementation of the HACCP program by the fresh and processed seafood industry, in *HACCP in Meat, Poultry and Fish Processing* (eds A.M. Pearson and T.R. Dutson), Blackie Academic & Professional, Chapman & Hall, London, pp. 109-33.

Genigeorgis, C.A. (1989) Present state of knowledge on staphylococcal intoxication. *International Journal of Food Microbiology*, **9** 327-60.

Gilmour, A. and Harvey, J. (1990) Staphylococci in milk and milk products. *Journal of Applied Bacteriology Symposium Supplement*, **69** 147S-166S.

Goepfert, J.M., Spira, W.M. and Kim, H.U. (1972). *Bacillus cereus*: food poisoning organism: a review. *Journal of Milk Food Technology*, **35** 213-27.

Gomez-Lucia, E., Goyache, J., Orden, J.A., Blanco, J.L., Ruiz-Santa-Quiteria, J.A., Dominguez, L. and Suarez, G. (1988) Production of enterotoxin by supposedly nonenterotoxigenic *Staphylococcus aureus* strains. *Applied and Environmental Microbiology*, **55** 1447-51.

Gould, G.W. (1984) Injury and repair mechanisms in bacterial spores, in *The Revival of Injured Microbes* (eds M.H.E. Andrew and A.D. Russel), Academic Press, London, p. 199.

Granum, P.E. (1994) *Bacillus cereus* and its toxins. *Journal of Applied Bacteriology Symposium Supplement*, **76** 61S-66S.

Granum, P.E., Brynestad, S., O'Sullivan, K. and Nissen, H. (1993) The enterotoxin from *Bacillus cereus*: production and biochemical characterisation. *Netherlands Milk Dairy Journal*, **47** 63-70.

Granum, P.E., Tomas, J.M. and Alouf, J.E. (1995) A survey of bacterial toxins in food poisoning: a suggestion for bacterial food poisoning toxin nomenclature. *International Journal of Food Microbiology*, **28** 129-44.

Hallis, B., James, B.A. and Shone, C.C. (1996) Development of novel assays for botulinum type A and B neurotoxins based on their endopeptidase activities. *Journal of Clinical Microbiology*, **34** 1934-38.

Hardt-English, P., York, G., Stier, R. and Cocotas, P. (1990) Staphylococcal food poisoning outbreaks caused by canned mushrooms from China. *Food Technology*, **44** (12) 74-77.

Hatheway, C.L. (1990) Toxigenic clostridia. *Clinical Microbiology Reviews*, **3** (3) 66-98.

Hatheway, C.L. (1995) Botulism: the present status of the disease, in *Clostridial neurotoxins* (ed. C. Montecucco), Springer, Berlin, pp. 55-75.

Hauschild, A.H.W. (1989) *Clostridium botulinum*, in *Foodborne Bacterial Pathogens* (ed. M.P. Doyle), Marcel Dekker, New York, pp. 111-89.

Hauschild, A.H.W. (1992) Epidemiology of human foodborne botulism, in *Clostridium botulinum. Ecology and Control in Foods* (eds A.H.W. Hauschild and K.L. Dodds), Marcel Dekker, New York, pp. 69-104.

Hirooka, E.Y., Muller, E.E., Freitas, J.C., Vicente, E., Yoshimoto, Y. and Bergdoll, M.S. (1988) Enterotoxigenicity of *Staphylococcus intermedius* of canine origin. *International Journal of Food Microbiology*, **7** 185-91.

Horiguchi, Y., Kozaki, S. and Sakaguchi, G. (1984) Determination of *Clostridium botulinum* toxin by reversed passive latex agglutination. *Japanese Journal of Veterinary Science*, **46** 487-91.

Huss, H.H. (1981) *Clostridium botulinum type E and Botulism*. Ministry of Fisheries, Technical University, Lyngby, Copenhagen, 58 pp.

Ibrahim, G.F., Radford, D.R., Baldock, A.K. and Ireland, L.B. (1981) Inhibition of growth of *Staphylococcus aureus* and enterotoxin production in cheddar cheese produced with induced starter failure. *Journal of Food Protection*, **44** 189-93.

ICMSF (International Commission on Microbiological Specifications for Foods) (1988) *Microorganisms in Foods. 4. Application of the Hazard Analysis Critical Control Point (HACCP) System to Ensure Microbiological Safety and Quality*. Blackwell Scientific Publications, Oxford, 357 pp.

Jackson, S.G., Goodbrand, R.B., Ahmed, R. and Kasatiya, S. (1995) *Bacillus cereus* and *Bacillus thuriengiensis* isolated in a gastroenteritis outbreak investigation. *Letters in Applied Microbiology*, **21** 103-105.

Jenson, I., Baird, L. and Delves-Broughton, J. (1994) The use of nisin as a preservative in crumpets. *Journal of Food Protection*, **57** 874-77.

Kim, J. and Foegeding, P.M. (1992) Principles of control, in *Clostridium botulinum. Ecology and Control in Foods* (eds A.H.W. Hauschild and K.L. Dodds), Marcel Dekker, New York, pp. 121-76.

Kneifel, W. and Berger, E. (1994) Microbiological criteria of random samples of spices and herbs retailed on the Austrian market. *Journal of Food Protection*, **57** 893-901.

Kovats, S.K., Doyle, M.P. and Tanaka, N. (1984) Evaluation of the microbiological safety of tofu. *Journal of Food Protection*, **47** 618-22.

Kramer, J.M. and Gilbert, R.J. (1989) *Bacillus cereus* and other *Bacillus* species, in *Foodborne Bacterial Pathogens* (ed. M.P. Doyle), Marcel Dekker, New York, pp. 21-70.

Kumar, P., Colston, J.T., Chambers, J.P., Rael, E.D. and Valdes, J.J. (1994) Detection of botulinum toxin using an evanescent wave immunosensor. *Biosensors and Bioelectronics*, **9** 57-63.

Leistner, L. (1978) Microbiology of ready-to-serve foods. *Die Fleischwirtschaft*, **58** 2008-11.

Lucke, F.-K. and Roberts, T.A. (1992) Control in meat and meat products, in *Clostridium botulinum. Ecology and Control in Foods* (eds A.H.W. Hauschild and K.L. Dodds), Marcel Dekker, New York, pp. 177-207.

Lund, B.M. (1990) Foodborne disease due to *Bacillus* and *Clostridium* species. *Lancet*, **336** 982-86.

Lund, B.M. and Notermans, S.H.W. (1992) Potential hazards associated with REPFEDs in *Clostridium botulinum. Ecology and Control in Foods* (eds A.H.W. Hauschild and K.L. Dodds), Marcel Dekker, New York, pp. 279-303.

Lund, B.M., George, S.M. and Franklin, J.G. (1987) Inhibition of type A and type B (proteolytic) *Clostridium botulinum* by sorbic acid. *Applied and Environmental Microbiology*, **53** 935.

Mansfield, J.M., Farkas, G., Wieneke, A.A. and Gilbert, R.J. (1983) Studies on the growth and survival of *Staphylococcus aureus* in corned beef. *Journal of Hygiene, Cambridge*, **91** 467-78.

Martin, S.T. and Beelman, R.B. (1996) Growth and enterotoxin production of *Staphylococcus aureus* in fresh packaged mushrooms (*Agaricus bisporus*). *Journal of Food Protection*, **59** 819-26.

McClure, P.J., Blackburn, C. de W., Cole, M.B., Curtis, P.S., Jones, J.E., Legan, J.D., Ogden, I.D., Peck, M.W., Roberts, T.A., Sutherland, J.P. and Walker, S.J. (1994a) Modelling the growth, survival and death of microorganisms in foods: the UK Food Micromodel approach. *International Journal of Food Microbiology*, **23** 265-75.

McClure, P.J., Cole, M.B. and Smelt, J.P.P.M. (1994b) Effects of water activity and pH on growth of *Clostridium botulinum*. *Journal of Applied Bacteriology Supplement*, **76** 105S-114S.

Melling, J. and Capel, B.J. (1978) Characteristics of *Bacillus cereus* emetic toxin. *FEMS Microbiology Letters*, **4** 133-35.

Meng, J. and Genigeorgis, C.A. (1994) Delaying toxigenesis of *Clostridium botulinum* by sodium lactate in *sous vide* products. *Letters in Applied Microbiology*, **19** 20-23.

Middlebrook, J.L. (1989) Cell surface receptors for protein toxins, in *Botulinum Neurotoxin and Tetanus Toxin* (ed. L.L. Simpson), Academic Press, New York, pp. 95-119.

Minor, T.E. and Marth, E.H. (1972) Loss of viability by *Staphylococcus aureus* in acidified media. Inactivation by several acids, mixtures of acids, and salts of acids. *Journal of Milk and Food Technology*, **35** 191-96.

Monk, J.D., Beuchat, L.R. and Doyle, M.P. (1995) Irradiation inactivation of foodborne microorganisms. *Journal of Food Protection*, **58** 197-208.

Montecucco, C. and Schiavo, G. (1993) Tetanus and botulism neurotoxins: a new group of zinc proteases. *Trends in Biochemical Sciences*, **18** 324-27.

Montecucco, C. and Schiavo, G. (1994) Mechanism of action of tetanus and botulinum neurotoxins. *Molecular Microbiology*, **13** 1-8.

Montecucco, C. and Schiavo, G. (1995) Structure and function of tetanus and botulinum neurotoxins. *Quarterly Reviews of Biophysics*, **28** 423-72.

Morissette, C., Goulet, J. and Lamoureux, G. (1991) Rapid and sensitive sandwich enzyme-linked immunosorbent assay for detection of staphylococcal enterotoxin B in cheese. *Applied and Environmental Microbiology*, **57** 836-42.

Norris, J.R., Berkeley, R.C.W., Logan, N.A. and O'Donnell, A.G. (1981) The genera *Bacillus* and *Sporolactobacillus*, in *The Prokaryotes—A Handbook on Habitats, Isolation and Identification of Bacteria*, vol. II (eds M.P. Starr, H. Stolp, H.G. Truper, A. Balows and G. Schlegel), Springer-Verlag, Berlin, pp. 1711-42.

Notermans, S.H.W. (1992) Control in fruits and vegetables, in *Clostridium botulinum. Ecology and Control in Foods* (eds A.H.W. Hauschild and K.L. Dodds), Marcel Dekker, New York, pp. 233-60.

Nychas, G.J.E. and Arkoudelos, J.S. (1990) Staphylococci in sausages. *Journal of Applied Bacteriology Symposium Supplement*, **69** 167S-188S.

O'Mahony, M.O., Mitchell, E., Gilbert, R.J., Hutchinson, D.N., Begg, N.T., Rodhouse, J.C. and Morris, J. E. (1990) An outbreak of foodborne botulism associated with contaminated hazelnut yoghurt. *Epidemiology and Infection*, **104** 389-95.

Osheroff, B.J., Slocum, G.G. and Decker, W.M. (1964) Status of botulism in the United States. *Public Health Reports (US)*, **79** 871-78.

Pace, P.J. and Krumbiegel, E.R. (1973) *Clostridium botulinum* and smoked fish production 1963–1972. *Journal of Milk and Food Technology*, **36** 42-49.

Park, C.E., Akhtar, M. and Rayman, M.K. (1993) Simple solutions to false-positive staphylococcal enterotoxin assays with seafood tested with an enzyme-linked immunosorbent assay kit (TECRA). *Applied and Environmental Microbiology*, **59** 2210-13.

Park, C.E., Akhtar, M. and Rayman, M.K. (1994) Evaluation of a commercial enzyme immunoassay kit (RIDASCREEN) for detection of SEs A, B, C, D and E in foods. *Applied and Environmental Microbiology*, **60** 677-81.

Park, C.E., Warburton, D., Laffey, P.J. *et al.* (1996) A collaborative study on the detection of SEs in foods with an enzyme immunoassay kit (TECRA). *Journal of Food Protection*, **59** 390-97.

Parry, J.M. and Gilbert, R.J. (1980) Studies on the heat resistance of *Bacillus cereus* spores and the growth of the organism in boiled rice. *Journal of Hygiene, Cambridge*, **84** 77-82.

Peck, M.W. and Fernandez, P.S. (1995) Effect of lysozyme concentration, heating at 90°C, and then incubation at chilled temperatures on growth from spores of non-proteolytic *Clostridium botulinum*. *Letters In Applied Microbiology*, **21** 50-54.

Peck, M.W., Lund, B.M., Fairbairn, D.A., Kaspersson, A.S. and Undeland, P.C. (1995) Effect of heat treatment on survival of, and growth from, spores of non-proteolytic *Clostridium botulinum* at refrigeration temperatures. *Applied and Environmental Microbiology*, **61** 1780-85.

Pereira, M.L., Carmo, L.S.D., Santos, E.J.D., Pereira, J.L. and Bergdoll, M.S. (1996) Enterotoxin H in staphylococcal food poisoning. *Journal of Food Protection*, **59** 559-61.

Podreshetnikova, N.A., Shapiro, B.M., Steblyanko, S.N. and Tryasina, S.G. (1970) Case of botulism due to canned vegetables. *Voprosy Pitanyi*, **29** 89.

Rasooly, L., Rose, N.R., Shah, D.B. and Rasooly, A. (1997) *In vitro* assay of *Staphylococcus aureus* enterotoxin A activity in food. *Applied and Environmental Microbiology*, **63** 2361-65.

Read, R.B. and Bradshaw, J.G. (1967) Gamma irradiation of staphylococcal enterotoxin B. *Applied Microbiology*, **15** 603-605.

Roblot, P., Roblot, F., Fauchere, J.L., Devilleger, A., Marechaud, R., Breux, J.P., Grollier, G. and Becq-Giraudon, B. (1994) Retrospective study of 108 cases of botulism in Poitiers, France. *Journal of Medical Microbiology*, **40** 379-84.

Rose, S.A., Modi, N.K., Tranter, H.S., Bailey, N.E., Stringer, M.F. and Hambleton, P. (1988) Studies on the irradiation of toxins of *Clostridium botulinum* and *Staphylococcus aureus*. *Journal of Applied Bacteriology*, **65** 223-29.

Sakaguchi, G., Ohishi, I. and Kozaki, S. (1981) Purification and oral toxicities of *Clostridium botulinum* progenitor toxins, in *Biomedical Aspects of Botulism* (ed. G.E. Lewis), Academic Press, New York, pp. 21-34.

Sakaguchi, G., Kozaki, S. and Ohishi, I. (1984) Structure and function of botulinum toxins, in *Bacterial Protein Toxins* (eds F.J. Fehrenbach, J.H. Freer and J. Jeljaszewicz), Academic Press, London, pp. 435-43.

Schantz, E.J. and Sugiyama, H. (1974) Toxic proteins produced by *Clostridium botulinum. Journal of Agricultural and Food Chemistry*, **22** 26-30.

Schmidt, K. (ed.) (1995) *WHO Surveillance Programme for Control of Foodborne Infections and Intoxications in Europe*, Federal Institute for Health Protection of Consumers and Veterinary Medicine (FAO/WHO Collaborating Centre for Research and Training in Food Hygiene and Zoonoses), Berlin, 340 pp.

Seals, J.E., Snyder, J.D., Edell, T.A., Hatheway, C.L., Johnson, C.J., Swanson, R.C. and Hughes, J.M. (1981) Restaurant-associated type A botulism: transmission by potato salad. *American Journal of Epidemiology*, **113** 436-44.

Shapton, D.A. and Shapton, N.F. (eds) (1991) *Principles and Practices for the Safe Processing of Foods*, Butterworth-Heinemann Ltd, Oxford, 457 pp.

Shinagawa, K., Otake, S., Matsusaka, N. and Sugii, S. (1992) Production of the vacuolation factor of *Bacillus cereus* isolated from vomiting-type food poisoning. *Journal of Veterinary Medical Science*, **54** 443-46.

Shone, C.C., Wilton-Smith, P., Appleton, N., Hambleton, P., Modi, N., Gatley, S. and Melling, J. (1985) Monoclonal antibody-based immunoassay for type A *Clostridium botulinum* toxin is comparable to the mouse bioassay. *Applied and Environmental Microbiology*, **50** 63-67.

Siegel, L.S. (1992) Destruction of botulinum toxins in food and water, in *Clostridium botulinum. Ecology and Control in Foods* (eds A.H.W. Hauschild and K.L. Dodds), Marcel Dekker, New York, pp. 323-41.

Siegel, L.S. and Metzger, J.F. (1979) Toxin production by *Clostridium botulinum* type A under various fermentation conditions. *Applied and Environmental Microbiology*, **38** 606-11.

Simini, B. (1996) Outbreak of foodborne botulism in Italy continues. *Lancet*, **348** 813.

Simpson, L.L. (1986) Molecular pharmacology of botulinum and tetanus toxin. *Annual Reviews of Pharmacology and Toxicology*, **26** 427-53.

Simpson, M.V., Smith, J.P., Dodds, K., Ramaswamy, H.S., Blanchfield, B. and Simpson, B.K. (1995) Challenge studies with *Clostridium botulinum* in a *sous vide* spaghetti and meat-sauce product. *Journal of Food Protection*, **58** 229-34.

Slater, P.E., Addiss, G., Cohen, A., Leventhal, A., Chassis, G., Zehavi, H., Bashari, A. and Costin, C. (1989) Foodborne botulism: an international outbreak. *International Journal of Epidemiology*, **18** 693-96.

Smith, L.D.S. and Sugiyama, H. (1988) *Botulism: the Organism, its Toxins, the Disease*, 2nd edn (ed. A. Balows), C.C. Thomas, Springfield, Illinois, 171 pp.

Sperber, W.H. (1982) Requirements of *Clostridium botulinum* for growth and toxin production. *Food Technology*, **36** 89-94.

St Louis, M.E., Peck, S.H.S., Bowering, D., Morgan, G.B., Blatherwick, J., Banerjee, S., Kettyls, G.D.M., Black, W.A., Milling, M.E., Hauschild, A.H.W., Tauxe, R.V. and Blake, P.A. (1988) Botulism from chopped garlic: delayed recognition of a major outbreak. *Annals of Internal Medicine*, **108** 363-68.

Strachan, N.J.C., John, P.G. and Millar, I.G. (1997) Application of a rapid automated immunosensor for the detection of *Staphylococcus aureus* enterotoxin B in cream. *International Journal of Food Microbiology*, **35** 293-97.

Su, Y.-C. and Wong, A.C.L. (1995) Identification and purification of a new staphylococcal enterotoxin, H. *Applied and Environmental Microbiology*, **61** 1438-43.

Su, Y.-C. and Wong, A.C.L. (1996) Detection of staphylococcal enterotoxin H by an enzyme-linked immunosorbent assay. *Journal of Food Protection*, **59** 327-30.

Su, Y.-C. and Wong, A.C.L. (1997) Current perspectives on detection of staphylococcal enterotoxins. *Journal of Food Protection*, **60** 195-202.

Tan, A., Heaton, S., Farr, L. and Bates, J. (1997) The use of *Bacillus* diarrhoeal enterotoxin (BDE) detection using an ELISA technique in the confirmation of the aetiology of *Bacillus*-mediated diarrhoea. *Journal of Applied Microbiology,* **82** 677-82.

Tatini, S.R. (1976) Thermal stability of enterotoxins in foods. *Journal of Milk and Food Technology,* **39** 432-38.

Tempelman, L.A., King, K.D., Anderson, G.P. and Ligler, F.S. (1996) Quantitating staphylococcal enterotoxin B in diverse media using a portable fibre-optic biosensor. *Analytical Biochemistry,* **233** 50-57.

Thayer, D.W. and Boyd, G. (1994) Control of enterotoxic *Bacillus cereus* on poultry or red meats and in beef gravy by gamma irradiation. *Journal of Food Protection,* **57** 758-64.

Tibana, A., Rayman, K., Aktar, M. and Szabo, R. (1987) Thermal stability of enterotoxins A, B and C in a buffered system. *Journal of Food Protection,* **50** 239-42.

Tolstoy, A. (1991) Practical monitoring of chill chain. *International Journal of Food Microbiology,* **13** 225-30.

Tranter, H.S. and Brehm, R.D. (1990) Production, purification and identification of the staphylococcal enterotoxins. *Journal of Applied Bacteriology Symposium Supplement,* **69** 109S-122S.

Turnbull, P.C.B. (1986) *Bacillus cereus* toxins, in *International Encyclopedia of Pharmacology and Therapeutics. Section 119: Pharmacology of Bacterial Toxins* (eds F. Dorner and J. Drews), Pergamon Press, Oxford, pp. 397-448.

van Netten, P., van de Moosdijk, A., van Hoensel, P., Mossel, D.A.A. and Perales, I. (1990) Psychrotrophic strains of *Bacillus cereus* producing enterotoxin. *Journal of Applied Bacteriology,* **69** 73-79.

Walls, I. and Scott, V.N. (1997) Use of predictive microbiology in microbial food safety risk assessment. *International Journal of Food Microbiology,* **36** 97-102.

Walls, I., Scott, V.N. and Bernard, D.T. (1996) Validation of predictive mathematical models describing growth of *Staphylococcus aureus*. *Journal of Food Protection,* **59** 11-15.

Weber, J.T., Hibbs, R.G., Darwish, A., Mishu, B., Corwin, A.L., Rakha, M. *et al.* (1993) A massive outbreak of type E botulism associated with traditional salted fish in Cairo. *Journal of Infectious Diseases,* **167** 451-54.

Wieneke, A.A., Roberts, D. and Gilbert, R.J. (1993) Staphylococcal food poisoning in the United Kingdom, 1969–90. *Epidemiology and Infection,* **110** 519-31.

Williams, A.P., Blackburn, C. de W. and Gibbs, P.A. (1992) Advances in the use of predictive techniques to improve the safety and extend the shelf-life of foods. *Food Science and Technology Today,* **6** 148-51.

Woolaway, M.C., Bartlett, C.L.R., Wieneke, A.A., Gilbert, R.J., Murrell, H.C. and Aureli, P. (1986) International outbreak of staphylococcal food poisoning caused by contaminated lasagne. *Journal of Hygiene,* **96** 67-73.

# 7 Mycotoxins

Keith A. Scudamore

## 7.1 Introduction

Mycotoxins are toxic secondary metabolites produced by certain species of fungi. They have a range of diverse chemical and physical properties and toxicological effects on man and animals. While many hundreds of such products have been identified, only 20 to 30 have been shown to be contaminants of human or animal food (Watson 1985). Many reviews of the subject have been published during the last 30 years and some of the most recent are Scudamore (1993), Smith *et al.* (1994), Miller (1995), Dutton (1996) and Moss (1996). The most important mycotoxins found in food are listed in Table 7.1 together with the principal fungal species responsible for their production. The Appendix provides further information about the toxicology of aflatoxins, ochratoxin A and fumonisins.

The presence of mycotoxins in raw commodities is only of concern for human health if they survive storage, processing and preparation of the food product as eaten by the consumer. Similarly, their occurrence in animal feeding stuffs only presents a risk for human health if they, or a toxic metabolite, are transferred to meat or animal products such as eggs, milk or dairy products, although they may impair animal health and affect productivity. A comprehensive reference work addressing the subject of mycotoxins in animal feeds is that by Smith and Henderson (1991).

It is of little surprise, when the diversity of chemical structures is considered, that mycotoxins exhibit a wide range of acute and chronic toxicological effects. The scourge of the Middle Ages in Europe, St Anthony's Fire, was caused by ergot alkaloids in cereals and many other animal and human diseases have been attributed to the presence of mycotoxins in food or the environment, although conclusive evidence for such associations is often difficult to obtain. Some mycotoxins are proven or suspected carcinogens, mutagens or teratogens, while others have been shown to challenge the immune systems of man and animals. This raises the possibility of increased susceptibility to other diseases without suspicion of mycotoxin involvement.

Most studies or surveys have targeted the presence of mycotoxins in human or animal foods but it has been demonstrated that intake of mycotoxins can occur as a result of their presence in fungal spores in the atmosphere (Canadian Public Health Association, 1987). This form of exposure may make a significant additional contribution to total intake under some circumstances, such as damp domestic housing (Flannigan *et al.*, 1991).

**Table 7.1**   Important mycotoxins that have been found in some food commodities and the fungi responsible

| Mycotoxin | Main fungal species | Foods infected |
|---|---|---|
| Aflatoxins $B_1$, $B_2$, $G_1$, $G_2$ | A. flavus, A. parasiticus[a] | Nuts, figs, dried fruit, spices, rice bran, maize |
| Aflatoxins $M_1$, $M_2$ | Metabolic products of aflatoxins $B_1$ and $B_2$ | Milk and dairy products |
| Sterigmatocystin | A. versicolor, A. nidulans | Cereals, cheese |
| Cyclopiazonic acid | A. flavus, P. commune | Cereals, pulses, nuts, cheese |
| Ochratoxin A | P. verrucosum, A. ochraceus | Cereals, coffee beans, field beans, beer, nuts |
| Citrinin | P. verrucosum | Cereals |
| Patulin | P. expansum, | Apple juice, fruits |
| Deoxynivalenol, nivalenol | F. graminearum, F. culmorum, F. crookwellense | Cereals |
| T-2 toxin | F. poae, F sporotrichioides | Cereals |
| Fumonisins $B_1$, $B_2$, $B_3$ | F. moniliforme, F. proliferatum | Maize, maize products |
| Zearalenone | F. graminearum, F. culmorum, F. crookwellense | Cereals |
| Moniliformin | Fusarium species | Cereals |
| Alternariol, alternariol monomethyl ether, tenuazonic acid | Alternaria alternata, A. tenuis | Fruit, tomatoes, oil seeds, cereals |

[a] aflatoxins $B_1$ and $B_2$ only.

Mycotoxins may be formed in the field before harvest following infection by any of a variety of fungal species, members of the genera *Fusarium*, *Alternaria* and *Aspergillus* being the most important. In the same way, crops are susceptible to fungal attack after harvest, during transport or when in storage, the main mycotoxigenic species being those of *Penicillium* and *Aspergillus*. There is a close relationship between fungal species and the secondary metabolites produced and it is thus important to have accurate taxonomic information based on correct identification of species according to criteria agreed internationally. Information on the fungi involved has sometimes been contradictory due to mis-identification of fungi at the species level or disagreement over the names applied to specific species. This has been especially true of the genus *Penicillium* (Frisvad, 1989). Extreme caution is required in attempting to relate fungal infection with the presence of mycotoxins as these substances can only occur if toxigenic strains of fungi are present and there are suitable conditions for fungal metabolism. Conversely, apparently mould-free products can still be contaminated with mycotoxins. The changing fungal flora throughout food production, together with the chemical stability of many of the mycotoxins, means that it is very unreliable to infer the presence or absence of mycotoxins by the fungi present at any stage in the food chain.

The production of mycotoxins is affected by many factors, including temperature, available moisture, oxygen levels, nutrients, trace elements, genetic variation between strains of specific species or competition with other organisms that may be present. The way in which fungi colonise and grow in crops in the field or infect food commodities during transport or storage, results in a highly heterogeneous distribution of any mycotoxins that subsequently develop. This has important implications when sampling: statistically based protocols are required to ensure that a representative sample is drawn. Several statistically based studies have been carried out to establish the distribution of mycotoxins in specific food commodities. The results of such studies are used to determine the number and size of samples required to be taken. Sometimes this may conflict with the practicalities involved in acquiring samples. Aflatoxins, for example, are controlled in the UK by the Aflatoxins in Nuts, Nut Products, Dried Figs and Dried Fig Product Regulations (Anon, 1992). These specify how nuts and figs should be sampled and involves taking a total sample of 10 kg of shelled peanuts comprising 30 sub-samples or 20 kg of whole figs from $20 \times 1$ kg sub-samples. This would normally be impracticable for application at retail outlets. Processed foods and drinks usually present less of a sampling problem as mycotoxins are likely be distributed in a much more homogeneous manner.

Detection of $\mu g/kg$ amounts of fungal products within a substrate that is composed of many natural products with similar chemical or physical properties presents a major challenge to the analytical chemist. Hence specific and precise analytical methods have been developed. Antibodies have been raised to most of the important mycotoxins and a range of immunologically based methods now complements, or has been incorporated into, chemically based methods such as thin-layer chromatography (TLC), high performance liquid chromatography (HPLC) and gas chromatography. Antibodies bound to activated Sepharose are commercially available as highly selective clean-up columns.

Many toxicological studies of the effects of mycotoxins in animals have been reported. However, the administration of a pure crystalline mycotoxin often leads to results at variance with those achieved when similar quantities of the crude product formed under natural conditions are given. The reason is that secondary fungal metabolism often leads to a cocktail of different metabolites which may act additively or synergistically. The use of animal and human cell lines for toxicological testing is increasingly used. Accumulation of toxicological data, and information on occurrence and food consumption, has enabled risk assessment to be carried out for the most important mycotoxins. This has led in some instances to recommended acceptable total daily intake values.

In view of the highly toxic nature of many of the mycotoxins, it is fortunate that their occurrence in food is spasmodic and often only in small amounts, at least in developed areas of the world. However, the potential for wide-scale problems exists should the appropriate circumstances arise. Low level contamination of foods by highly biologically active chemicals presents a major difficulty in assessing their true significance for man. Legislation is usually set on a national basis and is mainly restricted to the aflatoxins, of which aflatoxin $B_1$ is accepted as a potent liver carcinogen, although some countries have introduced limits for other selected mycotoxins (Food and Agriculture Organisation of the United Nations, 1997).

Fungi and mycotoxins, intimately associated with growing crops and stored foods, are difficult to eliminate, especially when they develop prior to harvest. Attention to good farming and storage practice are important factors in reducing the occurrence and amounts of mycotoxins. It is unfortunate that the less developed nations tend to have climatic conditions that encourage mould growth and mycotoxin formation and hence are faced with much greater problems, while at the same time having fewer resources to detect, control and reduce the extent of contaminated food.

In the production of food crops and consumer food products, the aim should be to reduce levels of mycotoxins to the lowest that can be technologically achieved within the existing economic constraints and with regard to risk assessment, where this has been carried out. The existence of a statutory limit requires instigation of structured sampling and analysis at agreed key points in trading and marketing.

Specific concerns often expressed by the food industry and other bodies include the means of observing legal limits, instigation of appropriate monitoring and control protocols, representative sampling, identification of products likely to be susceptible and the ability to respond to any public or media concern as, and if, the need arises. Study of mycotoxins should be carried out by a multi-disciplinary approach involving, for example, chemists, mycologists, toxicologists, veterinarians and statisticians.

## 7.2    Chemistry, toxicology and occurrence

### 7.2.1  Aflatoxins

*7.2.1.1 Chemical properties and natural occurrence.* Aflatoxins consist of a group of approximately 20 related fungal metabolites, although only aflatoxins $B_1$, $B_2$, $G_1$, $G_2$ and $M_1$ are normally found. The chemical structures of the most important aflatoxins and their derivatives are shown in Figure 7.1. Aflatoxins $B_2$ and $G_2$ are the dihydro derivatives of the parent compounds. They are produced by *Aspergillus flavus*, *A. parasiticus* and *A. nominus* and can occur in a wide range of important raw food commodities such as cereals, nuts, spices, figs and dried fruit. Although the highest concentrations are usually formed in food crops grown and stored in the warmer areas of the

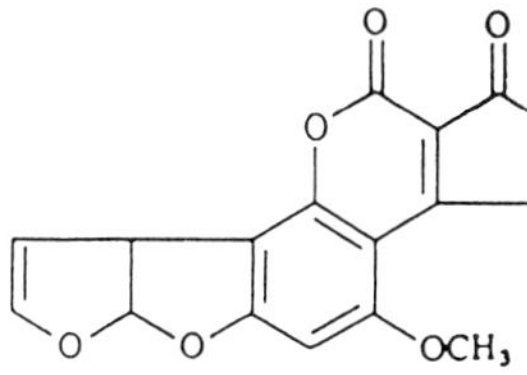

B$_1$

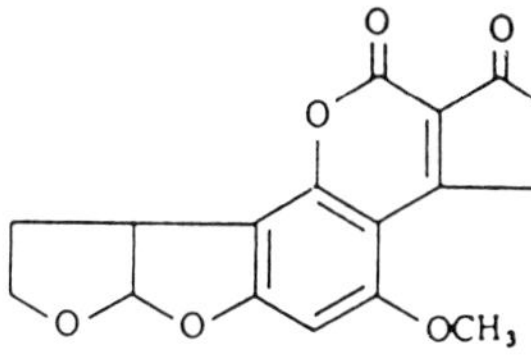

B$_2$

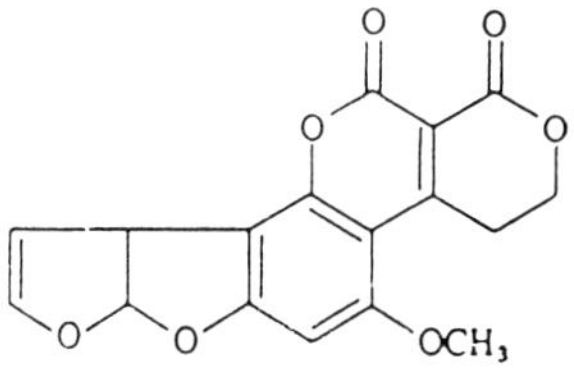

G$_1$

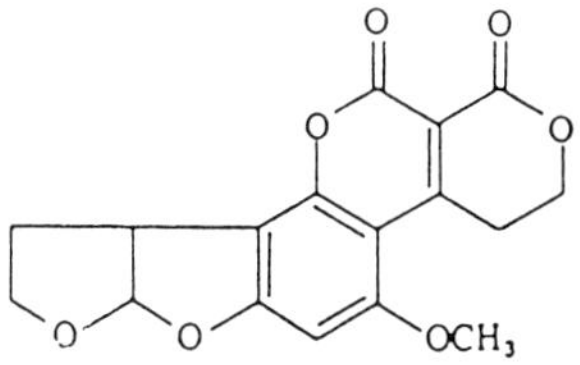

G$_2$

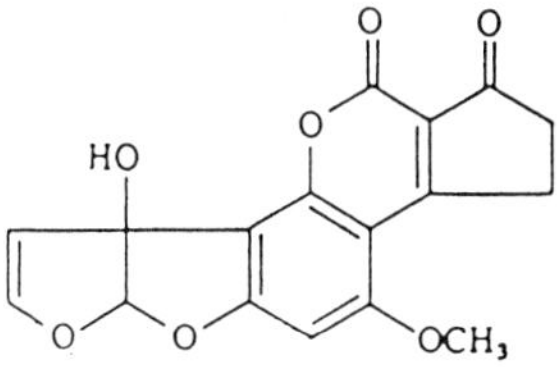

M$_1$

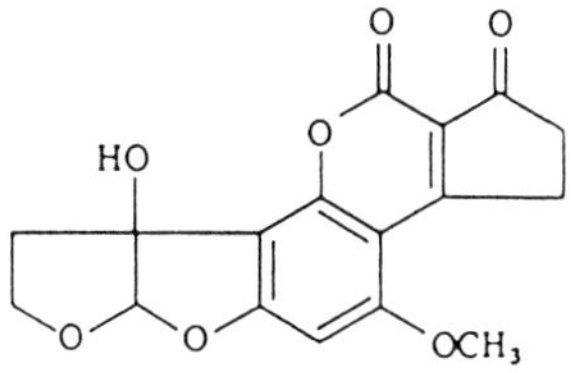

M$_2$

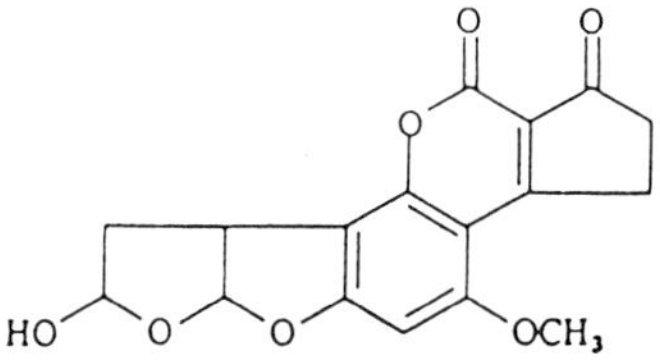

B$_{2a}$

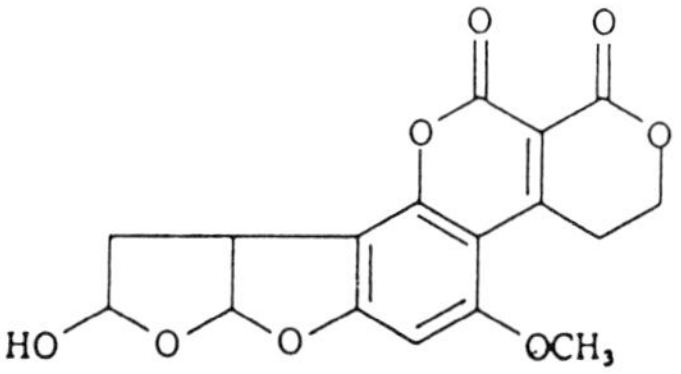

G$_{2a}$

world, the international trading of these important commodities ensures that aflatoxins are not only a problem for the producing nations but are also of concern for importing countries. Aflatoxins $M_1$ and $M_2$ are the hydroxylated metabolites of aflatoxins $B_1$ and $B_2$ and are produced when cows and other ruminants ingest feed contaminated with these mycotoxins. They are then excreted in milk and may contaminate other dairy products such as cheese and yoghurt.

Roberts (1974) reviewed the chemistry of the aflatoxins. Some of their important physical and chemical properties are given in Table 7.2. They are crystalline substances, freely soluble in moderately polar solvents such as chloroform, methanol and dimethyl sulphoxide and they dissolve in water to the extent of 10 to 20 mg/l. They fluoresce under UV irradiation, although aflatoxin $B_1$ and aflatoxin $G_1$ need derivatisation to enhance the fluorescence to a similar level to that of aflatoxins $B_2$ and $G_2$. This forms the basis for their detection by TLC or HPLC. On TLC plates the four substances are distinguished on the basis of their fluorescent colour, B standing for blue and G for green with subscripts relating to the relative chromatographic mobility. Aflatoxin $B_1$ is usually found in the highest concentration. Antibodies have been raised to the aflatoxins and immunological methods of detection based on these have been developed.

**Table 7.2**  Physical and chemical properties of some aflatoxins (WHO, 1979)

| Aflatoxin | Molecular formula | Molecular weight | Melting point | UV absorption maxima ($\varepsilon$) in methanol | |
|---|---|---|---|---|---|
| | | | | 265 nm | 360–362 nm |
| $B_1$ | $C_{17}H_{12}O_6$ | 312 | 268–269 | 12 400 | 21 800 |
| $B_2$ | $C_{17}H_{14}O_6$ | 314 | 286–289 | 12 100 | 24 000 |
| $G_1$ | $C_{17}H_{12}O_7$ | 328 | 244–246 | 9 600 | 17 700 |
| $G_2$ | $C_{17}H_{14}O_7$ | 330 | 237–240 | 8 200 | 17 100 |
| $M_1$ | $C_{17}H_{12}O_7$ | 328 | 299 | 14 150 | 21 250 (357) |
| $M_2$ | $C_{17}H_{14}O_7$ | 330 | 293 | 12 100 (264) | 22 900 (357) |
| Aflatoxicol | $C_{17}H_{14}O_6$ | 314 | 230–234 | 10 800 (261) | 14 100 (325) |

Crystalline aflatoxins are extremely stable in the absence of light and particularly UV radiation, even at temperatures in excess of 100°C. Solutions prepared in chloroform or benzene are stable for years if kept cold and in the dark. The purity and concentration of reference solutions can be calibrated using molar absorptivity data (Scott, 1990). The lactone ring makes aflatoxins susceptible to alkaline hydrolysis and processes involving ammonia or hypochlorite have been investigated as means for their removal from food commodities, although questions concerning the toxicity of the breakdown products have restricted the use of this means of eradicating aflatoxins from food and animal feeds. If alkaline treatment is mild, acidification will reverse the reaction to reform the original aflatoxin. In acid, aflatoxins $B_1$ and $G_1$ are converted to aflatoxins $B_{2a}$ and $G_{2a}$ by acid catalytic addition of water across the double bond of the furan ring. Oxidising reagents react and the molecules loss their fluorescence.

Aflatoxins are quite stable in many foods and are fairly resistant to degradation. Smith *et al.* (1994) have summarised the effectiveness of some processes in reducing concentrations of aflatoxins in food. This can be affected by many factors such as the presence of protein, pH, temperature and length of treatment.

Analytical methods have been developed mainly based on TLC, HPLC or enzyme-linked immunosorbent assay. Extraction with aqueous acetonitrile or methanol, followed by clean-up of the extract solutions using immunoaffinity columns, for example, provides sensitive and selective results for a wide range of foods and animal feeding stuffs (Sharman and Gilbert, 1991). Limits of detection below 1 μg/kg can be routinely achieved with an analytical precision of ±30%.

*7.2.1.2 Toxicology.* Aflatoxins are both acutely and chronically toxic. Aflatoxin $B_1$ is one of the most potent hepatocarcinogens known (Fishbein, 1979) and hence the long-term chronic exposure of extremely low levels of aflatoxins in the diet is an important consideration for human health. In the temperate, developed areas of the world, acute poisoning in animals is rare and in man is now extremely unlikely. The outbreak of so-called 'turkey-X disease', which caused the deaths of 100 000 turkeys and other poultry in the UK in 1960, was caused by extremely high concentrations of aflatoxins in imported groundnut meal (Allcroft and Carnaghan, 1962). This alerted industry and governments to the potentially devastating effects of mycotoxins, particularly the aflatoxins.

Acute aflatoxin toxicity has been demonstrated in a wide range of mammals, fish and birds; rabbits, dogs, primates, ducks, turkeys and trout are all highly susceptible. Age, sex and nutritional status all affect the degree of toxicity. Young animals are particularly susceptible and males more than females. For most species the $LD_{50}$ is between 0.5 and 10 mg/kg bodyweight (bw). The liver is the principal target organ although the site of the hepatic effect varies with species. Effects on the lungs, myocardium and kidneys have also been observed and aflatoxin can accumulate in the brain.

Teratogenic effects following administration of high doses of aflatoxin have been reported in some species. A high proportion of malformed, dead or resorbed foetuses was reported in hamsters following single intraperitoneal doses of 4 mg/kg aflatoxin $B_1$ on day 8 of gestation: only 50% of foetuses from the aflatoxin dams compared to 85% of the controls were normal (Elis and Di Paola, 1967). Teratogenic effects have also been reported in chicks and mice but no effects were reported in pigs given feed containing 0.45 mg/kg aflatoxin $B_1$.

Acute poisoning of man by aflatoxins does occur occasionally in some areas of the world. Cases of human aflatoxicosis have been reported sporadically, mainly in Africa or Asia. The majority of reported cases involve consumption of contaminated cereals, most frequently maize, rice or cassava, or cereal products such as pasta or peanut meal (see, for example, Oyelami *et al.*, 1996). A classic case occurred during a Chinese festival in Malaysia in which approximately 40 persons were affected and 13 children died (Chao *et al.*, 1991) after eating noodles highly contaminated with aflatoxin and boric acid. Symptoms included vomiting, diarrhoea, pyrexia and abdominal pain. A Reye-like symptom and coma occurred about 8 hours after ingestion and death between 2 and 9 days after onset. High levels of aflatoxin were found on autopsy in liver, lung, kidney, heart, brain and spleen. Aflatoxin may not always be the primary cause of death in these acute cases. Autopsy brain (cerebrum) specimens from 18 kwashiorkor children and 19 other children who had died from a variety of other diseases in Nigeria (Oyelami *et al.*, 1995) showed aflatoxin present in 81% of the cases (maximum total aflatoxin >100 µg/kg).

Aflatoxins have been implicated in sub-acute and chronic effects in humans. These effects include primary liver cancer, chronic hepatitis, jaundice, hepatomegaly and cirrhosis through repeated ingestion of low levels of aflatoxin. It is also considered that aflatoxins may play a role in a number of diseases including Reye's syndrome (Shank *et al.*, 1971), kwashiorkor (Coulter *et al.*, 1986) and hepatitis (Krishnamachari *et al.*, 1975; Ngindu *et al.*, 1982). Aflatoxins can also effect the immune system (Pier, 1991).

Aflatoxin $B_1$ is a potent mutagen causing chromosomal aberrations in a variety of plant, animal and human cells. It causes gene mutation in bacterial test systems following activation by rat or human S9 preparation and induces recessive lethal mutations in *Drosophila melanogaster*. The carcinogenicity of aflatoxins was first demonstrated in 1961 when rats fed the same peanut meal implicated in turkey-X disease developed hepatomas (Lancaster *et al.*, 1961). The carcinogenicity and mutagenicity of aflatoxins $B_1$, $G_1$ and $M_1$ are considered to arise as the result of the formation of a reactive epoxide at the 8,9 position of the terminal furan ring and its subsequent covalent binding to nucleic acid. The carcinogenicity of aflatoxin $B_1$ has been studied in at least 12 different species. Primary hepatocellular carcinomas were predominant, although primary tumours were also induced at the site of injection, colon, lung, kidney, skin (by topical application), Harderian gland in the hamster, nervous system, trachea, bones, pancreas, gall bladder and stomach (Sieber *et al.*, 1979; Busby and Wogan, 1984; Garner and Dingley, 1993). A linear dose–response relationship has been demonstrated for aflatoxin $B_1$ in at least two animal species down to doses of less than 0.1 µg/kg bw per day. Although aflatoxin $G_1$ has been tested less extensively, it appears to be toxicologically similar to aflatoxin $B_1$. It is a slightly less effective liver carcinogen but a slightly more potent kidney carcinogen.

The complete elimination of aflatoxins in human and animal food, while desirable, is extremely unlikely as they have the potential to arise in a wide range of agricultural products. Risk assessments have been carried out for aflatoxin (see, for example, IARC, 1993). Because aflatoxin $B_1$ is a geno-toxic carcinogen, most agencies, including the Joint Expert Committee on Food Additives (JECFA) and the US Food and Drug Administration, have not set a tolerable daily intake (TDI) figure. Kuiper-Goodman (1995) has discussed the application in Canada of a no-observed-adverse-effect level (NOAEL) to aflatoxin $B_1$ in order to give guidance on what is an acceptable intake for human consumers. In common with other dietary carcinogens, it is generally accepted that amounts in food should be reduced to the lowest levels that are technologically possible. Regulations have been set for human food and animal feed in many countries (Food and Agriculture Organisation of the United Nations, 1997). In the UK regulation of aflatoxin $B_1$ in animal feeding stuffs (Anon, 1982) has been effective in steadily reducing amounts of aflatoxin $M_1$ in milk, as shown by regular surveillance (Ministry of Agriculture, Fisheries and Food, 1980, 1987, 1993).

### 7.2.2  Sterigmatocystin

*7.2.2.1 Chemical properties and natural occurrence.* Sterigmatocystin is a toxic metabolite that is closely related in structure to the aflatoxins. It con-sists of a xanthone nucleus attached to a bifuran structure. Its structure and those of some related metabolites are shown in Figure 7.2. This mycotoxin is mainly produced by the fungi *Aspergillus nidulans* and *A. versicolor*. Sterigmatocystin has been found in mouldy grain, green coffee beans and cheese, although information on its occurrence in foods is limited. It appears to occur much less frequently than the aflatoxins, although analytical meth-ods for its determination are not as sensitive and it is likely that small con-centrations in food commodities may not always be detected.

| | $R_1$ | $R_2$ | $R_3$ |
|---|---|---|---|
| Sterigmatocystin | H | H | H |
| O-Methyl sterigmatocystin | $CH_3$ | H | H |
| Aspertoxin | $CH_3$ | OH | H |
| 5-Methoxy sterigmatocystin | H | H | $OCH_3$ |

**Figure 7.2**  Structures of sterigmatocystin and related compounds

Sterigmatocystin's physical properties are summarised in Table 7.3 together with those of several other mycotoxins reviewed in subsequent parts of this chapter. This particular mycotoxin crystallises as pale yellow needles and is readily soluble in methanol, ethanol, acetonitrile, benzene and chloroform. It reacts with hot ethanolic KOH and is methylated by methyl sulphate and methyl iodide. Methanol or ethanol in acid produces dihydro-ethoxysterigmatocystin.

*7.2.2.2 Toxicology.* The toxic effects of sterigmatocystin are much the same as those of aflatoxin $B_1$ (Ueno and Ueno, 1978). It is thus considered to be a potent carcinogen, mutagen and teratogen. The $LD_{50}$ in mice is in excess of 800 mg/kg. The 10 day $LD_{50}$ in Wistar rats is 166 mg/kg in males, 120 mg/kg in females and 60 to 65 mg/kg for intraperitoneal (ip) administration in males. The ip 10 day $LD_{50}$ for vervet monkeys is 32 mg/kg.

Chronic symptoms include induction of hepatomas in rats, pulmonary tumours in mice, and renal lesions and alterations in the liver and kidneys of African Green monkeys. Rats fed 5 to 10 mg/kg of sterigmatocystin for two years showed a 90% incidence of liver tumours (Ohtsubo *et al.*, 1978). It has been suggested that sterigmatocystin is about one tenth as potent a carcinogen as aflatoxin $B_1$. The acute toxicity, carcinogenicity and metabolism of sterigmatocystin have been compared with those for aflatoxin and several other hepatotoxic mycotoxins by Wannemacher *et al.* (1991).

Toxic effects of sterigmatocystin-fed laboratory animals have included kidney and liver damage and diarrhoea (Ciegler and Vesonder, 1983). Cattle exhibiting bloody diarrhoea, loss of milk production and in some cases death were found to have ingested feed containing *A. versicolor* and high levels of sterigmatocystin of about 8 mg/kg (Vesonder and Horn, 1985).

### 7.2.3 Cyclopiazonic acid

*7.2.3.1 Chemical properties and natural occurrence.* Cyclopiazonic acid is a toxic indole tetramic acid (Figure 7.3) that was first isolated from *Penicillium cyclopium* (Holzapfel, 1968) and subsequently from other *Penicillium* species, *Aspergillus flavus* (Luk *et al.*, 1977) and *A. versicolor* (Ohmono *et al.*, 1973). It has been detected in naturally contaminated mixed feeds, maize, peanuts, cheese and other foods and feeds. Methods for its detection are less sensitive than for mycotoxins such as aflatoxin $B_1$ and ochratoxin A. Cyclopiazonic acid is an optically active colourless crystalline compound that is soluble in chloroform, dichloromethane, methanol, acetonitrile and sodium bicarbonate. It reacts with 0.1 N sulphuric acid in methanol, gives a blue–violet Ehrlich colour reaction and an orange-red reaction with ferric chloride.

**Table 7.3** Physical properties of some mycotoxins

| Mycotoxin | Molecular formula | Molecular weight | Melting point | UV absorption (nm) |
|---|---|---|---|---|
| Sterigmatocystin | $C_{18}H_{12}O_6$ | 324 | 246 | 15 200 (325) benzene |
| Cyclopiazonic acid | $C_{20}H_{20}N_2O_3$ | 336 | 246 | 20 400 (282) methanol |
| Ochratoxin A | $C_{20}H_{18}ClNO_6$ | 403 | 169 | 36 800 (213), 6400 (332), ethanol |
| Citrinin | $C_{13}H_{14}O_5$ | 250 | 179 | 22 280 (222) 8279 (253) 4710 (319) ethanol |
| Patulin | $C_7H_6O_4$ | 154 | 111 | 14 600 (275) ethanol |
| Deoxynivalenol | $C_{15}H_{20}O_6$ | 296 | 131–135 | Maximum at 218 ethanol |
| T-2 toxin | $C_{24}H_{34}O_9$ | 466 | 150–151 | Maximum at 187 cyclohexane |
| Diacetoxyscirpenol | $C_{19}H_{26}O_7$ | 366 | 162–164 | None |
| Fumonisin $B_1$ | $C_{34}H_{59}NO_{15}$ | 721 | Powder | Low |
| Fumonisin $B_2$ | $C_{34}H_{59}NO_{14}$ | 705 | Powder | Low |
| Zearalenone | $C_{18}H_{22}O_5$ | 318 | 164 | 29 700 (236), 13910 (274), 6020, (316) ethanol |
| Moniliformin | $C_4HO_3Na$ | 120 | | |
| Tenuazonic acid | $C_{10}H_{15}NO_3$ | 197 | Oil | 5000 (218), 12 500 (277) acid methanol; 11 500 (240), |
| | | | | 14 500 (280) methanol |
| Altenuene | $C_{15}H_{16}O_6$ | 292 | 190–191 | 30 000 (240), 10000 (278), 6600 (319) ethanol |
| Alternariol | $C_{14}H_{10}O_5$ | 258 | 350 | 38 000 (258) ethanol |
| Alternariol monomethyl ether | $C_{15}H_{12}O_5$ | 272 | 267 | |

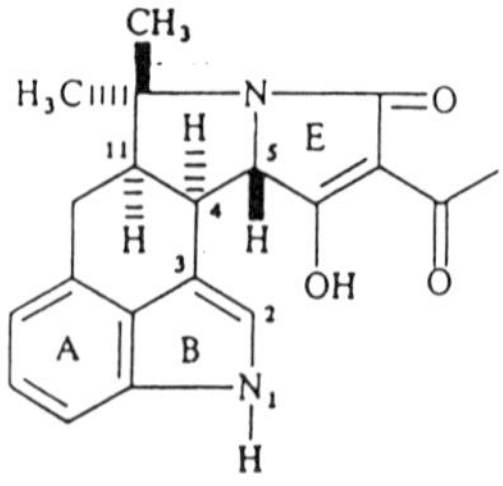

Cyclopiazonic acid

**Figure 7.3**  Structure of cyclopiazonic acid

*7.2.3.2 Toxicology.* Cyclopiazonic acid only appears to be toxic when present in high concentrations. Purchase (1971) found that cyclopiazonic acid was a neurotoxin when injected intraperitoneally into rats; the $LD_{50}$ in male rats was 2.3 mg/kg. Oral administration produced no convulsions, $LD_{50}$ values for rats were 36 mg/kg and 63 mg/kg for males and females respectively, and lesions in the liver, kidney, spleen and other organs were observed (Purchase, 1971). Effects reported include decreased weight gain, diarrhoea, dehydration, depression hyperaesthesia, hypokinesis, convulsion and death. It has been found mutagenic for *Salmonella typhimurium* TA98 and TA100 in the Ames assay.

Cyclopiazonic acid can co-occur with aflatoxins (Takashi *et al.*, 1992) and may enhance the overall toxic effect when this happens (Cole, 1986). There is a dearth of human exposure data. This precludes an assessment of possible health effects. However, 'Kodua' poisoning in India resulting from ingestion of contaminated millet seeds has been linked to this toxin. It has similar pharmacological properties to the anti-psychotic drugs chlorpromazine and reserpine in mice and rabbits. Near-lethal doses of 11 to 14 mg/kg bw induce continuous involuntary tremors and convulsions. It may be able to produce similar effects in humans.

*7.2.4  Ochratoxin A*

*7.2.4.1 Chemical properties and natural occurrence.* The ochratoxins are a group of structurally related compounds of which ochratoxin A is the most important and most commonly occurring. They consist of a polyketide-derived dihydroiso-coumarin moiety linked through the 12-carboxy group to phenylalanine (Figure 7.4). Ochratoxin A is produced by certain strains of

*Aspergillus ochraceus* and related species, and by *Penicillium verrucosum*. There are literature reports of other *Penicillia* producing ochratoxin A but most of these are probably as the result of mis-identification. *A. ochraceus* occurs principally in tropical climates while *P. verrucosum* is a common storage fungus in temperate areas such as Canada, eastern Europe, Denmark, parts of South America and the UK. Ochratoxin A often occurs in stored cereals and has been found in other foods including coffee (Tsubouchi *et al.*, 1988), beer (Payen *et al.*, 1983), dried fruit (Ozay and Alperden, 1991), wine (Zimmerli and Dick, 1996), cocoa (Ministry of Agriculture, Fisheries and Food, 1980) and nuts (Cooper *et al.*, 1982). A comprehensive review of the literature on the world-wide occurrence of ochratoxin has been carried out by Speijers and van Egmond (1993). Sensitive and reliable analytical methods have been developed with detection limits better than 1 µg/kg.

Ochratoxin A is a colourless crystalline compound, exhibiting blue fluorescence under UV light. It crystallises from benzene to give a product melting at 90°C containing one molecule of benzene. This can be removed under vacuum at 120°C to give a product melting at 168°C. It crystallises in a pure form from xylene. The sodium salt is soluble in water. As the acid, it is moderately soluble in polar organic solvents such as chloroform, methanol and acetonitrile, and dissolves in dilute aqueous sodium bicarbonate. On acid hydrolysis it yields phenylalanine and an optically active lactone acid, ochratoxin α. Reaction in methanol and hydrochloric acid yields the methyl ester, while methylation with diazomethane gives the *o*-methyl methyl ester. It can be stored in ethanol for at least a year under refrigeration and protected from light.

Ochratoxin A is a moderately stable molecule and will survive most food processing to some extent. This has been reviewed by Scott (1996) and in a series of papers covering its fate during malting and brewing (Baxter, 1996), during breadmaking (Subirade, 1996), during processing in cereals (Alldrick, 1996), during processing of coffee (Viani, 1996), during processing of meat products (Gareis, 1996) and during processing in animal feed (Scudamore, 1996). In biological systems, it will bind to serum albumin.

*7.2.4.2 Toxicology.* Ochratoxin A is a potent toxin affecting mainly the kidneys, in which it can cause both acute and chronic lesions. However, its dechloro derivative, ochratoxin B, is non-toxic. Ochratoxin acts principally on the first part of the proximal tubules in the kidney and induces a defect in the anion transport mechanism on the brush order of the proximal convoluted tubular cells and basolateral membranes (Endou *et al.*, 1986). A nephrotoxic effect has been demonstrated in all mammalian species tested to date (Harwig *et al.*, 1983). In acute toxicity studies $LD_{50}$ values vary greatly in different species, the dog being especially susceptible (Table 7.4).

**Table 7.4**  LD$_{50}$ values for ochratoxin A in various species
(Kuiper Goodman and Scott, 1989)

| Species | LD$_{50}$ values, (mg/kg bw) | | |
| --- | --- | --- | --- |
| | Oral | ip | iv |
| Mouse | 46–58.3 | 22–40.1 | 25.7–33.8 |
| Rat | 20–30.3 | 12.6 | 12.7 |
| Rat neonate | 3.9 | — | — |
| Dog | 0.2 | — | — |
| Pig | 1 | — | — |
| Chicken | 3.3 | — | — |

Many feeding trials lasting up to 90 days or more have examined the progressive effects of ochratoxin A on kidney function and damage through prolonged exposure. The sub-acute and sub-chronic effects in these trials have been summarised by Kuiper-Goodman and Scott (1989).

It is now well established that ochratoxin A is a potent teratogen in mice, rats, hamsters and chickens, but not in pigs when fed to sows during early pregnancy. The central nervous system is one of the most susceptible targets and is affected at the time of early organogenesis. The results of teratogenic and reproductive studies have been summarised by Kuiper-Goodman and Scott (1989).

Several studies have shown that ochratoxin A affects the immune system in a number of mammalian species. Studies on swine fed a diet containing 2.5 mg/kg ochratoxin A for 35 days led the authors to conclude that it may suppress cell-mediated immune response in growing pigs (Harvey *et al.*, 1992). Stormer and Lea (1995) studied the effects of ochratoxin A on early and late event human T-cell proliferation. They concluded that the low impact of the toxin on protein synthesis in activated cells may indicate that mechanisms other than just a general inhibition of protein synthesis are operating.

There is now mounting evidence that ochratoxin A is a genotoxic carcinogen (Dirheimer, 1996). Creppy *et al.* (1985) showed that ochratoxin A causes DNA single-strand breaks in mouse spleen cells. These breaks were also found *in vivo* in rat kidney and liver after gavage treatment for 12 weeks at a level equivalent to dietary concentrations of 2 mg/kg in food (Kane *et al.*, 1986). Other recent studies have further demonstrated genotoxicity (Pfohl-Leszkowicz *et al.*, 1993; Degen *et al.*, 1994; Föllmann *et al.*, 1995).

Human exposure to ochratoxin A has been clearly demonstrated by its detection in blood (Bauer *et al.*, 1986; Breitholtz *et al.*, 1991) and breast milk (Miraglia *et al.*, 1993). Risk assessments have been carried out by Kuiper-Goodman and Scott (1989), Kuiper-Goodman *et al.* (1993), Kuiper-Goodman (1996) and by a Nordic group on food toxicology (The Nordic Working Group on Food Toxicology and Risk Evaluation, 1991). The presence of ochratoxin A in foodstuffs is clearly undesirable, although few countries have introduced statutory control to date (Food and Agriculture Organisation of the United Nations, 1997).

### 7.2.5 Citrinin

*7.2.5.1 Chemical properties and natural occurrence.* Citrinin was first isolated as a pure compound from a culture of *Penicillium citrinum* in 1931. Its structure is shown in Figure 7.4. Since 1931 a number of species of *Penicillium* have been reported to produce citrinin (Frisvad, 1989) including *P. verrucosum*. Hence, citrinin often occurs together with ochratoxin A, but is not always detected. This may not be the real situation as citrinin is more readily lost in analytical procedures and is sought much less frequently. In addition, *Aspergillus terreus, A. carneus* and *A. niveus* may also produce this mycotoxin. Citrinin has mainly been found in rice and other cereals.

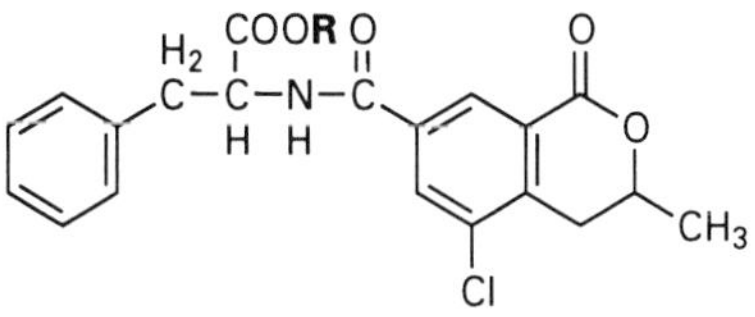

| | R |
|---|---|
| Ochratoxin A | H |
| Ochratoxin A methyl ester | $CH_3$ |
| Ochratoxin A ethyl ester | $CH_2CH_3$ |

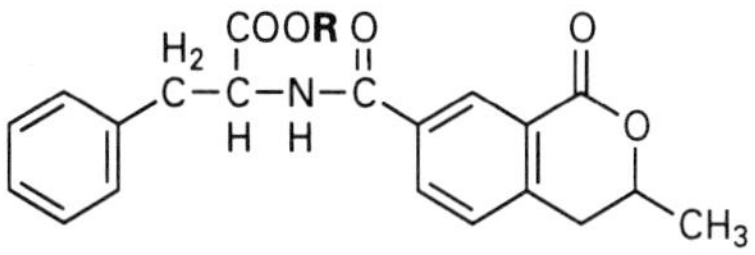

| | R |
|---|---|
| Ochratoxin B | H |
| Ochratoxin B methyl ester | $CH_3$ |
| Ochratoxin B ethyl ester | $CH_2CH_3$ |

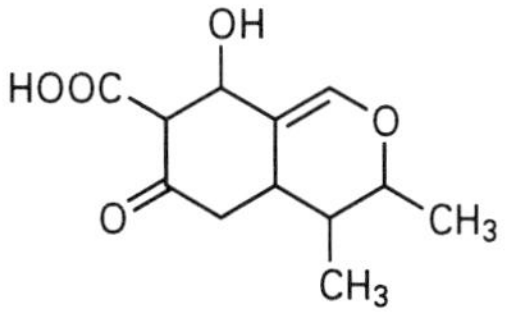

Citrinin

**Figure 7.4** Structures of ochratoxin A and B, related compounds and citrinin.

Citrinin crystallises as lemon-coloured needles melting at 172°C. It is sparingly soluble in water but soluble in dilute sodium hydroxide, sodium carbonate or sodium acetate, in methanol, acetonitrile, ethanol and most other polar organic solvents. Some photodecomposition occurs in fluorescent light both in solution and in the solid state. It can be degraded in acid or alkaline solution. Colour reactions include brown with ferric chloride, green with titanium chloride and deep wine-red with hydrogen peroxide followed by alkali. Mono-acetate, diethyl, methyl ester and dihydro derivatives can be prepared.

There is little information on the fate of citrinin during processing but it is likely to be degraded by heat and alkali. However, even though citrinin may be destroyed, toxic breakdown products have been demonstrated (Trivedi *et al.*, 1993).

*7.2.5.2 Toxicology.* The $LD_{50}$ of citrinin was reported as about 50 mg/kg for oral administration to the rat, 35 to 58 mg/kg (ip) to the mouse and 19 mg/kg (ip) to the rabbit. Citrinin causes kidney damage and mild liver damage in the form of fatty infiltration. A review of citrinin toxicity is given by Scott (1977). Citrinin often co-occurs with ochratoxin and has been implicated in mycotoxic nephropathy of pigs (Krogh *et al.*, 1973). It seems unlikely that citrinin presents much risk to humans.

*7.2.6 Patulin*

*7.2.6.1 Chemical properties and natural occurrence.* Patulin is a polyketide lactone (Figure 7.5) produced by certain species of *Penicillium, Aspergillus* and *Byssochlamys* growing on fruit, including apples, pears, grapes and melons. In whole fruits, visual inspection will usually identify poor quality items. The principal risk arises when unsound fruit is used for the production of juices and other processed products. It has also been reported in vegetables, cereal grains and silage. *P. expansum* appears to be the mould usually responsible for patulin in apple juice.

Patulin

**Figure 7.5**   Structure of patulin.

Patulin can be isolated as colourless to white crystals from ethereal abstracts that have no optical activity. It melts at about 110°C and sublimes in high vacuum at 70 to 100°C. It is soluble in water, methanol, ethanol, acetone and ethyl or amyl acetate, and less soluble in diethyl ether and benzene. It undergoes all the reactions expected of a secondary alcohol, reduces warm Fehling's solution and decolourises potassium permanganate. It is stable in acid solutions but can be decomposed by boiling in 2 N sulphuric acid for 6 hours. It is susceptible to alkaline hydrolysis, reduced by sulphur dioxide and by fermentation. Thus when sulphur dioxide is used as a food preservative in fruit juice or other foods, patulin will be broken down. It is not usually found in alcoholic beverages or vinegar but has been found in 'sweet' cider in which unfermented apple juice is added to the cider. In acid conditions, it is relatively stable to heat processes up to about 100°C. Chloroform is preferred for storage of patulin solutions as it tends to decompose in distilled water.

Analysis of patulin is usually by HPLC. The small molecular size of patulin has hindered the raising of antibodies; rapid tests based on immunological principles have not been developed to date for this mycotoxin.

*7.2.6.2 Toxicology.* Patulin possesses wide-spectrum antibiotic properties and has been tested in humans to evaluate its ability to treat the common cold. However, its effectiveness has never been proven and its use to treat medical conditions has not been pursued because it irritates the stomach, causing nausea and vomiting. In acute and short-term studies patulin causes gastrointestinal hyperaemia, distension haemorrhage and ulceration.

For patulin, the $LD_{50}$ for the rat has been reported as 15 mg/kg bw (Broom *et al.*, 1944) and 25 mg/kg after subcutaneous injection (Katzman *et al.*, 1944). Death was usually caused by pulmonary oedema. Lungs were oedematous, with the alveoli filled with protein-rich fluid and many leucocytes. The pulmonary vessels were congested but haemorrhages were few. Hepatic and intestinal blood vessels were congested and in sections of the kidneys there was slight congestion, mild degeneration of the tubular epithelium and a few loci of haemorrhages. Patulin injected in large amounts over a two month period was carcinogenic, resulting in induction of sarcomas at the injection site (Dickens and Jones, 1961). In long-term studies at lower dose levels these effects were not observed. Patulin has also been shown to be immunotoxic and neurotoxic. The International Agency for Research on Cancer (IARC, 1986) concluded that no evaluation could be made of the carcinogenicity of patulin to humans and that there was inadequate evidence in experimental animals. Based on reproduction and long-term carcinogenicity studies in rats and mice the Joint Expert Committee on Food Additives allocated a Provisional Tolerable Weekly Intake of 7 μg/kg bw.

Patulin is not usually covered by statutory regulation but quality is sometimes controlled by the setting of a 'guideline' or a 'recommended' maximum concentration. This is commonly set at 50 µg/l or µg/kg.

### 7.2.7 Trichothecenes

*7.2.7.1 Chemical properties and natural occurrence.* The 12,13-epoxytrichothecenes (Figure 7.6) are a group of related and biologically active mycotoxins produced by certain species of *Fusarium*, such as *F. poae*, *F. sporotrichioides*, *F. culmorum* and *F. graminearum*. They are often classified as Group A and Group B compounds depending on whether they have a side chain on the C-7 atom. The most commonly reported Group A trichothecenes include T-2 toxin, HT-2 toxin, neosolaniol, monoacetoxyscirpenol and diacetoxyscirpenol (DAS; Figure 7.6). These are highly soluble in ethyl acetate, acetone, chloroform, methylene chloride and diethyl ether. The Group B trichothecenes, deoxynivalenol (commonly called DON or vomitoxin), nivalenol, 3-acetyldeoxynivalenol, 15-acetyldeoxynivalenol, fusarenone-X, scirpentriol and T-2 tetraol are highly hydroxylated and relatively polar, being soluble in methanol, acetonitrile and ethanol.

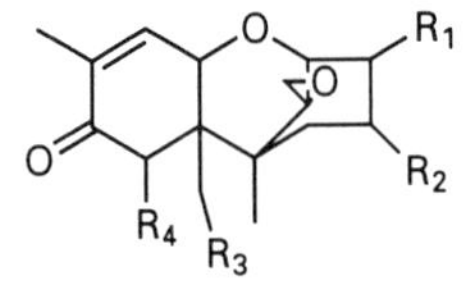

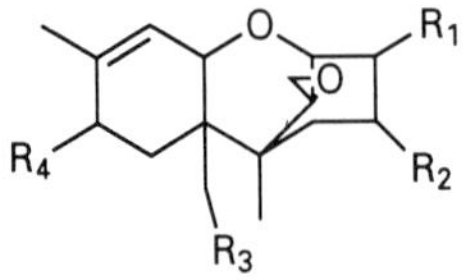

| Tricothecenes | $R_1$ | $R_2$ | $R_3$ | $R_4$ |
|---|---|---|---|---|
| nivalenol | OH | OH | OH | OH |
| deoxynivalenol | OH | H | OH | OH |
| Fusarenon | OH | OAc | OH | OH |
| T-2 toxin | OH | OAc | OAc | OC(O)CH₂CHMe₂ |
| HT-2 toxin | OH | OH | OAc | OC(O)CH₂CHMe₂ |
| DAS | OH | OAc | OAc | H |
| neosolaniol | OH | OAc | OAc | OH |

**Figure 7.6**  Structures of some trichothecene mycotoxins.

Another group of trichothecenes that are generally more acutely toxic than T-2 toxin is known as the macrocyclic trichothecenes. These are produced by mould species such as *Stachybotrys atra* and include the satratoxins, verrucarins and roridins, which may be produced in hay and straw stored under unsatisfactory conditions. However, there is little evidence that these compounds occur in human food, although the presence of macrocyclic trichothecenes in airborne fungal spores may contribute to some forms of sick building syndrome (Croft *et al.*, 1986).

All trichothecenes containing an ester group are hydrolysed to their respective parent alcohols when treated with alkali. A dilute solution of potassium carbonate, sodium hydroxide or ammonium hydroxide hydrolyses T-2 toxin and neosolaniol to T-2 tetraol and diacetoxy- and monoacetoxy-scirpenol to scirpentriol. Many of the alcohols are unaffected, even by hot dilute alkali. Trichothecenes are thus chemically stable and can persist for long periods once formed. Prolonged boiling in water or under highly acidic conditions causes a skeletal rearrangement due to opening of the epoxide ring. Owing to the hindered nature of the epoxide and stability of the ring system, reactions of the trichothecenes usually proceed in a manner predictable from sound chemical principles. For example, primary and secondary hydroxyl groups are easily oxidised to the aldehyde and ketone derivatives by reagents such as $CrO_3$-$H_2SO_4$ in acetone, $CrO_3$-pyridine and $CrO_3$-acetic acid.

Most trichothecenes, with the exception of some of the macrocyclics such as roridin A and verrucarin, possess little absorption in the UV, other than end absorption. Because of this, together with the complexity of mixtures that can occur naturally, the analytical method of choice is often gas chromatography/mass spectrometry. Both HPLC and TLC can be used but are much less selective and sensitive. Concentrated sulphuric acid and *p*-anisaldehyde are often used to give characteristic colours which can be used for detection by TLC (Mirocha *et al.*, 1977).

Trichothecenes occur in cereals and other food commodities. There are many reports of deoxynivalenol and nivalenol in cereals although T-2 toxin and diacetoxyscirpenol are found much less frequently. Surveillance commonly targets deoxynivalenol only although other trichothecenes are likely to be present.

*7.2.7.2 Toxicology.* The acute toxicity of the trichothecenes varies considerably (Table 7.5). T-2 toxin and the macrocyclic mycotoxins are far more toxic than deoxynivalenol but fortunately are not often found in food. Acute trichothecene toxicity is characterised by gastrointestinal disturbances, such as vomiting, diarrhoea and inflammation, dermal irritation, feed refusal, abortion, anaemia and leukopenia. This group of toxins is acutely cytotoxic and strongly immunosuppressive.

**Table 7.5**    LD$_{50}$ values for mice (intraperitoneal route)
            for some trichothecenes

| Trichothecene | LD$_{50}$ (mg/kg bw) |
| --- | --- |
| Deoxynivalenol | 70 |
| Diacetoxyscirpenol | 23 |
| Neosolaniol | 14.5 |
| HT-2 toxin | 9.0 |
| T-2 toxin | 5.2 |
| Nivalenol | 4.1 |
| Verrucarin A | 0.5 |

When given orally or by intraperitoneal injection the trichothecenes are acutely toxic at low concentrations. Dosed animals become listless or inactive and develop diarrhoea and rectal haemorrhaging. Necrotic lesions may develop in the mouth parts, the mucosal epithelium of the stomach and small intestine erodes, accompanied by haemorrhage, which may develop into severe gastroenteritis, followed by death. In larger animals, massive haemorrhages develop in the lumen of the small intestine (Pier *et al.*, 1980). The cells of the bone marrow, lymph nodes and intestines undergo a pathological degeneration. The trichothecenes have not been shown to be mutagenic or carcinogenic but do inhibit DNA and protein synthesis.

Deoxynivalenol is a common contaminant of cereals and causes vomiting in pigs at relatively low concentrations. However, pigs are very sensitive to its presence and will reject contaminated feed, effectively limiting any further toxic effects. Deoxynivalenol is, however, immunosuppressive in low concentrations and this may be more important than its low acute toxicity. Because of the number of closely related metabolites likely to occur in combination in foods or animal feeds, the toxicology is complex with both synergistic and antagonistic effects. This has been discussed by Miller (1995).

Alimentary toxic aleukia (ATA) is the most common human trichothecene mycotoxicosis. T-2 toxin is thought to have contributed to the epidemiology of ATA in Russia which was responsible for widespread disease and many deaths. Continuous exposure to trichothecenes results in skin rashes, which may proceed to necrotic lesions.

### 7.2.8  Fumonisins

*7.2.8.1 Chemical properties and natural occurrence.* The fumonisins (Figure 7.7) are a group of closely related mycotoxins that often occur in maize, the most important compound being fumonisin B$_1$. They are polar metabolites obtained from several species of *Fusarium*, including *F. moniliforme, F. proliferatum, F. nygamai, F. anthophilum, F. dlamini* and *F. napiforme*. Their structures are based on a long hydroxylated hydrocarbon chain. Two hydroxyl groups are esterified to two propane-1,2,3-tricarboxylic acids.

Fumonisin $B_1$ differs from fumonisin $B_2$ in that it has an extra hydroxyl group at the 10 position. Fumonisins contain four free carboxyl groups and an amino group, which enables their solubility in water and polar organic solvents such as methanol. Aqueous methanol or acetonitrile can be used for extraction from maize and maize products. Their insolubility in many organic solvents partly explains the difficulty in their original identification.

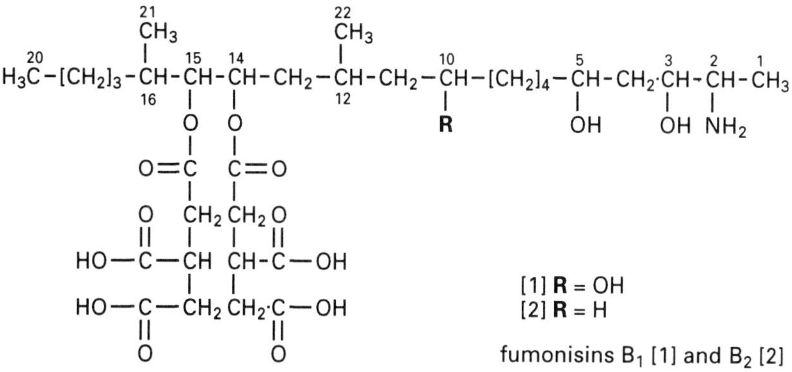

fumonisins $B_1$ [1] and $B_2$ [2]

[1] R = OH
[2] R = H

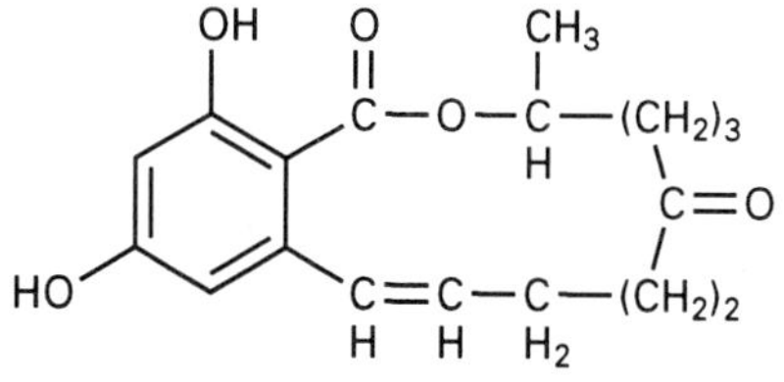

Zearalenone

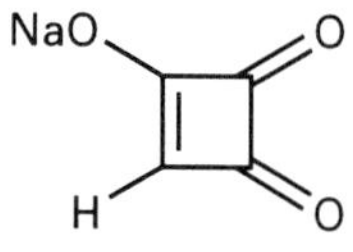

Monoliformin

**Figure 7.7** Structures of fumonisins, zearalenone and moniliformin

Fumonisins $B_1$ and $B_2$ are stable in methanol if stored at $-18°C$ but steadily degrade at $25°C$ and above. In acetonitrile they were found to be stable over a six-month period at $25°C$ (Visconti *et al.*, 1993). Lack of a suitable chromophore in the molecule means that it must be derivatised with reagents such as *p*-anisaldehyde, fluorescamine or *o*-phthaldialdehyde to allow detection by HPLC. A recent review of the occurrence and toxicity of the fumonisins is that of Dutton (1996).

Fumonisins are quite stable and are not broken down by moderate heat (Bordson *et al.*, 1995). However, no fumonisins were detected in tortilla flour made by treatment with calcium hydroxide (nixtamilisation) and it has been suggested that this process degrades fumonisins (Sydenham *et al.*, 1991). Scott and Lawrence (1994) succeeded in obtaining about 80% reduction by heating at higher temperatures. However, caution is required as it has been reported that a breakdown product (hydrolysed fumonisin) is just as toxic as the parent compound (Hopkins and Murphy, 1993).

*7.2.8.2 Toxicology.* Although fumonisins were not formally identified until 1988 (Bezuidenhout *et al.*, 1988; Gelderblom *et al.*, 1988), the effects of these compounds have been observed in a sporadic fatal disease in horses and related species called equine leucoencephalomalacia (ELEM). On a weight for weight basis, fumonisins are far less acutely toxic than the aflatoxins. However, fumonisins commonly occur in concentrations of parts per million in maize (Shephard *et al.*, 1996), at up to 300 mg/kg (Fazekas and Tothe, 1995), whereas aflatoxins are usually measured at concentrations of parts per billion in foods.

Fumonisins are thought to be toxic due to their effects on sphingolipid synthesis (Riley *et al.*, 1993). Alteration in sphingolipid base ratios occurs almost immediately after exposure because fumonisin inhibits ceramide synthetase (Wang *et al.*, 1992). This property is indicative of fumonisin exposure in a number of species including horses and pigs. Animal studies with $^{14}C$-labelled fumonisin $B_1$ generally show the uptake to be poor and elimination rapid. The effect of fumonisins on mammals appears to be species related. A long documented disease in horses, ELEM, was first linked to the presence of *F. moniliforme* in feed and more recently to the presence of fumonisins. Affected animals commonly lose appetite, become lethargic and develop neurotoxic effects after a period of ingesting contaminated feed. Autopsy shows oedema in the brain and liquefaction of areas within the cerebral hemispheres. The liver is also generally affected and, in severe cases, gross liver lesions may be seen with fibrosis of the centrilobular areas. In pigs, fumonisins induce pulmonary oedema and hydrothorax, with thoracic cavities filled with a yellow liquid. There may also be respiratory problems and foetal mortality.

When rats were fed material from *F. moniliforme* cultures, primary hepatocellular carcinomas were produced (Gelderblom *et al.*, 1988; Gelderblom and Snyman, 1991). These results were reproduced using purified fumonisins $B_1$, $B_2$ and $B_3$ (Gelderblom *et al.*, 1993, 1994). However, experimental carcinogenicity studies have been hampered by lack of pure standards.

Lebepe-Mazur *et al.* (1995a,b) showed that fumonisin $B_1$ affected the foetus in pregnant rats, causing low litter weights and foetal bone development as compared with controls.

In humans, there appears to be a link in some maize-consuming areas of the world between fumonisin toxicity and the occurrence of oesophageal cancer. Further epidemiological studies are required to define more precisely the role of *F. moniliforme* and its metabolites in oesophageal cancer. The incidence of this form of cancer is high in the Transkei, China and in northern Italy. Many studies of the toxicology of fumonisins are in progress. The full significance of fumonisins in maize for human and animal health still remains to be determined.

### 7.2.9 Zearalenone

*7.2.9.1 Chemical properties and natural occurrence.* Zearalenone (Figure 7.7) is a phenolic resorcyclic acid lactone produced by a number of species of *Fusarium* including *F. culmorum*, *F. graminearum* and *F. crookwellense*. In fungal cultures a number of closely related metabolites are formed but there is only limited evidence that these occur in foodstuffs, although there is experimental evidence for some transmission of zearalenone and α- and β-zearalenols into the milk of sheep, cows and pigs fed high concentrations (Mirocha *et al.*, 1981).

Zearalenone is a white crystalline compound that exhibits blue–green fluorescence when excited by long wavelength UV light (360 nm) and a more intense green fluorescence when excited with short wavelength UV light (260 nm). In methanol, UV absorption maxima occur at 236 nm ($\varepsilon = 29\,700$), 274 nm ($\varepsilon = 13\,909$) and 316 nm ($\varepsilon = 6020$). Maximum fluorescence in ethanol occurs with irradiation at 314 nm and with emission at 450 nm. Solubility in water is about 0.002 g per 100 ml. Zearalenone is slightly soluble in hexane and progressively more so in benzene, acetonitrile, methylene chloride, methanol, ethanol and acetone. It is also soluble in aqueous alkali.

A variety of food-grade grains (Table 4.4) and other foods have been found to contain zearalenone. These include corn products (Williams, 1985) such as corn beer (Lovelace and Nyathi, 1977), wheat flour (Tanaka *et al.*, 1985) and walnuts (Jemmali and Mazerand 1980). The presence of zearalenone in whole plants and parts of maize used for silage making has been investigated in Germany (Oldenberg, 1993). In that work, zearalenone was detected at concentrations up to 300 μg/kg and mainly accumulated at the end of the ripening process, with subsequent contamination of the silage.

Zearalenone is only partly decomposed by heat. Approximately 60% of zearalenone remained unchanged in bread while about 50% survived the production of noodles (Matsuura and Yoshizawa, 1981). In dry milling of maize, concentrations in the main food-producing fractions including flour and grits, were reduced by 80 to 90% although increased concentrations were found in bran and germ (Bennett *et al.*, 1976). Its distribution in wet-milled corn products is reviewed by Bennett and Anderson (1978).

*7.2.9.2 Toxicology.* The most important effect of zearalenone is on the reproductive system. In New Zealand zearalenone in pasture is a recognised cause of infertility in sheep (Towers and Sprosen, 1992). Its acute toxicity is low, $LD_{50}$ values (mg/kg bw) for oral and intraperitoneal administration are, respectively: >2000 and >500 in the mouse, >4000–10 000 and >5500 in the rat, and >15 000 for oral administration in chickens.

The ability of zearalenone to cause hyperestrogenism, particularly in swine, has been known for many years. Two comprehensive reviews of this have been published by Mirocha *et al.* (1971) and Mirocha and Christensen (1974). Several of a number of closely related metabolites of zearalenone produced by *Fusarium* spp. also possess similar properties, although few have been proven to occur naturally. Gareis (1993) reported that swine fed a diet containing 50 mg/kg of pure zearalenone suffered abortion and still-births, while levels above 10 mg/kg reduced the litter size and reduced the weight of piglets. Trial feeding of female pigs demonstrated that a concentration of 0.25 mg/kg, or even less, produced distinct redness and swelling of the vulva, slight swelling of the mammae and numerous vesicular follicles and some cystic follicles on the ovaria (Bauer *et al.*, 1987). It was also found that these effects could be produced by lower levels of zearalenone in swine fed naturally contaminated feed. Although swine have been found to be the most sensitive domesticated animal to zearalenone, calves have been reported to show earlier sexual maturity, dairy cows have been reported to have vaginitis, prolonged oestrus and infertility (Palti, 1978) and sheep are reported to become sterile (Towers and Sprosen, 1992). The effective dose for sheep may be approximately 1 mg/kg.

Sub-acute and sub-chronic toxicity studies, of up to 14 weeks' duration, have been completed using several species and results have been summarised by Kuiper-Goodman *et al.* (1987). Most effects were due to the oestrogenicity of zearalenone, which in mice caused atrophy of seminal vesicles and testes, squamous metaplasia of the prostate gland, osteoperosis, myelofibrosis of bone marrow, cytoplasmic vacuolisation of the adrenal gland, hyperkeratosis of the vagina and endometrial hyperplasia. Makela *et al.* (1995) compared the oestrogenic potency of zearalenone with that of other plant-derived oestrogens in MCF-7 or T-47D breast cancer cells and concluded that in comparison with 17-β-oestradiol it is one of the most potent natural xenoestogens.

In a review by the International Agency for Research on Cancer (IARC, 1993) it was concluded that there was limited evidence in experimental animals for the carcinogenicity of zearalenone. Evidence for genotoxicity has been contradictory but Pfohl-Leskowicz *et al.* (1995) showed that zearalenone is genotoxic in mice.

A risk assessment of the mycotoxin has been carried out (Kuiper-Goodman *et al.*, 1987) and that paper provides a comprehensive review. The authors concluded that no adverse human health effects would be anticipated from zearalenone contamination of corn in Canada but expressed concern that other unidentified sources might add to the oestrogenic burden. Since publication of that work there has been increasing awareness of the potential effects of such natural compounds.

### 7.2.10 Moniliformin

*7.2.10.1 Chemical properties and natural occurrence.* Moniliformin is formed by a number of *Fusarium* species and occurs as the sodium or potassium salt of 1-hydroxycyclobut-1-ene-3,4-dione (Figure 7.7). It is soluble in water and polar solvents. On heating to 360°C moniliformin decomposes without melting. UV maxima are 229 nm and 260 nm in methanol.

Data on the occurrence of moniliformin in food are scarce. Thiel *et al.* (1982) showed that levels up to 12 mg/kg occurred in maize intended for human consumption in the Transkei. More recently analysis of imported maize-milled products destined for incorporation into animal feeding stuffs in the UK showed that 60% of samples were contaminated with concentrations up to 4.6 mg/kg (Scudamore *et al.*, 1997). Moniliformin has also been shown to occur in other cereals such as wheat and rice. There is only limited information on its degradation during processing.

*7.2.10.2 Toxicology.* There are a limited amount of data on the effects of moniliformin on mammalian species. The oral $LD_{50}$ in rodents is approximately 50 mg/kg and for day-old cockerels 4 mg/kg. The ip $LD_{50}$ values were 21 and 29 mg/kg, respectively, for female and male mice. In acute studies, the main lesion appears to be intestinal haemorrhage but in sub-acute and chronic studies, in a variety of avian species and laboratory rodents, the principal target was the heart. Moniliformin is a potent inhibitor of mitochondrial pyruvate and ketoglutarate oxidation. Data on the effects of moniliformin on reproduction and the foetus, and its mutagenic and carcinogenic potential are negative but extremely limited. In humans, moniliformin has casually been linked with Keshan disease, which is endemic in some areas of China.

Contaminated maize may contain a cocktail of toxic *Fusarium*-derived residues such as fumonisins, zearalenone and trichothecenes (Thiel *et al.*,

1982; Scudamore *et al.*, 1998). Thus some of the published data in which maize containing moniliformin has been fed to animals may need re-evaluation.

### 7.2.11 Alternaria *toxins*

*7.2.11.1 Chemical properties and natural occurrence. Alternaria* is a common genus that usually invades crops at the pre-harvest stage and under suitable conditions may lead to production of certain mycotoxins (Magan *et al.*, 1984). The mycotoxins that occur most frequently are tenuazonic acid, alternariol monomethyl ether and alternariol (Figure 7.8). Altenuene, iso-altenuene and altertoxins I and II may occur occasionally. This type of contamination is normally associated with fruits, vegetables and oilseeds (Stinson *et al.*, 1981). Occurrence of *Alternaria* species and their mycotoxins in oilseeds has been reported by a number of workers, e.g. in sunflower seed (Chulze *et al.*, 1995) and in oilseed rape and sunflower seed meal (Nawaz *et al.*, 1997). Mycotoxins produced by *Alternaria* have also been reported in apples, olives, tomato products and cereals such as sorghum, wheat and rye (Visconti *et al.*, 1986; Grabarkiewicz-Szczesna *et al.*, 1989; Ansari and Shrivastava, 1990; Bottalico and Logrieco, 1992).

Tenuazonic acid is a colourless, viscous oil and is a monobasic acid with $pK_a$ 3.5. It is soluble in methanol and chloroform. On standing, heating or treatment with a base, optical activity is lost and crystallisation may occur as a result of formation of isotenuazonic acid. It forms complexes with calcium, magnesium, copper, iron and nickel ions. Tenuazonic acid is usually stored as its copper salt. Alternariol and alternariol monomethyl ether crystallise from ethanol as colourless needles, with melting points with decomposition of 350 and 267°C, respectively. They sublime in a high vacuum without decomposing at 250°C and 180 to 200°C. They are soluble in most organic solvents and give a purple colour reaction with ethanolic ferric chloride. Altenuene crystallises as colourless prisms melting at 190 to 191°C. Altertoxin I is an amorphous solid melting at 180°C and fluoresces bright yellow under UV light.

*7.2.11.2 Toxicology. Alternaria* toxins exhibit both acute and chronic effects. The $LD_{50}$ values for alternariol monomethyl ether, alternariol, altenuene and altertoxin I in mice are 400, 400, 50 and 0.2 mg/kg bw respectively. Those for tenuazonic acid are 162 and 115 mg/kg bw (by the intravenous route) for male and female mice, respectively.

*Alternaria* toxins have been implicated in animal and in human health disorders (Woody and Chu, 1992). During investigation into outbreaks of suspected mycotoxicoses, Gruber-Schley and Thalmann (1988) showed that cereal samples collected from affected farms in Germany were more frequently contaminated with *Alternaria* mycotoxins than samples from farms with healthy animals. Deaths in rabbits and poultry have been reported as a result of toxic action of *Alternaria* species found in the fodder and feed (Forgacs *et al.*, 1958; Wawrzkiewicz *et al.*, 1989). *Alternaria* spp. were also detected in cereal samples in which *Fusarium* spp. were implicated as the likely cause for an outbreak of alimentary toxic aleukia in Russia (Joffe, 1960).

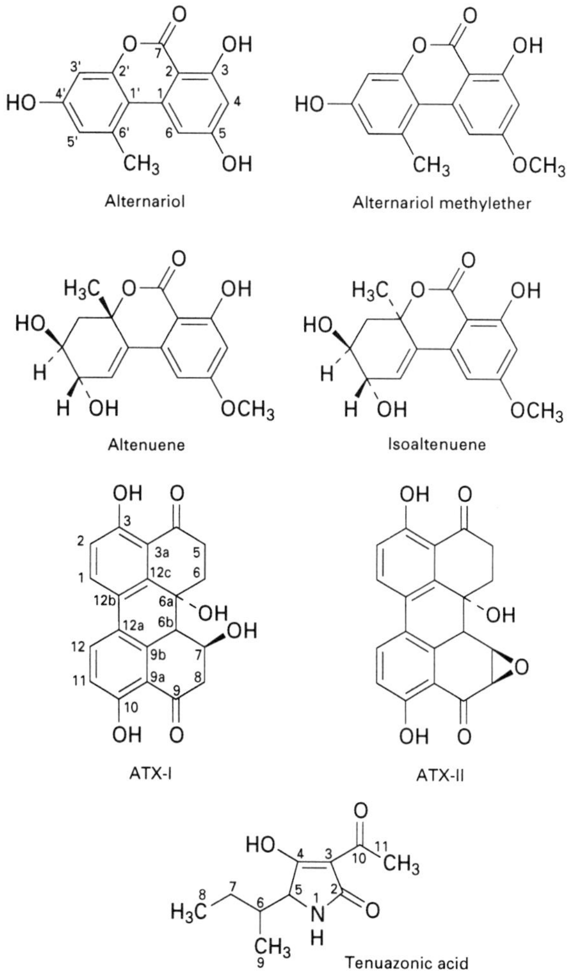

**Figure 7.8**  Structures of *Alternaria* mycotoxins.

Tenuazonic acid has been most studied of the *Alternaria* toxins. Its principal mode of action appears to be the inhibition of protein synthesis by suppressing the release of newly formed proteins from ribosomes into supernatant fluid (Shigeura and Gordon, 1963). It exhibits antitumour, antiviral and antibacterial activity. Alternariol and alternariol monomethyl ether show foetotoxic and teratogenic effects in mice, including a synergistic effect when a combination of the toxins was administered (Pero *et al.*, 1973). Most *Alternaria* mycotoxins exhibit considerable cytotoxic activity, including mammalian toxicity. The altertoxins are of particular concern because of their mutagenic activity (Scott and Stoltz, 1980; Chu, 1981; Stack and Prival, 1986). Stack and Prival (1986) showed that altertoxin III exhibits mutagenic activity that is approximately one-tenth that of aflatoxin $B_1$, while altertoxins I and II showed less mutagenicity.

### 7.2.12 Miscellaneous mycotoxins

There are many other mycotoxins that occur from time to time in animal feeds and forage and there is limited evidence for their presence in human food. As such, they fall outside the scope of this chapter.

Smith *et al.* (1994) reviewed mycotoxins in human health and the reader is recommended to consult this and other works for more information on the following lengthy, but incomplete, list: toxins from *Aspergillus fumigatus* and *A. clavatus*, citreoviridin, ergot alkaloids, fusarin C, gliotoxin, lolitrem B, mycophenolic acid, 3-nitropropionic acid, penicillic acid, PR-toxin, roquefortine C, rubratoxin A, satratoxins G and H, sporidesmin, viomellein, vioxanthin and xanthomegnin.

### References

Allcroft, R. and Carnaghan, R.B.A. (1962) Groundnut toxicity. *Aspergillus flavus* toxin (aflatoxin) in animal products: preliminary communication. *Veterinary Record*, **74** 863-64.

Alldrick, A.J. (1996) The effects of processing on the occurrence of ochratoxin A in cereals. *Food Additives and Contaminants*, **13** (suppl.) 27-28.

Anon (1982) The Feeding Stuffs (Sampling and Analysis) Regulations 1982, Statutory Instrument 1982 No. 1144, HMSO, London.

Anon (1992) Aflatoxins in Nuts, Nut Products, Dried Figs and Dried Fig Products Regulations 1992, Statutory Instrument 1992 No. 3236, HMSO, London.

Ansari, A.A. and Shrivastava, A.K. (1990) Natural occurrence of *Alternaria* mycotoxins in sorghum and ragi from North Bihar, India. *Food Additives and Contaminants*, **7** 815-20.

Bauer, J., Gareis, M. and Gedek, B. (1986) Incidence of ochratoxin A in blood serum and kidneys of man and animals, in *Proceedings of the 2nd World Congress on Foodborne Infections and Intoxications*, Berlin, 26–30 May 1986, p. 907.

Bauer, J., Heinritzi, K., Gareis, M., and Gedek, B. (1987) Veränderungen am Genitaltrakt des weiblichen Schweines nach Verfütterung praxisrelevanter Zearalenonmengen. *Tierärztliche Praxis*, **15** 33-36.

Baxter, E.D. (1996) The fate of ochratoxin A during malting and brewing. *Food Additives and Contaminants*, **13** (suppl.) 23-24.

Bennett, G.A., and Anderson, R.A. (1978) Distribution of aflatoxin and/or zearalenone in wet-milled corn products: a review. *Journal of Agricultural Food Chemistry*, **26** 1055-60.

Bennett, G.A., Peplinski, A.J., Brekke, O.L., and Jackson, L.K. (1976) Zearalenone: distribution in dry-milled fractions of contaminated corn. *Cereal Chemistry*, **53** 299-307.

Bezuidenhout, S.C., Gelderblom, W.C.A., Gorst-Allman, C.P., Horak, R.M., Marasas, W.F.O., Spiteller, G. and Vleggaar, R. (1988) Structure elucidation of the fumonisins, mycotoxins from *Fusarium moniliforme. Journal of the Chemical Society, Chemical Communications*, 743-45.

Bordson, G.O., Meerdink, G.L., Bauer, J.K. and Tumbleson, M.E. (1995) Effects of drying temperature on fumonisin recovery from feeds. *Journal of the Association of Official Analytical Chemists International*, **78** 1183-88.

Bottalico, A. and Logrieco, L. (1992) *Alternaria* plant disease in Mediterranean countries and associated mycotoxins, in *Alternaria—Biology, Plant Disease and Metabolites* (eds J. Chelkowski and A. Visconti), Elsevier, Amsterdam, pp. 209-32.

Breitholtz, A., Olsen, M., Dahlbäck, Å. and Hult, K. (1991) Plasma ochratoxin A levels in three Swedish populations surveyed using an ion-pair HPLC technique. *Food Additives and Contaminants*, **8** 183-92.

Broom, W.A., Bulbring, E., Chapman, C.J., Hampton, J.W.F., Thomson, A.M., Ungar, J., Wien, R. and Woolfe, G. (1944) The pharmacology of patulin. *British Journal of Experimental Pathology*, **25** 195-207.

Busby, W.F., and Wogan, G.N. (1984) Aflatoxins. *Chemical Carcinogens*, 2nd edn, American Chemical Society Monographs, vol. 2, 945-1136.

Canadian Public Health Association (1987) Significance of fungi in indoor air: report of a Working Group. *Canadian Journal of Public Health*, **78** S1-S14,

Chao, T.C., Maxwell, S.M., and Wong, S.Y. (1991) An outbreak of aflatoxicosis and boric acid poisoning in Malaysia. *Journal of Pathology*, **164** 225-33.

Chu, F.S. (1981) Isolation of altenuisol and altertoxin I and II, minor mycotoxins elaborated by *Alternaria. Journal of the American Oil Chemists Society*, **58** 1006A-1008A.

Chulze, S.N., Torres, A.M., Dalcero, A.M., Etcheverry, M.G., Ramírez, M.L. and Farnochi, M.C. (1995) *Alternaria* mycotoxins in sunflower seeds: incidence and distribution of the toxins in oil and meal. *Journal of Food Protection*, **58** 1133-35.

Ciegler, A.C., and Vesonder, R.F. (1983) Microbial food and toxicants: fungal toxins, in *CRC Series in Nutrition and Food* (ed. M. Recheigl, Jr), CRC Press, Boca Raton, Florida, p. 135.

Cole, R.J. (1986) Etiology of turkey-X disease in retrospect: a case for the involvement of cyclopiazonic acid. *Mycotoxin Research*, **2** 3.

Cooper, S.J., Wood, G.M., Chapman, W.B. and Williams, A.P. (1982) Mycotoxins occurring in mould-damaged foods, in *Proceedings of the Fifth International IUPAC Symposium on Mycotoxins and Phycotoxins*, September 1-3 1982, Vienna, Austria, IUPAC, pp. 64-67.

Coulter, J.B.S., Hendrickse, R.G., Lamplugh, S.M., Macfarlane, S.B.J., Moody, J.B., Omer, M.I.A., Sulliman, G.I. and Williams, T.E. (1986) Aflatoxins and kwashiorkor: clinical studies in Sudanese children. *Transactions of the Royal Society of Tropical and Medical Hygiene*, **80** 945-51.

Creppy, E.E., Kane, A., Dirheimer, G., Lagarge-Frayssinet, C., Mousset, F. and Frayssinet, C. (1985) Genotoxicity of ochratoxin A in mice: DNA single-strand break evaluation in spleen, liver and kidney. *Toxicology Letters*, **28** 29-35.

Croft, W.A., Jarvis, B.B. and Yatawara, C.S. (1986) Airborne outbreak of trichothecene toxicosis. *Atmospheric Environment*, **20** 549-52.

Degen, G., Gerber, M.M., Obrecht, S., Pfohl-Leszkowicz, A. and Dirheimer, G. (1994) Genotoxicity and cytotoxicity of ochratoxin A in ovine seminal vesicle cells culture. *Frühjahrstagung der Deutchen Gemeinschaft Pharmakologie und Toxikologie*, Mainz, Germany.

Dickens, F. and Jones, H.E.H. (1961) Carcinogenic activity of a series of reactive lactones and related substances. *British Journal of Cancer*, **15** 85-100.

Dirheimer, G. (1996) Mechanistic approaches to ochratoxin toxicity. *Food Additives and Contaminants*, **13** (suppl.) 45-48.

Dutton, M. (1996) Fumonisins, mycotoxins of increasing importance: their nature and their effects. *Pharmacology and Therapeutics*, **70** 137-61.

Elis, J. and Di Paola, J.A. (1967) Aflatoxin B₁. *Archives of Pathology*, **83** 53-57.

Endou, H., Koseki, C., Yamada, H. and Obara, T. (1986) Evaluation of nephrotoxicity using isolated nephron segments. *Developments in Toxicological and Environmental Science*, **14** 207-16.

Fazekas, B. and Tothe, H.E. (1995) Incidence of fumonisin B₁ in maize cultivated in Hungary. *Magy. Allatorv. Lapja*, **50** 515-18.

Fishbein, L. (1979) Range of potency of carcinogens in animals, in *Potential Industrial Carcinogens and Mutagens*, Elsevier Scientific, Amsterdam, Oxford and New York, p. 1.

Flannigan, B., Mccabe, E.M. and Mcgarry, F. (1991) Allergenic and toxigenic microorganisms in houses, in *Pathogens in the Environment* (ed. B. Austin), Journal of Applied Bacteriology Symposium Supplement, no. 20, 615-735.

Föllmann, W., Hillebrand, I.E., Creppy, E.E. and Bolt, H.M. (1995) Sister chromatid exchange frequency in cultured isolated porcine urinary bladder epithelial cells (PUBEC) treated with ochratoxin A and alpha. *Archives of Toxicology*, **69** 280-86.

Food and Agriculture Organisation of the United Nations (1997) *Worldwide Regulations for Mycotoxins, 1995, a Compendium*, FAO Food and Nutrition Paper, Food and Agriculture Organisation, Rome.

Forgacs, J., Koch, H., Carll, W.T. and White-Stevens, R.H. (1958) Additional studies on the relationship of mycotoxicoses to poultry haemorrhagic syndrome. *American Journal of Veterinary Research*, **19** 744-53.

Frisvad, J.C. (1989) The connection between the *Penicillia* and *Aspergilli* and mycotoxins with emphasis on misidentified isolates. *Archives of Environmental Contamination and Toxicology*, **18** 452-67.

Gareis, M. (1993) *Fusarium* mycotoxins an animal feeds and effects on livestock, in *Proceedings of the UK Workshop on Occurrence and Significance of Mycotoxins, Slough, Central Science Laboratory, MAFF 21–23 April 1993* (ed. K.A Scudamore), MAFF, London, pp. 7-15.

Gareis, M. (1996) Fate of ochratoxin A on processing of meat products. *Food Additives and Contaminants*, **13** (suppl.) 35-38.

Garner, R.C., and Dingley, K.H. (1993) Human exposure to aflatoxin, in *Proceedings of the UK Workshop on Occurrence and Significance of Mycotoxins, Slough, Central Science Laboratory, MAFF 21–23 April 1993* (ed. K.A Scudamore), MAFF, London, pp. 91-95.

Gelderblom, W.C.A. and Snyman, S.D. (1991) Mutagenicity of potentially carcinogenic mycotoxins produced by *Fusarium moniliforme*. *Mycological Research*, **7** 46-50.

Gelderblom, W.C.A., Jaskiewicz, K., Marasas, W.F.O., Thiel, P.G., Horak, R.M., Vleggaar, R. and Kriek, N.P.J. (1988) Fumonisins—novel mycotoxins with cancer-promoting activity produced by *Fusarium moniliforme*. *Applied Environmental Microbiology*, **54** 1806-11.

Gelderblom, W.C.A., Cawood, M.E., Snyman, S.D., Vleggaar, R. and Marasas, W.F. (1993) Structure–activity relationship in short-term carcinogenesis and cytotoxicity assays. *Food Chemistry and Toxicology*, **31** 407-414.

Gelderblom, W.C.A., Cawood, M.E., Snyman, S.D., and Marasas, W.F. (1994) Fumonisin B₁ dosimetry in relation to cancer initiation in rats. *Carcinogenesis*, **15** 209-214.

Grabarkiewicz-Szczesna, J., Chelkowski, J. and Zajkowski, P. (1989) Natural occurrence of *Alternaria* mycotoxins in the grain and chaff of cereals. *Mycotoxin Research*, **5** 77-80.

Gruber-Schley, S. and Thalmann, A. (1988) The occurrence of *Alternaria* spp. and their metabolites in grain and possible connection with illness in farm animals. *Landwirtschaftliche Forschung Sonderheft*, **41** 11-29.

Harvey, R.B., Elissalde, M.H., Kubena, L.F., Weaver, E.A., Corrier, D.E. and Clement, B.A. (1992) Immunotoxicity of ochratoxin A to growing gilts. *American Journal of Veterinary Research*, **53** 1966-70.

Harwig, J., Kuiper-Goodman, T. and Scott, P.M. (1983) Microbial food toxicants: ochratoxins, in *Handbook of Foodborne Diseases of Biological Origin* (ed. M. Rechcigl, Jr), CRC Press, Boca Raton, Florida, pp. 193-238.

Holzapfel, C.W. (1968) The isolation and structure of cyclopiazonic acid, a toxic metabolite of *Penicillium cyclopium. Tetrahedron,* **24** 2101-19.

Hopkins, E.C. and Murphy, P.A. (1993) Detection of fumonisins $B_1$, $B_2$, $B_3$ and hydrolyzed fumonisin $B_1$ in corn-containing foods. *Journal of Agricultural and Food Chemistry,* **41** 1655-58.

IARC (1986) Patulin. *IARC Monographs,* **40** 83-98.

IARC (1993) *Some Naturally Occurring Substances: Food Items and Constituents. Heterocyclic Aromatic Amines and Mycotoxins,* IARC Monographs on the Evaluation of Carcinogenic Risks to Humans, V.56, IARC, Lyon, France.

Jemmali, M. and Mazerand, C. (1980) Présence de zéaralénone ou $F_2$ dans les noix de commerce. *Annules de Microbiologie (Paris),* **B131** 319-21.

Joffe, A.Z. (1960) Mycoflora of overwintered cereals and its toxicity. *Bulletin of the Research Council of Israel,* Section D, **9** 101-26.

Kane, A., Creppy, E.E., Roth, A., Röschenthaler, R. and Dirheimer, G. (1986) Distribution of the [3H]-label from low doses of radioactive ochratoxin A ingested by rats, and evidence for DNA single-strand breaks caused in liver and kidneys. *Archives of Toxicology,* **58** 219-24.

Katzman, P.A., Hays, E.E., Cain, C.K., Van Wyk, J.J., Reithel, F.J., Thayer, S.A., Doisy, E.A., Gaby, W.L., Carroll, C.J., Muir, R.D., Jones, L.R. and Wade, N.J. (1944) Clavacin, an antibiotic substance from *Aspergillus clavatus. Journal of Biological Chemistry,* **154** 475-86.

Krishnamachari, K.A.V.R., Bhat, R.V., Nagarajan, V. and Tilak, T.B.G. (1975) Hepatitis due to aflatoxicosis. An outbreak in Western India. *Lancet,* **i** 1061-63.

Krogh, P., Hald, B. and Pedersen, E.J. (1973) Occurrence of ochratoxin A and citrinin on cereals associated with porcine nephropathy. *Acta Pathologica et Microbiologica Scandanavica,* Section B, **81** 689-95.

Kuiper-Goodman, T. (1995) Mycotoxins: risk assessment and legislation. *Toxicology Letters,* **82/83** 853-59.

Kuiper-Goodman, T. (1996) Risk assessment of ochratoxin A: an update. *Food Additives and Contaminants,* **13** (suppl.) 53-57.

Kuiper-Goodman, T. and Scott, P.M. (1989) Risk assessment of the mycotoxin ochratoxin A. *Biomedical and Environmental Sciences,* **2** 179-248.

Kuiper-Goodman, T., Scott, P.M. and Watanabe, H. (1987) Risk assessment of the mycotoxin zearalenone. *Regulatory Toxicology and Pharmacology,* **7** 253-306.

Kuiper-Goodman, T., Omininski, K., Marquardt, R.R., Malcolm, S., Mcmullen, E., Lombaert, G.A. and Morton, T. (1993) Estimating human exposure to ochratoxin A in Canada, in *Human Ochratoxicosis and its Pathologies* (eds E.E. Creppy, M. Castegnaro and G. Dirheimer), John Bibbey Eurotext, Montrouge, France, pp. 167-74.

Lancaster, M.C., Jenkins, F.P. and Philip, J.M. (1961) Toxicity associated with certain samples of groundnuts. *Nature,* **192** 1095.

Lebepe-Mazur, S., Bal, H., Hopmans, E., Murphy, P. and Hendrich, S. (1995a) Fumonisin $B_1$ is fetotoxic in rats. *Vet. Human Toxicol.,* **37** 126-30.

Lebepe-Mazur, S., Wilson, T. and Hendrich, S. (1995b) *Fusarium proliferatum* fermented corn stimulates development of placental glutathione S-transferase-positive altered hepatic foci in female rats. *Vet. Human Toxicol.,* **37** 39-45.

Lovelace, C.E.A. and Nyathi, C.B. (1977) Estimation of the fungal toxins zearalenone and aflatoxin, contaminating opaque maize beer in Zambia. *J. Sci. Food Agric.,* **28** 288-92.

Luk, K.C., Kobbe, B. and Townsend, J.M. (1977) Production of cyclopiazonic acid by *Aspergillus flavus* Link. *Applied Environmental Microbiology,* **33** 211-12.

Magan, N., Cayley, G.R. and Lacey, J. (1984) Effect of water activity and temperature on mycotoxin production by *Alternaria alternata* in cultures and on wheat grain. *Applied Environmental Microbiology,* **47** 1113-17.

Makela, S., Poutanen, M., Lehtimaki, J., Kostian, M.L., Santti, R. and Vihko, R. (1995) Estrogen-specific 17β-hydroxysteroid oxidoreductase type 1 (E.C. 1.1.1.62) as a possible target for the action of phytoestrogens. *P.S.E.B.M.,* **208** 51-59.

Matsuura, Y. and Yoshizawa, T. (1981) Effect of food additives and heating on the decomposition of zearalenone in wheat flour. *Journal of the Food Hygiene Society of Japan*, **22** 293-98.

Miller, J.D. (1995) Fungi and mycotoxins in grain: implications for stored product research. *Journal of Stored Product Research*, **31** 1-16.

Ministry of Agriculture, Fisheries and Food (1980) *Surveillance of mycotoxins in the United Kingdom*. The fourth report of the Steering Group on Food Surveillance, The Working Party on Mycotoxins, Food Surveillance Paper No. 4, HMSO, London.

Ministry of Agriculture, Fisheries and Food (1987) *Mycotoxins*, the eighteenth report of the Steering Group on Food Surveillance, The Working Party on Naturally Occurring Toxicants in Food: Sub-Group on Mycotoxins, Food Surveillance Paper No. 18, HMSO, London.

Ministry of Agriculture, Fisheries and Food (1993) *Mycotoxins: Third Report*, the thirty-sixth report of the Steering Group on Chemical Aspects of Food Surveillance, Sub-Group on Mycotoxins, Food Surveillance Paper No. 36, HMSO, London.

Miraglia, M., Brera, C., Corneli, S. and De Dominics, R. (1993) Ochratoxin A in Italy: status of knowledge and perspectives, in *Human Ochratoxicosis and its Pathologies* (eds E.E. Creppy, M. Castegnaro and G. Dirheimer), John Bibbey Eurotext, Montrouge, France, pp. 129-40.

Mirocha, C.J. and Christensen, C.M. (1974) Oestrogenic mycotoxins synthesised by *Fusarium*, in *Mycotoxins* (ed. I.F.H. Purchase), Elsevier, Amsterdam, pp. 129-48.

Mirocha, C.J., Christensen, C.M. and Nelson, G.H. (1971) *Microbial Toxins*, Chapter 4, Academic Press, New York.

Mirocha, C.J., Pathre, S.V. and Christensen, C.M. (1977) Chemistry of *Fusarium* and *Stachybotrys* mycotoxins, in *Mycotoxic, Fungi, Mycotoxins and Mycotoxicoses*, vol. 1 (eds T.D. Wyllie and L.G. Morehouse), Marcel Dekker, New York.

Mirocha, C.J., Pathre, S.V. and Robison, T.S. (1981) Comparative metabolism of zearalenone and transmission into bovine milk. *Food Cosmet. Toxicol.*, **19** 25-30.

Moss, M.O. (1996) Mycotoxins—centenary review. *Mycological Research*, **100** 513-23.

Nawaz, S., Scudamore, K.A. and Rainbird, S.C. (1997) Mycotoxins in ingredients of animal feeding stuffs: I. Determination of *Alternaria* mycotoxins in oilseed rape meal and sunflower seed meal. *Food Additives and Contaminants*, **14** 249-62.

Ngindu, A., Johnson, B.K., Kenya, P.R., Ngira, J.A., Ocheng, D.M., Nandwa, H. and Omondi, T.N. (1982) Outbreak of acute hepatitis caused by aflatoxin poisoning in Kenya. *Lancet*, **ii** 346-48.

Ohmono, S., Sugita, M. and Abe, M. (1973) Isolation of cyclopiazonic acid, cyclopiazonic acid imine and bissecodehydrocyclopiazonic acid from the cultures of *Aspergillus versicolor*. *J. Agric. Chem. Soc. Japan*, **47** 57-63.

Ohtsubo, K., Saito, M., Kimura, H. and Tsuruta, O. (1978) High incidence of hepatic tumours in rats fed mouldy rice contaminated with *Aspergillus versicolor* and sterigmatocystin. *Food Cosmet. Toxicol.*, **16** 143-50.

Oldenberg, E. (1993) Occurrence of zearalenone in maize. *Mycotoxin Research*, **9** 72-78.

Oyelami, O.A., Maxwell, S.M., Adelusola, K.A., Aladekoma, T.A. and Oyelese, A.O. (1995) Aflatoxins in the autopsy brain tissue of children in Nigeria. *Mycopathologia*, **132** 35-38.

Oyelami, O.A., Maxwell, S.M. and Adeoba, E. (1996) Aflatoxins and ochratoxin A in the weaning food of Nigerian children. *Annals of Tropical Paediatrics*, **16** 137-40.

Ozay, G. and Alperden, I. (1991) Aflatoxin and ochratoxin A contamination of dried figs (*Ficus carina* L.) from the 1988 crop. *Mycotoxin Research*, **7** 85-91.

Palti, J. (1978) Toxigenic fusaria, their distribution and significance as causes of disease in animal and man. *Acta Phytomed.*, **6** 110 pp.

Payen, J., Girard, T., Gaillardin, M. and Lafont, P. (1983) Sur la présence de mycotoxines dans des bières. *Microbiol. Aliments Nutr.*, **1** 143-46.

Pero, R.W., Porner, H., Blois, M., Harvan, D. and Spalding, J.W. (1973) Toxicity of metabolites produced by the 'Alteria'. *Environmental Health Perspectives*, June, 87-94.

Pfohl-Leszkowicz, A., Grosse, Y., Kane, A., Castegnaro, M., Creppy, E.E. and Dirheimer, G. (1993) Preponderance of DNA-adducts in kidney after ochratoxin A exposure, in *Human Ochratoxicosis and its Pathologies* (eds E.E. Creppy, M. Castegnaro and G. Dirheimer), Eurotext No. 231, John Libbey, Montrouge, France, pp. 199-207.

Pfohl-Leszkowicz, A., Chekir-Ghedir, L. and Bacha, H. (1995) Genotoxicity of zearalenone, an oestrogenic mycotoxin: DNA adduct formation in female mouse tissues. *Carcinogenesis*, **16** 2315-20.

Pier, A.C. (1991) The influence of mycotoxins on the immune system, in *Mycotoxins and Animal Foods* (eds J.E. Smith and R.S. Henderson), CRC Press, Boca Raton, Florida, pp. 489-97.

Pier, A.C., Richard, J.L. and Cysewski, S.J. (1980) The implications of mycotoxins in animal disease. *Journal of the American Veterinary and Medical Association*, **176** 719.

Purchase, I.F.H. (1971) The acute toxicity of the mycotoxin cyclopiazonic acid to rats. *Toxicology and Applied Pharmacology*, **18** 114-23.

Riley, R.T., An, S., Showker, A.L., Yoo, H.S., Norred, W.P., Chamberlain, W.J., Wang, E., Merrill, A.H., Motelin, G., Beasley, V.R. and Haschek, W.M. (1993) Alteration of tissue and serum sphinganine to sphingosine ratio: an early biomarker of exposure to fumonisin containing feeds in pigs. *Toxicology and Applied Pharmacology*, **118** 105-12.

Roberts, J.C. (1974) Aflatoxins and sterigmatocystin. *Fortschr. Chem. Org. Naturst.*, **31** 119-51.

Scott, P.M. (1977) *Penicillium* mycotoxins, in *Mycotoxic, Fungi, Mycotoxins and Mycotoxicoses*, Vol. 1 (eds T.D. Wyllie and L.G. Morehouse), Marcel Dekker, New York, pp. 283-356.

Scott, P.M. (1990) Natural poisons, 971.22 standards for aflatoxins. *AOAC Official Methods of Analysis*, AOAC, pp. 1186-87.

Scott, P.M. (1996) Effects of processing and detoxification treatments on ochratoxin A: introduction. *Food Additives and Contaminants*, **13** (suppl.) 19-22.

Scott, P.M. and Lawrence, G.A. (1994) Stability and problems in recovery of fumonisins added to corn-based foods. *Journal of the Association of Official Analytical Chemists*, **77** 541-45.

Scott, P.M. and Stoltz, D.R. (1980) Mutagens produced by *Alternaria alternata*. *Mutation Research*, **78** 33-40.

Scudamore, K.A. (1993) The occurrence of mycotoxins in food and animal feedstuffs in the UK, in *Proceedings of the UK Workshop on Occurrence and Significance of Mycotoxins, Slough, Central Science Laboratory, MAFF 21–23 April 1993* (ed. K.A Scudamore), MAFF, London, pp. 172-85.

Scudamore, K.A. (1996) The effects of processing on the occurrence of ochratoxin A in cereals. *Food Additives and Contaminants*, **13** (suppl.) 39-42.

Scudamore, K.A., Nawaz, S. and Hetmanski, M.T. (1998) Mycotoxins in ingredients of animal feeding stuffs: II. Determination of mycotoxins in maize and maize products. *Food Additives and Contaminants* (in press).

Shank, R.C., Bourgeois, C.H., Keschamaras, N. and Chandavimol, P. (1971) Aflatoxins in autopsy specimens from Thai children with an acute disease of an unknown aetiology. *Food Cosmet. Toxicol.*, **9** 61-69.

Sharman, M. and Gilbert, J. (1991) Automated aflatoxin analysis of foods and animal feeds using immunoaffinity column clean-up and high-performance liquid chromatographic determination. *Journal of Chromatography*, **543** 220-25.

Shephard, G.S., Thiel, P.G., Stockenström, S. and Sydenham, E.W. (1996) Worldwide survey of fumonisin contamination of corn and corn-based products. *Journal of the Association of Official Analytical Chemists International*, **79** 671-87.

Shigeura, H.T. and Gordon, C.N. (1963) The biological activity of tenuazonic acid. *Biochemistry*, **2** 1132-37.

Sieber, S.M., Correa, P., Dalgard, D.W. and Adamson, R.H. (1979) Induction of osteogenic sarcomas and tumors of the hepatobiliary system in non-human primates with aflatoxin $B_1$. *Cancer Research*, **39** 4545-54.

Smith, J.E. and Henderson, R.S. (1991) *Mycotoxins and Animal Foods*, CRC Press, Boca Raton, Florida.

Smith, J.E., Lewis, C.W., Anderson, J.G. and Solomons, G.L. (1994) A literature review carried out on behalf of the agro-industrial division, E2, of the European Commission Directorate-General

XII for scientific research and development. *Mycotoxins in Human Nutrition and Health*, European Commission.

Speijers, G.J.A. and van Egmond, H.P. (1993) World-wide ochratoxin A levels in food and feeds, in *Human Ochratoxicosis and its Pathologies* (eds E.E. Creppy, M. Castegnaro and G. Dirheimer), John Bibbey Eurotext, Montrouge, France, pp. 85-100.

Stack, M.E. and Prival, M.J. (1986) Mutagenicity of the *Alternaria* metabolites altertoxins I, II and III. *Applied Environmental Microbiology*, **52** 718-22.

Stinson, E.E., Osman, S.F., Heisler, E.G., Siciliano, J. and Bills, D.D. (1981) Mycotoxin production in whole tomatoes, apples, oranges and lemons. *J. Agric. Food Chem.*, **29** 790-92.

Stormer, F.C. and Lea, T. (1995) Effects of ochratoxin A upon early and late events in human T-cell proliferation. *Toxicology*, **95** 45-50.

Subirade, I. (1996) Fate of ochratoxin A during breadmaking. *Food Additives and Contaminants*, **13** (suppl.) 25-26.

Sydenham, E.W., Shephard, G.S., Thiel, P.G., Marasas, W.F.O. and Stockenström, S. (1991) Fumonisin contamination of commercial corn-based human foodstuffs. *J. Agric. Food Chem.*, **39** 2014-18.

Takashi, U., Trucksess, M.W., Beaver, W.R., Wilson, D.M., Dorner, J.W. and Dowell, F.E. (1992) Co-occurrence of cyclopiazonic acid and aflatoxin in corn and peanuts. *Journal of the Association of Official Analytical Chemists*, **75** 838.

Tanaka, T., Hasegawa, A., Matsuki, Y., Lee, U.-S. and Ueno, Y. (1985) Rapid and sensitive determination of zearalenone in cereals by high-performance liquid chromatography with fluorescence detection. *Journal of Chromatography*, **328** 271-78.

The Nordic Working Group On Food Toxicology and Risk Evaluation (1991) Health evaluation of ochratoxin A in food products. *Nordiske Seminar-og Arbejdsrapporter*, **545** 1-26.

Thiel, P.G., Meyer, C.J. and Mararas, W.F.O. (1982) Natural occurrence of moniliformin together with deoxynivalenol and zearalenone in Transkeian corn. *J. Agric. Food Chem.*, **30** 308-12.

Towers, N.R. and Sprosen, J.M. (1992) *Fusarium* mycotoxins in pastoral farming: zearalenone induced infertility in ewes, in *Recent Advances in Toxicology Research*, vol. 3 (eds P. Gopalakrishnakone and C.K. Tan), National University of Singapore, Singapore, pp. 272-84.

Trivedi, A.D., Hiroto, M., Dol, E. and Kitabatake, N. (1993) Formation of a new toxic compound, citrinin H1, from citrinin on mild heating in water. *Journal of the Chemical Society, Perkin Transactions*, **1** 2167-71.

Tsubouchi, H., Terada, H., Yamamoto, K., Hisada, K. and Sakabe, Y. (1988) Ochratoxin A found in commercial roast coffee. *J. Agric. Food Chem.*, **36** 540-42.

Ueno, Y. and Ueno, I. (1978) Toxicology and biochemistry of mycotoxins, in *Toxicology, Biochemistry and Pathology of Mycotoxins* (eds K. Uraguchi and M. Yamazaki), John Wiley, New York, pp. 107-55.

Vesonder, R.F. and Horn, B.W. (1985) Sterigmatocystin in dairy cattle feed contaminated with *Aspergillus versicolor. Applied Environmental Microbiology*, **49** 234-35.

Viani, R. (1996) Fate of ochratoxin A (OTA) during processing of coffee. *Food Additives and Contaminants*, **13** (suppl.) 29-34.

Visconti, A., Logrieco. A. and Bottalico, A. (1986) Natural occurrence of *Alternaria* mycotoxins in olives—their production and possible transfer into the oil. *Food Additives and Contaminants*, **3** 323-30.

Visconti A., Doko, M.B., Bottalico, C., Schurer, B. and Boenke, A. (1993) The stability of fumonisins (fumonisin $B_1$ and fumonisin $B_2$) in solution, in *Proceedings of the UK Workshop on Occurrence and Significance of Mycotoxins, Slough, Central Science Laboratory, MAFF 21–23 April 1993* (ed. K.A Scudamore), MAFF, London, pp. 196-99.

Wang, E., Ross, F., Wilson, T.M., Riley, R.T. and Merrill, A.H. (1992) Increases in serum sphingosine and sphinganine and decreases in complex sphingolipids in ponies given feed containing fumonisins, mycotoxins produced by *Fusarium moniliforme. Journal of Nutrition*, **122** 1706-16.

Wannemacher, R.W., Bunner, D.L. and Neufeld, H.A. (1991) Toxicity of trichothecenes and other related mycotoxins in laboratory animals, in *Mycotoxins and Animal Foods* (eds J.E. Smith and R.S. Henderson), CRC Press, Boca Raton, Florida, pp. 499-552.

Watson, D.H. (1985) Toxic fungal metabolites in food. *CRC Critical Reviews in Food Science and Nutrition*, **22** 177-98.

Wawrzkiewicz, K., Gluch, A., Rubaj, B. and Wrobel, M. (1989) *Alternaria* spp., an opportunist pathogen. *Medycyna Weterynary*, **45** 27-30.

Williams, B.C. (1985) Mycotoxins in foods and feedstuffs, in *Mycotoxins: a Canadian Perspective* (eds P.M. Scott, H.L. Trenholm and M.D. Sutton), National Research Council Canada, Ottawa, pp. 49-53.

Woody, M.A. and Chu, F.S. (1992) Toxicology of *Alternaria* mycotoxins, in *Alternaria—Biology, Plant Disease and Metabolites* (eds J. Chelkowski and A. Visconti), Elsevier, Amsterdam, pp. 409-33.

Zimmerli, B. and Dick, R. (1996) Ochratoxin A in table wine and grape-juice: occurrence and risk assessment. *Food Additives and Contaminants*, **13** 655-68.

# 8 Phycotoxins in seafood

John W. Leftley and Fiona Hannah

## 8.1 Introduction

Contamination of seafood with phycotoxins and the resultant effects on human health is a world-wide problem and research into all aspects of these compounds is being conducted in many countries. Consequently, there is a plethora of data and it is possible here to give only a brief account of the most important phycotoxins. In addition to the literature cited in this chapter, the reader is referred to two comprehensive publications (Hallegraeff *et al.*, 1995; Andersen, 1996) produced by the Intergovernmental Oceanographic Commission (see the note at the end of this chapter) which amplify most of the topics covered below.

## 8.2 Causative and vector organisms

The organisms that produce the phycotoxins described here are certain genera of unicellular algae, usually photosynthetic, which may be planktonic (free floating or swimming) or benthic, i.e. live on surfaces of, for example, plants and corals, or in or on marine sediments. With the exception of the diatoms that cause amnesic shellfish poisoning, most are dinoflagellates (Table 8.1). Detailed accounts of the taxonomy of the algae implicated in phycotoxin poisoning have been given by Steidinger (1993), Hallegraeff *et al.* (1995) and Andersen (1996). The phycotoxins can be regarded as secondary metabolites and their taxonomic distribution, biosynthesis and significance in the food chain have been reviewed by Shimizu (1996).

Seafood poisoning is often associated with the occurrence of algal 'blooms', where the microscopic algae may reach sufficient density to produce a visible discoloration of the water. These blooms, not necessarily toxic, are a natural phenomenon and occur when there is a particular combination of physical and chemical conditions that allows rapid growth of the organisms (Boney, 1989). Blooms of harmful algae are often confusingly referred to as 'red tides', although the colour of the water may actually be either red, brown or green (Anderson, 1994). The incidence of harmful algal blooms appears to be increasing all over the world (Hallegraeff, 1995), but it remains to be established whether this apparent increase is owing to increased vigilance by the many countries that have monitoring programmes (see below) or is a genuine phenomenon caused by as yet unknown factors, or is a combination of both.

Bivalve shellfish are the most common vectors of phycotoxins other than in ciguatera fish poisoning (Table 8.1). This is because they are filter feeders and naturally ingest any phytoplankton or particles to which they may be attached and thereby concentrate any toxins in their tissues. The shellfish that have been most studied as regards accumulation of algal toxins are those consumed directly by humans, such as clams and mussels (Shumway *et al.*, 1995). However, the importance of carnivorous gastropods and crustaceans as vectors should not be ignored. Shumway (1995) has provided comprehensive data on the occurrence of phycotoxins in these organisms.

## 8.3 Paralytic shellfish poisoning

Paralytic shellfish poisoning (PSP) is caused by the ingestion of one or more of a group of basic, water-soluble, nitrogenous toxins originating from dinoflagellates belonging to the genera *Alexandrium*, *Gymnodinium* and *Pyrodinium* (Table 8.1). PSP has been recognized for centuries but its cause was first understood only this century (Kao, 1993). On a global scale PSP is the most common and widespread of the phycotoxin syndromes, as is the occurrence of PSP toxins in seafood (Figure 8.1a). Up to 1993 there were about about 2500 cases of human intoxication recorded throughout the world (Kao, 1993) and more cases are reported each year. The consequences of PSP can be very severe. For example, in Guatemala in 1987 about 186 people were admitted to hospital after ingesting PSP toxins, 26 of whom subsequently died. A detailed account of all aspects of PSP can be found in Kao (1993).

Although dinoflagellates are undoubtedly the source of the PSP toxins, certain bacteria are also known to produce these compounds and the possible role of prokaryotes in PSP has come under scrutiny. Some photosynthetic cyanobacteria, for example, are a source of the PSP toxin saxitoxin as well as other unrelated toxins (see below). It has been found that some marine bacteria produce PSP toxins, including bacteria associated with dinoflagellates that produce similar toxins (Franca *et al.*, 1996; Gallacher *et al.*, 1996, 1997; Levasseur *et al.*, 1996; Shimizu *et al.*, 1996). The exact relationship between these bacteria and dinoflagellates as regards toxin production remains to be determined (Shimizu *et al.*, 1996).

### 8.3.1  The PSP toxins
More than 20 PSP toxins are known to exist at present, all of which are water-soluble. The basic molecule is a tetrahydropurine substituted at various positions, as shown in Figure 8.2. The specific toxicity of these compounds varies. For example, the most potent are the carbamate toxins (saxitoxin, neosaxitoxin and the gonyautoxins GTX1 to GTX4) which are 10 to 100 times more toxic than the N-sulphocarbamoyl derivatives, the B

**Table 8.1** Phycotoxin poisoning causative and vector organisms, clinical symptoms and treatment. After Hallegraeff (1995) with additional information taken from Andersen (1996), Cembella et al. (1995), Fleming et al. (1995) and Quilliam and Wright (1995)

| Paralytic shellfish poisoning (PSP) | Diarrhetic shellfish poisoning (DSP) | Amnesic shellfish poisoning (ASP) | Neurotoxic shellfish poisoning (NSP) | Ciguatera fish poisoning (CFP) |
|---|---|---|---|---|
| *Causative organisms*<br>Dinoflagellates:<br>Alexandrium catenella<br>Alexandrium minutum<br>Alexandrium tamarense<br>Gymnodinium catenatum<br>Pyrodinium bahamense | Dinoflagellates:<br>Dinophysis acuminata<br>Dinophysis acuta<br>Dinophysis fortii<br>Dinophysis norvegica<br>Prorocentrum lima | Diatoms:<br>Nitzschia actydrophila<br>Pseudo-nitzschia australis<br>Pseudo-nitzschia pseudo-delicatissima<br>Pseudo-nitzschia pungens<br>f. multiseries<br>Pseudo-nitzschia seriata | Dinoflagellates:<br>Gymnodinium breve<br>(= Ptychodiscus brevis)<br>G. cf. breve (New Zealand)<br><br>Raphidophytes [a]<br>Fibrocapsa japonica<br>Heterosigma akashiwo | Dinoflagellates:<br>Gambierdiscus toxicus<br>? Prorocentrum lima |
| *Vector organisms*<br>Shellfish and crustaceans such as mussels, clams, oysters and lobsters, e.g. Cardium edule, Mytilus edulis, Pecten maximus | Shellfish, e.g. mussels | Shellfish, e.g. blue mussels and crabs | Shellfish, e.g. mussels and clams. Humans may also be affected by direct contact with the toxic algae via sea spray or swimming | Carnivorous fishes, mainly barracudas, groupers, jacks, sea bass, snappers and surgeon fish which feed on herbivorous fish that inhabit coral reefs |

[a] Brevetoxins have been detected in these algae but they have not yet been implicated in NSP.

| *Effect and symptoms* | | | | |
| --- | --- | --- | --- | --- |
| Neurotoxic | Gastrointestinal disturbance | Neurotoxic | Neurotoxic | Complex, primarily neurotoxic |
| *Mild case* | | | | |
| Within 30 min: tingling sensation or numbness around lips, gradually spreading to face and neck; prickly sensation in fingertips and toes; headache, dizziness, nausea, vomiting and diarrhoea | After 30 min to a few hours (seldom more than 12 h): Diarrhoea, nausea, vomiting, abdominal pain | After 3 to 5 h: nausea, vomiting, diarrhoea, abdominal cramp | After 3 to 6 h: chills, headache, diarrhoea, muscle weakness; muscle and joint pain; nausea and vomiting; irritation to eyes and nasal membranes where direct contact with algae | Symptoms develop within 12 to 24 h of eating fish. Gastro-intestinal symptoms: diarrhoea, abdominal pain, nausea, vomiting |
| *Extreme case* | | | | |
| Muscular paralysis; pronounced respiratory difficulty, choking sensation; death, through respiratory paralysis may occur within 2 to 24 h after ingestion | Chronic exposure may promote tumour formation in the digestive system | Decreased reaction to deep pain; dizziness, hallucinations, confusion; short-term memory loss, sometimes permanent; seizure; damage to hippocampus in brain; coma; death in some extreme cases | Paraesthesia; altered perception of hot and cold; difficulty in breathing; double vision; trouble in talking and swallowing | Neurological symptoms: numbness and tingling of hands and feet; cold objects feel hot to touch; difficulty in balance; low heart rate and blood pressure; rashes; death in some extreme cases through respiratory failure |
| *Average fatality rate* | | | | |
| 1–14% | 0% | 3% | 0% | <1% |
| *Treatment* | | | | |
| Patient has stomach pumped and is given artificial respiration. No lasting effects | Intravenous infusion of electrolytes. Recovery after three days irrespective of medical treatment | None at present other than life support systems if required | Support as required | No antidote or specific treatment is available; neurological symptoms may last for months and years; calcium and mannitol may help relieve symptoms |

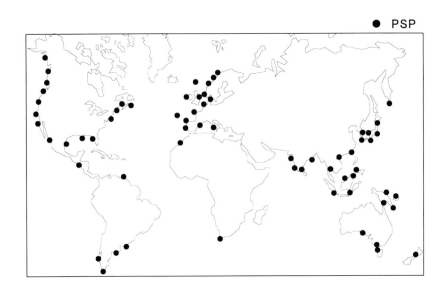

**Figure 8.1a**    See Figure 8.1e for legend.

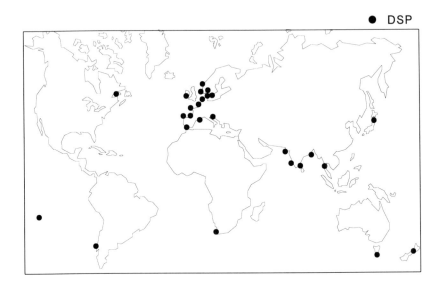

**Figure 8.1b**    See Figure 8.1e for legend.

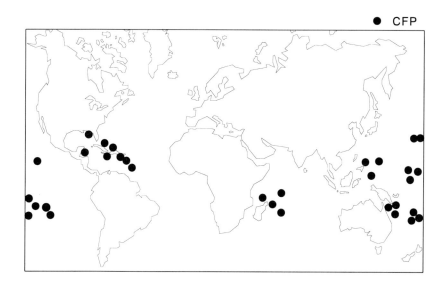

**Figure 8.1c**    See Figure 8.1e for legend.

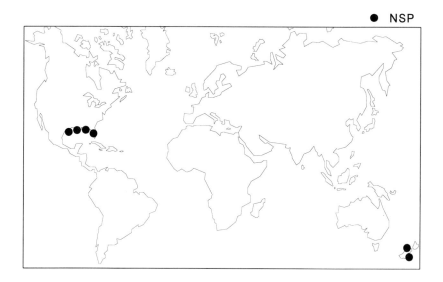

**Figure 8.1d**    See Figure 8.1e for legend.

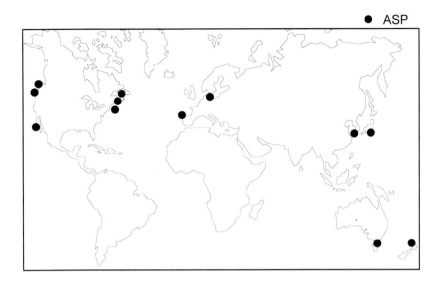

**Figure 8.1e**    Global distribution of the reported occurrence of (a) paralytic shellfish poisonings, (b) diarrhetic shellfish poisonings, (c) ciguatera fish poisonings, (d) neurotoxic shellfish poisonings and (e) amnesic shellfish poisonings and of the occurrence of each of these toxins in seafood or phytoplankton (from Hallegraeff, 1995; and Andersen, 1996). Black dots ● indicate the location of reported occurrences.

and C toxins (Cembella *et al.,* 1993; Wright, 1995). PSP toxins may form up to 0.2% of the wet weight of PSP-toxic dinoflagellates and the most predominant toxins are usually the sulphated derivatives (Laycock *et al.*, 1994). However, some of these compounds may undergo degradation or biotransformation after being assimilated by shellfish and other organisms (Cembella *et al.*, 1994; Oshima, 1995a; Wright, 1995; Bricelj *et al.*, 1996) and novel derivatives are occasionally reported (Gago-Martinez *et al.*, 1996). Intoxicated shellfish that grow in cold or temperate waters most commonly contain the sulphated C toxins GTX2 and 3 and also saxitoxin (Wright, 1995).

## 8.3.2  Toxic effects

The symptoms of PSP poisoning in humans are very characteristic and range from a tingling sensation or numbness as a result of mild intoxication to death through respiratory paralysis in extreme cases (Table 8.1). At the biochemical level the effect of the PSP toxins, especially saxitoxin, is well understood. They act by blocking neuronal and muscular sodium channels, thereby affecting transmission of nerve impulses and muscle contraction (Table 8.2). Detailed accounts of the mechanism of action of saxitoxin and other PSP toxins can be found in Baden and Trainer (1993) and Kao (1993).

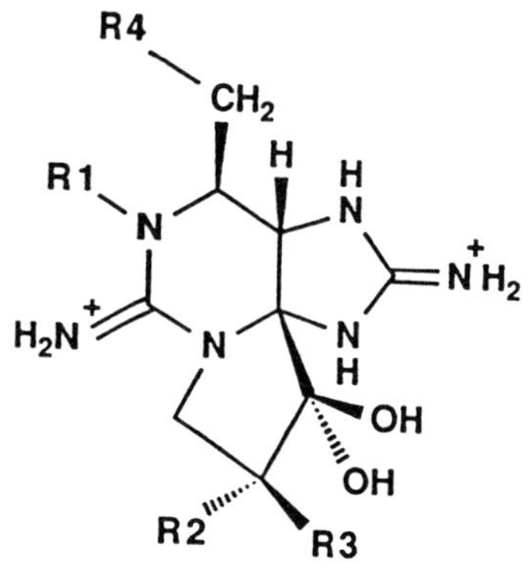

| R1 | R2 | R3 | O<br>‖<br>R4: -OCNH₂ | O<br>‖<br>R4: -OCNH·SO₃⁻ | R4: -OH | R4: -H |
|---|---|---|---|---|---|---|
| H | H | H | STX | B1 (GTX5) | *dc* STX | *do* STX |
| OH | H | H | neoSTX | B2 (GTX6) | *dc* neoSTX | * |
| OH | OSO₃⁻ | H | GTX1 | C3 | *dc* GTX1 | * |
| H | OSO₃⁻ | H | GTX2 | C1 | *dc* GTX2 | *do* GTX2 |
| H | H | OSO₃⁻ | GTX3 | C2 | *dc* GTX3 | *do* GTX3 |
| H | H | OSO₃⁻ | GTX4 | C4 | *dc* GTX4 | * |

STX = Saxitoxin     *dc* = decarbamoyl
GTX = Gonyautoxin     *do* = deoxycarbamoyl

**Figure 8.2** Chemical structure of the PSP toxins (after Oshima, 1995b).

## 8.4 Diarrhetic shellfish poisoning

Three disparate groups of lipophilic polyether compounds make up the family of diarrhetic shellfish toxins: okadaic acid (OA) and the dinophysistoxins (DTXs), the pectenotoxins (PTXs) and yessotoxin (YTX) and its derivatives. The collective term 'diarrhetic shellfish toxins' is a misnomer since only okadaic acid and DTXs are actually diarrhetic, whereas the compounds in the other groups have different physiological effects (Table 8.1) and perhaps should be reclassified (Aune and Yndestad, 1993; Draisci *et al.*, 1996). Diarrhetic shellfish poisoning (DSP) in humans is caused primarily by eating shellfish, such as mussels and clams contaminated with OA and/or DTXs which originate mainly from certain *Dinophysis* species (Table 8.1).

**Table 8.2** Sites of action and primary physiological effects of phycotoxins. After Baden and Trainer (1993) with additional information from Cembella *et al.* (1995)

| Toxin | Biochemical site of action | Primary physiological effects |
|---|---|---|
| PSP toxins | Site 1 on voltage-dependent sodium channels | Block sodium ion influx in neuronal and muscular sodium channel. Prevents propagation of the action potential essential for conduction of nerve impulses and contraction of muscles. Periphe[ral] nervous system particularly affected in vertebrates |
| DSP toxins | | |
| *Okadaic acid and derivatives* | Catalytic subunit of protein phosphorylase phosphatases type1 and 2A | Inhibit protein phosphorylase phosphatases |
| *Pectenotoxins* | Not known | Hepatotoxic |
| *Yessotoxin* | Not known | Damages heart muscle |
| NSP toxins | Site 5 on voltage-dependent sodium channels | Induce channel-mediated sodium ion influx; depolarizes isolated muscle and nerve cells |
| Ciguatera toxins | | |
| *Ciguatoxin* | Site 5 on voltage-dependent sodium channels | Opening of sodium channels at resting potential and inability of open channels to be inactivated during subsequent depolarizatio[n] |
| *Maitotoxin* | Calcium channels | Calcium ion influx, which may lead to cell death |
| Domoic acid | Glutamate receptors in central nervous system | Binds to glutamate receptors, i.e. competes with glutamate; receptor-induced depolarization and excitation |

The global distribution of poisonings and the occurrence of DSP toxins in shellfish are shown in Figure 8.1b. This is the second most widespread intoxication of humans and shellfish caused by algae. As regards OA and the DTXs, the predominant toxin may vary according to geographic region. For example, OA is normally the major toxin in most of Europe whereas DTX-1 usually predominates in Japanese and Canadian shellfish, and in Ireland DTX-2 predominates (Quilliam and Wright, 1995; Carmody *et al.*, 1996). The pectenotoxins have so far been detected in shellfish and in *Dinophysis* species in Japan (Yasumoto *et al.*, 1989), and in natural samples of *Dinophysis fortii* collected from the Adriatic (Draisci *et al.*, 1996). YTXs have been found in shellfish in Japan (Murata *et al.*, 1987; Satake *et al.*, 1996), the Adriatic (Ciminiello *et al.*, 1997) and also in Norway where YTX occurred simultaneously with DTX-1 in mussels (Lee *et al.*, 1988). A detailed account of all aspects of DSP has been given by Aune and Yndestad (1993).

### 8.4.1 The DSP toxins

*8.4.1.1 Okadaic acid and the dinophysis toxins.* Okadaic acid and dinophysis toxins, the latter so named because they occur in the dinoflagellate genus *Dinophysis* (see Table 8.1), are acidic compounds (Figure 8.3a). The most important of this group of acidic toxins as regards shellfish contamination are OA, DTX-1 and DTX-2, which may occur singly or together. The polyether backbone of OA, DTX-1 and DTX-2 may be acylated in the digestive glands of shellfish to produce a mixture of compounds with diarrhetic activity, collectively known as 'DTX-3', which have fatty acid side chains (Quilliam and Wright, 1995; Wright 1995). A number of other okadaic acid derivatives are known to occur, including diol esters that do not inhibit protein phosphatases (see below). These esters are labile and might undergo chemical or biochemical transformation to toxic derivatives (Quilliam and Wright, 1995). Two sulphated derivatives of DTX, DTX-4 and DTX-5, which are unusual in being water-soluble, have been isolated from the benthic dinoflagellate *Prorocentrum lima* (Hu *et al.*, 1995a,b; Quilliam *et al.*, 1996) but the significance of these toxins in shellfish poisoning is presently unknown.

*8.4.1.2 Pectenotoxins.* The pectenotoxins are a group of neutral macrolide polyether lactones. Seven PTXs have been isolated from algae or shellfish and four, PTX-1, -2, -3 and -6, have so far been chemically characterized (Figure 8.3b). PTX-2 has only ever been found in the dinoflagellate *Dinophysis fortii* and never in shellfish. It has been suggested that all other PTXs are derived from it by metabolic reactions in the hepatopancreas of shellfish (Yasumoto *et al.*, 1989; Draisci *et al.*, 1996).

(a)

| R1 | R2 | R3 | |
|----|----|----|---|
| CH₃ | H | H | Okadaic acid |
| CH₃ | CH₃ | H | Dinophysistoxin-1 (DTX-1) |
| H | CH₃ | H | DTX-2 |
| H or CH₃ | | Acyl | DTX-3 |

(b)

| R | |
|---|---|
| CH₂OH | Pectenotoxin-1 (PTX-1) |
| CH₃ | PTX-2 |
| CHO | PTX-3 |
| COOH | PTX-6 |

(c)

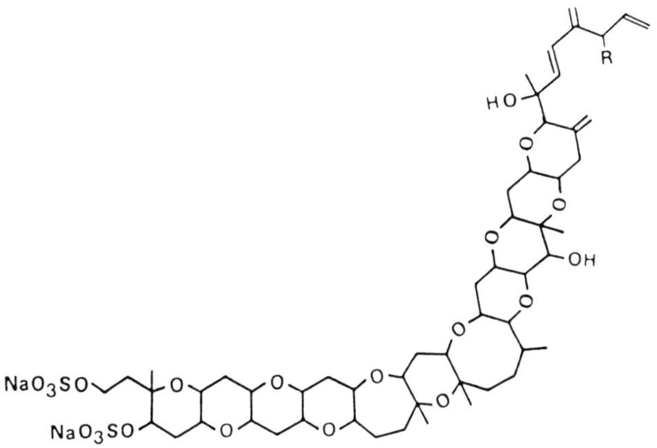

| R | |
|---|---|
| H | Yessotoxin (YTX) |
| OH | 45-hydroxyyessotoxin (45-OHYTX) |

**Figure 8.3**     (a) Chemical structure of okadaic acid and some related compounds (from Quilliam and Wright, 1995). (b) Chemical structure of the pectenotoxins. (c) Chemical structure of yessotoxin and related compounds.

*8.4.1.3 Yessotoxins.* Yessotoxin, so called because it was originally isolated from the scallop *Patinopecten yessoensis*, resembles the brevetoxins and ciguatoxins in that it has contiguously fused ether rings (Figure 8.3c) but differs in that it has a longer backbone of 47 carbon atoms, a terminal side chain of nine carbons, two sulphate esters and lacks carbonyl groups (Murata *et al.*, 1987; Takahashi *et al.*, 1996). Two derivatives of YTX have been described, 45-hydroxy YTX and 45,46,47 trinorYTX (Yasumoto *et al.*, 1989; Satake *et al.*, 1996).

*8.4.2 Toxic effects*
The symptoms of DSP in humans are summarized in Table 8.1. Gastrointestinal disturbance is the main effect and the symptoms usually disappear within three days. Studies on the pathological effects of the DSP group (OA, DTXs, PTXs and YTX) have been confined mainly to suckling and adult mice and to rats—detailed accounts can be found in Terao *et al.*

(1990, 1993) and in Aune and Yndestad (1993). Intraperitoneal (ip) and oral doses of OA and DTXs cause marked changes in the small intestine, such as fluid accumulation and distension. Ultrastructural changes include degeneration of the intestinal absorptive epithelium. Terao *et al.* (1990, 1993) also observed liver damage in rats and mice given ip and oral doses of OA and DTX-1. PTX-1 had no effect on the intestines of suckling mice but there was extensive liver damage. Similar results were obtained with adult mice and extensive necrosis of hepatocytes was observed after 24 hours. YTX also had no effect on the intestines of mice but caused severe cardiac damage including the swelling of cardiac muscle cells and also of cells of the endothelial lining of capillaries. Desulphated YTX caused minimal damage to heart muscle but liver damage was observed.

The effects of purified OA, DTX-1, PTX-1 and YTX on freshly prepared rat hepatocyte cells have been observed using light and electron microscopy (Aune *et al.*, 1991). OA and DTX-1 produced dose-dependent changes including 'blebbing' of the cell surface and overall irregular shape. PTX-1 caused the smoothing of the external surface of the cells due to loss of the external microvilli but the normal overall rounded shape was retained. The hepatocytes were least affected by YTX, which retained a normal rounded shape but small blebs formed on the cell surface. Zhou *et al.* (1994) studied the effect of PTX-1 on chick embryo liver cells and found that it caused actin accumulation at the cell peripheries and cytoplasm, due to disruption of actin microfilaments within myofibrils, and microtubules were reduced in number and lost their radial arrangement. The damage was reversible if the cells were exposed to < 0.5 µg/ml PTX-1 for less than 4 hours. Treatment of cultured human intestinal epithelial cells with OA changes their permeability, which may contribute to the diarrhetic symptoms in humans (Tripuraneni *et al.*, 1997).

At a biochemical level OA and DTXs are powerful inhibitors of protein phosphatases PP1 and PP2 and 2A, which are important in regulating many important metabolic processes in eukaryotic cells (Table 8.2). This has been used as an assay to detect these toxins (Table 8.3). OA and DTXs are also potent tumour promoters but the possible effects of chronic exposure to these toxins in humans has still to be established (Aune and Yndestad, 1993; van Egmond *et al.*, 1993). The sites of action of PTXs and YTXs at the molecular level are presently unknown.

## 8.5   Ciguatera fish poisoning

Ciguatera fish poisoning (CFP) in humans is caused by ingestion of a complex group of polyether toxins, the ciguatoxins (CTXs), that accumulate in the flesh of fish living on and around tropical coral reefs. The name ciguatera is derived from the Spanish word *cigua*, the common name given to the

**Table 8.3** Summary of assays and analytical methods used to detect phycotoxins[a]

| Toxin group | In vivo assays | In vitro assays | Chemical analyses |
|---|---|---|---|
| PSP | Mouse[b] | Cultured mouse neuroblastoma cells[®][c]<br>Immunoassay[®]<br>Receptor binding | HPLC; capillary electrophoresis (both of these may be interfaced to a mass spectrometer [MS]) |
| DSP | Mouse[b] (four variants) Rat | Cultured cells: Buffalo Green Monkey cells[d], human carcinoma cells[e], mouse and rat intestinal epithelial cells[e]; freshly prepared rat hepatocytes; inhibition of protein phosphatases PP1 and 2A[f]<br>Immunoassay[®] | HPLC; HPLC-MS; Micellar electrokinetic chromatography[g] |
| PTX | Mouse[b] | | |
| YTX | Mouse[b] | | |
| ASP | Mouse (has been used but insensitive) | Receptor binding | HPLC[b]; HPLC-MS; capillary electrophoresis[h] |
| NSP | Mouse[b] | Cultured mouse neuroblastoma cells<br>Immunoassay[®] (brevetoxins) Receptor binding | HPLC-MS[i]; electrokinetic capillary chromatography[j] |
| Ciguatera |  |  |  |
| Ciguatoxin | Mouse[b] | Immunoassay[®]<br>Receptor binding | HPLC; HPLC-MS[k] |
| Maitotoxin | Mouse[b] | Receptor binding | HPLC; HPLC-MS |

a   Except where indicated, details of all the above methods, including practical protocols, can be found in Hallegraeff et al. (1995) and see also Falconer (1993) and Yasumoto et al. (1995).
b   Accepted standard test.
c   ® = Test kits commercially available.
d   Croci et al. (1997).
e   Blay and Poon (1995).
f   Honkanen et al. (1996a); Honkanen et al. (1996b); Nunez and Scoging (1997).

g   Bouaicha et al. (1997).
h   Zhao et al. (1997).
i   Hua et al. (1996).
j   Shea (1997).
k   Lewis and Jones (1997).

Andersen, 1996). The occurrence of CFP toxins in fish in a specific area is often sporadic; the same species of fish caught simultaneously at the same locality may not all be toxic (Andersen, 1996).

CFP is concentrated mainly in tropical and subtropical areas, especially islands, in a band between latitudes 35°N and 35°S (Figure 8.1c), and is a serious public health problem in those countries, where fish constitute the main source of dietary protein. With the advent of rapid air transport CFP may occasionally occur in countries outside those latitudes where the fish are imported by specialist seafood restaurants or symptoms may develop in tourists after they have returned home. About 20 000 people are affected by CFP each year but it is rarely fatal. For detailed accounts of CFP see Bagnis (1993), Lewis and Holmes (1993) and Yasumoto and Satake (1996).

### 8.5.1 The CFP toxins

*8.5.1.1 Ciguatoxins.* The structures of some ciguatoxins (CTX) are shown in Figure 8.4. They are lipophilic polyethers. Gambiertoxin-4, isolated from the dinoflagellate *Gambierdiscus toxicus*, is probably the parent compound (Lewis and Holmes, 1993). Ciguatoxins have been isolated and purified from relatively few organisms so it is likely that the CTX molecules that occur in carnivorous fish are modified during their passage through the food chain and many more variants may exist. This could explain the wide range of clinical symptoms that has been observed (Bagnis, 1993; Wright, 1995). At present eight ciguatoxinsfrom the Pacific area have been fully characterized. There are at least 11 oxidized ciguatoxins (Lewis and Jones, 1997). At least four new ciguatoxins have been identified from the Caribbean area but have yet to be structurally defined (Vernoux and Lewis, 1997). Detailed information on the isolation and structure of CTXs can be found in Legrand *et al.* (1992), Lewis *et al.* (1991, 1994), Lewis and Jones (1997), and Yasumoto and Satake (1996).

*8.5.1.2 Maitotoxin.* Maitotoxin (MTX) is a water-soluble compound that is often associated with CTXs in the viscera of herbivorous fish. It is one of the most potent marine toxins known, with an $LD_{50}$ in mice of 0.17 µg/kg (Baden and Trainer, 1993). Murata *et al.* (1994) isolated MTX from cultures of the dinoflagellate *G. toxicus* and determined its structure and partial stereochemistry. It is a large and complex bisulphated molecule (molecular weight = 3422) containing 32 ether rings, not all of which are contiguous. The complete structure and stereochemistry of MTX have been determined by Nonomura *et al.* (1996) and Zheng *et al.* (1996). Relatives of MTX, MTX-2 and -3, have been identified by mass spectrometry (Lewis *et al.*, 1994). MTX is thought to play only a minor role in CFP in humans since it has not been detected in significant quantities in the muscle tissue of either

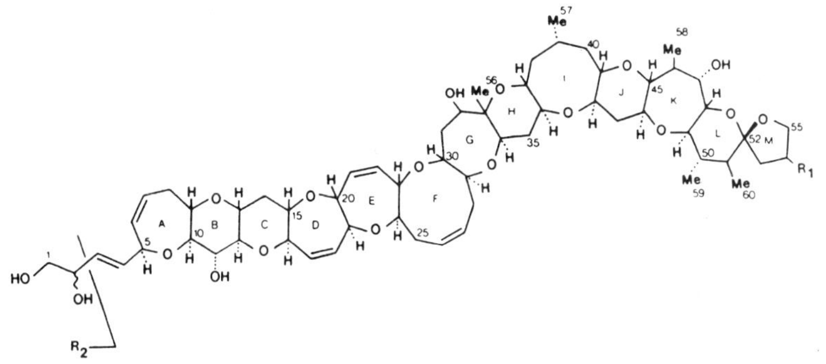

| R1 | R2 | |
|----|----|--|
| OH | | Ciguatoxin-1 (CTX-1) |
| H | | CTX-2 (= 52 *epi*-CTX-3) |
| H | | CTX-3 |
| H | CH₂ = CH - | Gambiertoxin-4B |

**Figure 8.4**   Chemical structure of the major ciguatoxins and gambiertoxin (from Lewis, 1995). Note that CTX-1, -2 ands -3 occur in the flesh of some carnivorous fish. Gambiertoxin-4B occurs in the dinoflagellate *Gambierdiscus toxicus* and some herbivorous reef fish.

most potent marine toxins known, with an $LD_{50}$ in mice of 0.17 µg/kg (Baden and Trainer, 1993). Murata *et al.* (1994) isolated MTX from cultures of the dinoflagellate *G. toxicus* and determined its structure and partial stereochemistry. It is a large and complex bisulphated molecule (molecular weight = 3422) containing 32 ether rings, not all of which are contiguous. The complete structure and stereochemistry of MTX have been determined by Nonomura *et al.* (1996) and Zheng *et al.* (1996). Relatives of MTX, MTX-2 and -3, have been identified by mass spectrometry (Lewis *et al.*, 1994). MTX is thought to play only a minor role in CFP in humans since it has not been detected in significant quantities in the muscle tissue of either herbivorous or carnivorous fishes (Bagnis, 1993; Lewis and Holmes, 1993).

### 8.5.2  Toxic effects

The symptoms produced by CFP toxins are complex and the effects may be long lasting (Table 8.1). Comparatively little is known about the effects of these toxins at an ultrastructural level. CTXs cause microscopic oedema of neural tissue (Bagnis, 1993) and CTX-1b appears to cause nodal swelling in isolated frog nodes of Ranvier (Benoit *et al.*, 1996). CTXs act by binding to and activating voltage-sensitive sodium channels. The high toxicity of MTX is explained by the fact that it activates both voltage-sensitive and receptor-operated calcium channels in the plasma membrane of cells, resulting in calcium influx and ultimately cell death due to calcium overload. The biochemical and physiological effects of CTXs are summarized in Table 8.2. Further details can be found in Baden and Trainer (1993) and Yasumoto and Satake (1996).

## 8.6   Neurotoxic shellfish poisoning

Neurotoxic shellfish poisoning (NSP), sometimes also referred to as neurological shellfish poisoning (Cembella *et al.*, 1995), is caused by ingestion of a group of lipophilic polyether toxins, the brevetoxins (PbTXs), produced by the naked dinoflagellate *Gymnodinium breve* (= *Ptychodiscus brevis*). As well as being present in shellfish, the PbTXs may also affect humans directly through contact with the algae (Table 8.1). Dense blooms of this alga may also cause large-scale fish kills.

Until recently the incidence of NSP was restricted to the Gulf of Mexico and the east coast of Florida, where 'red tides' due to blooms of *G. breve* are a common occurrence. In 1987, however, a bloom of *G. breve* originating in Florida was spread by the Gulf Stream to North Carolina where incidents of poisoning were reported (Morris *et al.*, 1991) and it has since continued to be present there (Hallegraeff, 1995). An outbreak of NSP occurred in New Zealand in 1993 and affected 180 people. The causative organism was similar but not identical to *G. breve* (Jasperse, 1993; Hallegraeff, 1995). Species similar or closely related to *G. breve* have been reported in Spain and Japan (Chou *et al.*, 1985) but there have been no reports of poisonings in these regions. The geographic distribution of NSP and the occurrence of the toxins is shown in Figure 8.1d.

### 8.6.1   The NSP toxins: the brevetoxins
The brevetoxins (PbTXs) are a group of lipophilic polyethers that is  similar in some ways to ciguatoxins. The PbTXs are grouped as types 1 or 2, based on the backbone structures, as shown in Figure 8.5. One type-1 and eight type-2 PbTXs have been described (Baden and Trainer, 1993). As well as PbTXs, *G. breve* has also been found to produce two phosphorus-containing ichthytoxins (Premazzi and Volterra, 1993). Brevetoxins have also been discovered in algae other than dinoflagellates, the chloromonads *Fibrocapsa japonica* and *Hetrosigma akashiwo*, both of which belong to the class Raphidophyceae (Khan *et al.* 1996, 1997), but these have not been implicated in human poisonings.

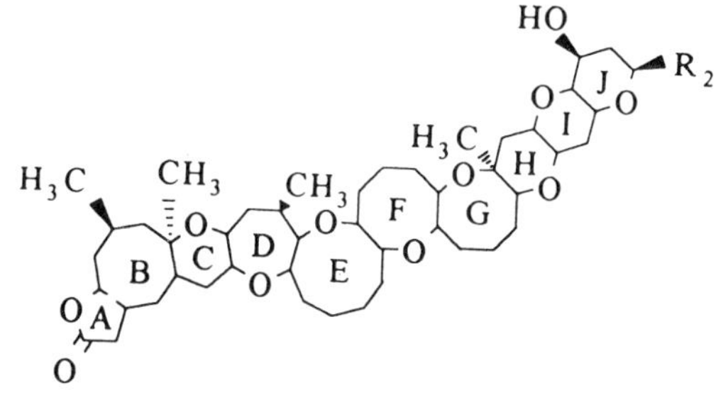

PbTX-1 type

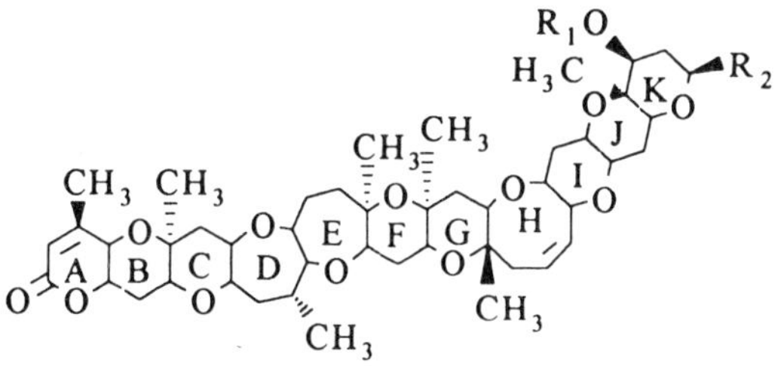

PbTX-2 type

**Figure 8.5**    Chemical structure of the brevetoxins. The basic structures are shown for PbTX-1 and PbTX-2 types, which are derivatized at $R_1$ and $R_2$ (after Baden and Trainer, 1993).

### 8.6.2  Toxic effects

Some of the symptoms of NSP are similar to those seen in mild cases of PSP and usually resolve within a few days (Table 8.1). The physiological action of brevetoxins is well understood and is similar to that of ciguatoxins. They act specifically on site-5 voltage-dependent sodium channels and induce influx of sodium ions into affected cells (Table 8.2). Detailed descriptions of the pharmacological action of the PbTxs can be found in Baden and Trainer (1993) and Premazzi and Volterra (1993).

## 8.7  Amnesic shellfish poisoning

Amnesic shellfish poisoning (ASP) is the most recently discovered toxic shellfish syndrome. It was first recognized in 1987 on Prince Edward Island, on the east coast of Canada, when a serious incident occurred in which there were four human fatalies and over 100 cases of acute poisoning following the consumption of blue mussels (*Mytilus edulis*). ASP gets its name from the fact that one of the recognized symptoms of the poisoning is loss of memory (Table 8.1). Several of the severely affected cases during the initial incident still suffered memory loss five years later (Todd, 1993). The toxin responsible was identified as domoic acid, a water-soluble, non-protein amino acid that was found to originate from the diatom *Pseudonitzschia multiseries* (= *Pseudo-nitzschia pungens* f. *multiseries*) (Ravn, 1995; Wright, 1995). This was the first recorded incidence of a diatom species being implicated in shellfish intoxication and other diatoms known to produce domoic acid are listed in Table 8.1.

Another, less serious, outbreak affecting humans occurred near Monterey Bay, California, in 1991. It was traced to razor clams. Prior to this incident the deaths of cormorants and pelicans in the area had been shown to be due to the consumption of anchovies that had accumulated domoic acid after feeding on a bloom of diatoms composed of *Pseudo-nitzschia australis* (Wright, 1995).

To date reports of domoic acid in seafood products have been mainly confined to North America (Alaska, Bay of Fundy, British Columbia, California, Oregon, Prince Edward Island and Washington) while less significant concentrations have been found in Australia, Europe, Japan and New Zealand (Hallegraeff, 1995; and see Figure 8.1e).

Following the initial outbreaks in Canada and the US the regulatory authorities in those countries introduced monitoring and control measures and since then no serious cases of ASP have been reported. For a comprehensive review of domoic acid and shellfish poisoning see Todd (1993).

### 8.7.1 The ASP toxins: domoic acid and its isomers
Domoic acid is a water-soluble, acidic, non-protein amino acid (Figure 8.6). A number of isomers of domoic acid have been isolated from the diatom *P. pungens* f. *multiseries* and from mussel tissues but these are less toxic than domoic acid (Wright, 1995; Wright and Quilliam, 1995).

### 8.7.2 Toxic effects
The major symptoms of ASP are summarized in Table 8.1. Necrosis of the hippocampal region in rat brain has been observed as well as a number of physiological effects on neurones (Baden and Trainer, 1993). At a biochemical level domoic acid acts competitively with glutamic acid as a neurotransmitter and has an antagonistic effect at several types of glutamate receptors (Table 8.2). For further details see Baden and Trainer (1993) and Wright (1995).

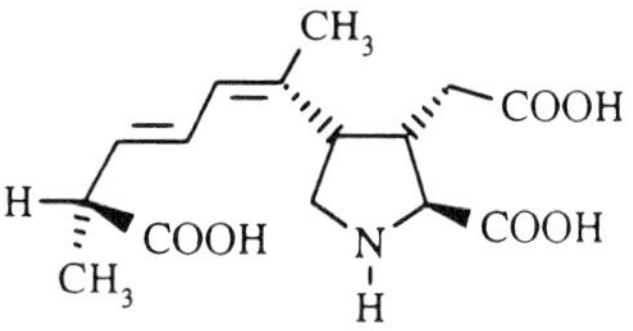

**Figure 8.6** Chemical structure of domoic acid (from Wright and Quilliam, 1995).

## 8.8 Some other phycotoxins

### 8.8.1 Cyanobacterial toxins

Various cyanobacteria (blue–green algae) are known to produce a number of potent toxins. The main ones are the microcystins and nodularin, which are hepatotoxic peptides, anatoxin-a, an alkaloid neurotoxin, anatoxin-a(s), a guanidinium phosphate ester that inhibits the enzyme cholinesterase, and PSP toxins such as saxitoxin, neosaxitoxin, C toxins and gonyautoxins (Carmichael and Falconer, 1993; Negri and Jones, 1995). Blooms of toxic cyanobacteria are predominantly a freshwater phenomenon, although they may also occur in estuarine and marine environments. Such blooms have caused illness and death in livestock. For example, an extensive bloom of PSP-toxic *Anabena* in the Australian Darling River in 1990 caused the deaths of about 1600 cattle and sheep that had drunk contaminated water. The effects of cyanobacterial toxins on human health through potable water supplies and recreational use of affected fresh water are well documented (Carmichael and Falconer, 1993; Codd, 1994; Ressom *et al.*, 1994 ).

The potential for intake of cyanobacterial toxins with food exists but there are no clinical reports of such poisoning (Falconer, 1996). Measurement of cyanobacterial toxins in foodstuffs is recommended, however, particularly in crustaceans and shellfish harvested from waters with high cyanobacterial concentrations (Falconer, 1993). Falconer *et al.* (1992) found cyanobacterial toxins present in edible mussels harvested in an estuary containing toxic *Nodularia* species. In an experimental study Vasconelos (1995) found that mussels (*Mytilus galloprovincialis*) could accumulate microcystin when exposed to the toxic estuarine cyanobacterium *Microcystis aeruginosa*. Microcystins have also been found in the freshwater mussel *Anodonta cygnea* (Eriksson *et al.*, 1989). Marine mussels are also known to accumulate these toxins (Chen *et al.*, 1993).

When a strain of *Anabaena circinalis*, which synthesises PSP gonyau-toxins and C toxins, was fed to the Australian freshwater mussel *Alathyria condola*, these PSP toxins accumulated in the tissues of the bivalve. It was concluded that bioaccumulation of the toxins by natural populations might pose a risk to human health (Negri and Jones, 1995). In a study of PSP tox-icity in the gastropod *Haliotis tuberculata*, in Galician coastal waters (Spain), Bravo *et al.* (1996) detected gonyautoxins in *Rivularia* species but the toxicity in the molluscs could not be attributed directly to this cyanobac-terium.

The recent discovery that chronic exposure to some cyanobacterial tox-ins may promote tumour production (Falconer, 1991; Falconer and Humpage, 1996; Yu, 1994) will increase awareness of these toxins, although the main risk is through freshwater rather than food.

### 8.8.2 *Macrocycle lactones*

Examples of toxic macrocycle lactones are prorocentrolide (PC), prorocen-trolide-B (Torigoe *et al.*, 1988; Hu *et al.*, 1996) and gymnodinine. PC co-occurs with okadaic acid and DTX-1 in the dinoflagellate *Prorocentrum lima* but it has an entirely different skeleton, which includes an imine group. PC was found to be lethal to mice at a dose of 400 μg/kg (ip).

Gymnodinine has been isolated from oysters in New Zealand and the dinoflagellate *Gymnodinium* sp. (Seki *et al.*, 1995, 1996; Mackenzie *et al.*, 1996). The molecule is composed of a 16-membered carbocyclic ring, a butenolide ring and a cyclic imine. Its lethality to mice is 450 μg/kg (ip) but it is not thought to constitute a hazard to human health.

### 8.8.3 *Miscellaneous phycotoxins*

There are many other toxic compounds that are known to occur in marine microalgae, for example cooliatoxin (Holmes *et al.*, 1995), palytoxin ana-logues (Usami *et al.*, 1995) and amphidinol-2 (see Shimizu, 1996). Although these toxins have not yet been directly implicated in human poi-sonings they may be present in the food chain. Some of these compounds are ichthytoxic and algal blooms have been responsible for the large-scale mortality of both wild and cultured fish (Andersen, 1996). The structure and occurrence of most of these phycotoxins have been reviewed by Yasumoto (1990), Premazzi and Volterra (1993) and Shimizu (1996).

### 8.9   Detection of phycotoxins in algae and seafood

Only a brief overview of the methodology of detection (summarized in Table 8.3) is provided here. In-depth coverage of all the topics touched upon can be conveniently found in a single volume (Hallegraeff *et al.*, 1995), which gives both theoretical and practical details. Another useful source of information is the annual review of methods for detecting toxins in seafood published by the Association of Official Analytical Chemists (see Quilliam, 1995, 1996, 1997).

### 8.9.1 Assays and analyses

Sullivan (1993) has drawn a useful distinction between assays and analyses for toxins. An assay is a method that produces a single response from the collective responses of all the individual components. Thus it indicates over-all toxicity but does not identify which toxins are present and their relative abundance. An example is the mouse bioassay discussed below. An analysis is a method that attempts to differentiate the various specific components present in a mixture and to quantify them individually, for example the separation and quantification of PSP and DSP toxins by high performance liquid chromatography.

### 8.9.2 Mammalian bioassays

The mouse bioassay is presently the mainstay for detecting phycotoxins and is recognized as the standard test for PSP, DSP, NSP and ciguatera toxins in most countries that carry out monitoring for phycotoxins. The basic procedure involves intraperitoneal injection of an extract of the sample containing the toxin and observing the symptoms. There are recommended strains and weights of mice, and the protocol varies depending on the toxins being assayed (van Egmond et al., 1992, 1993; Sullivan, 1993; Cembella et al., 1995; Lewis, 1995). Four variants of the mouse bioassay for DSP are in use and a rat bioassay is also employed for the detection of these toxins (Cembella et al., 1995).

8.9.2.1 *Disadvantages of the mouse bioassay.* The mouse bioassay has a number of disadvantages, which have been summarized by Sullivan (1993):

(i) *Presence of multiple toxins:* Samples often contain more than one member of a family of toxins, each of which may have a different degree of toxicity, as is normally the case with PSP, DSP, NSP and ciguatera toxins. The bioassay therefore provides only a measure of the *total* toxicity, which is expressed relative to the effects of a reference toxin. This is adequate for toxicity monitoring but can provide no indication of the relative amounts of individual toxins in the sample. An additional problem that has been recognized is the presence of 'side toxins', i.e. toxins that have been extracted that may cause symptoms in mice, or are detected by other bioassays, but which are not related to the toxin(s) actually being assayed (Luu et al., 1993; Zhao et al., 1993; Amzil et al., 1996; Mackenzie et al., 1996).

(ii) *Inherent variability:* This can exceed ±20% of the true value compared to chromatographic techniques, which have a variability <10%.

*(iii) Route of administration of the toxin:* Intraperitoneal injection bypasses the gastro-intestinal tract, the normal route exposure to phy-cotoxins in humans, and its functions (absorption, metabolism and distribution), which may be important in decreasing or increasing the toxicity of the food.

*(iv) Public opposition:* There is growing public opposition, including mil-itant action, to the use of animals for experimental purposes.

It has been recognized internationally for some time that there is an urgent need to replace mouse bioassays for phycotoxins with other methods. What are needed for monitoring seafoods for public health reasons are rapid, specific and relatively inexpensive assays that can be used to screen large numbers of samples, ideally 'at the dock-side', and can be undertaken by relatively unskilled personnel. Such assays can be validated as necessary by accurate and precise instrumental analyses. Much has been done in recent years towards achieving these goals, but relatively few methods have been developed to a stage where they have gained international acceptance The determination of domoic acid by high performance liquid chromatography (HPLC) is a notable exception.

### 8.9.3 *Instrumental analysis*

Instrumental analyses for phycotoxins have been developed using such methods as HPLC. This is usually with sensitive fluorescence detection (Table 8.3) or the HPLC apparatus may be interfaced with a mass spec-trometer (MS), especially where confirmation of the structure of a particu-lar molecule is required. There are standard HPLC analyses for PSP and DSP toxins using fluorescence detection and for domoic acid using UV detection.

There are a number of problems associated with instrumental analyses, for example the high initial capital cost of the equipment, especially for MS. Lengthy clean-up procedures are usually required, especially for lipophilic toxins, and this limits daily sample throughput. For fluorescence detection the appropriate fluorescent derivatives must be prepared. These may be unstable unless they are maintained under constant conditions or the deriva-tization reagents themselves may be unstable. There is a lack of pure ana-lytical standards for some phycotoxins, which makes quantitation difficult. Details of analytical protocols and discussions of associated problems can be found in Oshima (1995b), Quilliam and Wright (1995), and Wright and Quilliam (1995).

### 8.9.4 In vitro *assays*

8.9.4.1 *Cytotoxicity assays.* Cytotoxicity assays using tissue culture microplate techniques have been developed for PSP, NSP and CFP toxins and for the DSP toxins okadaic acid and DTX-1. The PSP, NSP and CFP assays use mouse neuroblastoma cells. Various DSP assays use Buffalo Green Monkey (BGM) cells, mouse intestinal epithelial cells, rat hepatocytes or human carcinoma cells (Table 8.3).

The cytotoxicity method for PSP is based on the fact that cultured neuroblastoma cells will swell and die if incubated in the presence of ouabain, an Na/K ATPase inhibitor, and veratridine, which causes depolarization of membranes. Both of these substances allow uncontrolled influx of sodium into the cells, causing death. PSP toxins, or other sodium channel blockers, counteract this effect and the cells remain viable. Dead cells lose adhesion to the plastic surface on which they grow and during staining with crystal violet, rinsing and fixing of the cells the dead cells are washed away. Absorbance at 595 nm, measured automatically with a microplate reader, is proportional to the number of viable cells and therefore to the quantity of PSP toxins in the sample. The cytotoxicity assays for NSP and CFP toxins measure the effect of sodium channel activators. They are similar to the PSP method in that they use the same cell line and inhibitors, and similar equipment. The assays measure the ability of the cells to reduce a tetrazolium dye to a coloured compound (Cembella et al., 1995). Various end points are used for the DSP cytotoxicity assays: direct observation of morphological changes (cell rounding and vacuolization) caused by okadaic acid with BGM cells (Croci et al., 1997), morphological changes and leakage of the enzyme lactate dehydrogenase with rat hepatocytes, and reduction of a tetrazolium dye to a coloured product by human intestinal cells (Blay and Poon, 1995; Cembella et al., 1995). Although such assays are best carried out in a fully equipped tissue-culture laboratory, kits are available commercially for the PSP assay that require less rigorous conditions (Cembella et al., 1995).

One problem with cytotoxicity assays is that they can respond to non-specific inhibitors. Tissue extracts are 'dirty' and may contain substances that affect the assay. For example, zinc in some mussel extracts can be toxic to mice and is presumably also so to cultured cells (Sullivan, 1993). Manger et al. (1995) observed non-specific toxic effects with crab viscera extracts but the problem was overcome by dilution. Another problem is that these assays may respond to unknown 'side toxins' in the sample (see above).

*8.9.4.2 Receptor binding assays.* The PSP, NSP, ASP and CFP toxins all share a common property in that they bind very specifically to certain receptor sites (Table 8.2). A number of binding assays for these toxins have been developed that exploit this property. They use synaptosome preparations from animal brains and usually measure competition for the specific binding sites between a radioactive substrate and the toxin(s) in the sample (Table 8.3). The objection to using animal preparations may be overcome by using cloned receptor proteins (Goldin et al., 1986; Quilliam, 1996).

Binding assays are sensitive, specific and represent an integrated measure of the potencies of a mixture of a family of toxins such as PSP. Good correlations have been obtained between the standard mouse bioassay and binding assays for PSP toxins and the NSP toxin, brevetoxin (Cembella *et al.*, 1995).

*8.9.4.3 Immunoassays.* A number of immunoassays have been developed for some of the PSP, DSP and NSP toxins and ciguatoxin (Table 8.3) and some of these are available commercially. Cembella *et al.* (1995) have discussed some of the problems encountered in developing these assays, such as the lack of pure toxins for conjugation and the low antigenicity of some of the lower molecular weight toxin molecules. Also, antibodies are usually prepared from a single purified toxin, such as saxitoxin, whereas natural samples may usually contain several closely related derivatives and the antibody may show limited cross-reactivity to these compounds. Both monoclonal and polyclonal antibodies have been produced to various toxins and these have been visualized using techniques such as enzyme-linked immunosorbent assays. 'Dip-stick' type tests have been developed for saxitoxin and ciguatoxins. In general, imunnoassays for phycotoxins are many times more sensitive than instrumental methods. If problems of low cross-reactivity and false positives can be overcome, this type of assay may prove useful for initial rapid screening of suspect samples.

*8.9.4.4 Enzyme inhibition assays for DSP toxins.* Enzyme inhibition assays have been developed for okadaic acid and DTX-1 based on the fact that they are potent inhibitors of protein phosphatases PP1 and PP2A. A radioisotope assay involving $^{32}$P and PP1 and PP2A has been developed by Holmes (1991). It involves liquid chromatography (LC) prior to the assay to resolve phosphatase inhibitors into discrete fractions, since the assay responds to all phosphatase inhibitors. The method can quantify OA and DTX-1. Luu *et al.* (1993) subsequently applied Holmes' assay to identify DSP toxins in cultures of the dinoflagellate *Prorocentrum lima* in natural populations of phytoplankton and in mussels obtained both from Holland and from Canada. The most interesting result was that at least six phosphatase inhibitors distinct from known DSP toxins were found in mussel extracts. These did not include pectenotoxins and yessotoxin, which were found to be inactive against PP1 and 2A. A protein phosphatase assay for OA and DTX-1 in shellfish extracts using PP2A and $^{32}$P has been described by Honkanen *et al.* (1996a,b) who point out the problems involved in using $^{32}$P and PP2A. A non-radioactive colourimetric assay using PP1 has been described that can detect OA and DTX-1 with a limit of about 1.5 ng total toxin per gram of mussel hepatopancreas (Nunez and Scoging, 1997). These enzyme assays can also be used to detect microcystins from cyanobacteria (see, for example, Boland *et al.*, 1993).

The main problem with protein phosphatase assays for OA and DTX-1 is that they respond to all phosphatase inhibitors in crude extracts. Two other problems are the use of $^{32}$P, which can be avoided by using a colourimetric end-point but with lower sensitivity, and the relative scarcity and expense of the enzymes; this may be overcome by genetic engineering.

## 8.10 Depuration of phycotoxins

### 8.10.1 Natural depuration

If shellfish contaminated with phycotoxins are left for sufficient time they will depurate (detoxify) themselves naturally once the causative algae are no longer present in the water. In order to speed up this process affected shellfish may be harvested and moved to a site where the water is free of toxic algae. However, this is not always a satisfactory solution as the rates of depuration vary greatly between species and on the type of toxin they carry, as well as physical factors. Shumway *et al.* (1995) have provided a comprehensive compilation of the approximate times taken for a number of phycotoxins to fall below either statutory limits or levels of detection in a wide range of shellfish. These times range from two days to more than two years.

There is a vast amount of literature dealing with depuration of PSP toxins in both bivalve and crustacean shellfish (e.g. Watson-Wright *et al.*, 1991; Haya *et al.*, 1992; Bricelj and Cembella, 1995; Desbiens and Cembella, 1995; Shumway *et al.*, 1995). In general, shellfish depurate PSP toxins relatively slowly and various methods of enhancing depuration have been tried with limited success, including variation in temperature or salinity, chlorination, ozonation and electrical stimulation (Shumway *et al.*, 1995).

Comparatively little information exists on depuration of DSP toxins and most of this concerns okadaic acid and DTXs. In many cases these toxins are eliminated relatively quickly (Marcaillou-Le Baut *et al.*, 1993; Quilliam *et al.*, 1993; Croci *et al.*, 1994; Bauder *et al.*, 1996; Poletti *et al.*, 1996) but they may persist for long periods (Carmody *et al.*, 1995; Dahl *et al.*, 1995; Shumway *et al.*, 1995).

For domoic acid, depuration times ranging from two days to more than two years have been reported (Shumway *et al.*, 1995). Intoxicated mussels transferred from field to laboratory conditions eliminated the toxin to residual levels within 72 hours (Novaczek *et al.*, 1992). However, in laboratory experiments where toxic diatoms were fed to mussels the depuration rate was about 17% per day and in scallops treated in the same way the rate was lower (Wohlgeschaffen *et al.*, 1992). A computer simulation model of the flux of domoic acid through a mussel population and comparison with field data indicated a possible link between high levels of accumulation of domoic acid and reduction in depuration rates (Silvert and Rao, 1992).

### 8.10.2 Depuration by cooking

Both domestic and commercial cooking have been studied as ways of reducing toxicity, primarily for bivalve shellfish contaminated with PSP toxins (Table 8.4). The main effect of boiling or pre-cooking with steam (e.g. domestic cooking and some commercial canning), seems to be to leach out and dilute the water-soluble PSP toxins in the tissues. Since a good proportion of the cooking liquor is discarded this lowers the total concentration of toxins in the shellfish (Quayle, 1969; Prakash *et al.*, 1971; Berenguer *et al.*, 1993). Cooking by retorting (110°C for 80 min or 122°C for 22 min) of PSP-contaminated clams was reported to reduce significantly the concentration of toxins in tissues, for example from >1800 µg STX-equivalents/100 g tissue to <9 µg STX-equivalents/100 g in the digestive gland (Noguchi *et al.*, 1980a,b). Shumway *et al.* (1995) point out that the effectiveness of canning as a means of reducing PSP toxin levels below the statutory limit depends on the initial toxicity and so must be used with caution.

Ohta *et al.* (1992) investigated the effect of extrusion processing on various tissues of contaminated clams mixed with defatted soya protein. Extrusion was carried out at 130°C and 170°C and at elevated pressures. This considerably reduced the toxin content of the mixture, by up to 82% at 130°C and up to 97% at 170°C. The reduction in moisture content of the mixture after heating was only 1 to 2% so the decrease in toxicity did not appear to be due to leaching. HPLC analysis of the uncooked mixture showed it contained gonyautoxins-1, -2, -3 and -4 and saxitoxin, but after processing at either of the two temperatures it contained only saxitoxin, which has a higher specific toxicity. Nagashima *et al.* (1991) examined the thermal stability of PSP toxins under various conditions. Scallop homogenates showed little residual toxicity after heating to 120°C for 2 hours, whereas the toxicity of oyster homogenates doubled when heated to100°C for up to 2 hours and then declined linearly on further heating. The increase in toxicity (as measured by the mouse bioassay) was attributed to chemical conversion of the toxins to more toxic derivatives.

The DSP toxins contained in mussel tissue are stable to cooking at >95°C for 15 min, as estimated by the mouse bioassay (Vernoux *et al.*, 1994). Comparison of raw and cooked meat showed that heating did not change the concentration of toxins or their partitioning between the digestive gland (the most toxic organ) and the rest of the meat. Prolonged boiling of mussels for 163 min, however, was found to reduce the concentration of okadaic acid by 50% (Edebo *et al.*, 1988).

Both CFP toxins in fish tissue and NSP toxins in shellfish are stable to cooking and boiling (Premazzi and Volterra, 1993; Lewis, 1995).

Domoic acid in the viscera of Dungeness crabs (*Cancer magister*) cooked by normal commercial processes in salt or fresh water could be reduced by up to 67% (Hatfield *et al.*, 1995). After cooking some domoic

**Table 8.4** The effects of cooking and freezing on the phycotoxin content of some shellfish

| Toxins | Organism | Process | Effect on toxin content in tissues | References |
|---|---|---|---|---|
| PSP | American lobster (*Homarus americanus*) | Cooking | Reduction | Lawrence *et al.* (1994) Watson-Wright *et al.* (1991) |
| | Butter clams (*Saxidomus giganteus*) | Cooking | Reduction | Quayle (1969) |
| | | Freezing | Minimal effect | Quayle (1969) |
| | Mediterranean cockle (*Acanthocardia tuberosum*) | Cooking | Reduction | Berenguer *et al.* (1993) |
| | Mussels (*Mytilus edulis*) | Cooking | Reduction | Prakash *et al.* (1971) |
| | Soft clams (*Mya arenaria*) | Cooking | Reduction | Prakash *et al.* (1971) |
| | Scallops (*Patinopecten yessoensis*) | Cooking | Reduction | Noguchi *et al.* (1980a,b) Ohta *et al.* (1992) |
| | Mussels (*Mytilus* sp.) | Freezing | Migration to other tissues | Noguchi *et al.* (1984) |
| | | Cooking | No reduction | Vernoux *et al.* (1994) |
| DSP | | | | |
| Domoic acid | Crab (*Cancer magister*) | Cooking | Reduction | Hatfield *et al.* (1995) |
| | | Chilling and freezing | Migration to other tissues | Hatfield *et al.* (1995) |

acid was detectable in the body or leg meats of raw crabs, although it was not originally present in these tissues. The majority of the toxin was extracted and diluted into the cooking liquor.

Shumway *et al.* (1995) have concluded that, with the possible exception of the cooking method described by Berenguer *et al.* (1993), '...there have been no useful methods devised for effectively reducing phycotoxins in contaminated shellfish. All methods tested to date have been either unsafe, economically unfeasible or yielded products unacceptable in appearance and taste'.

### 8.10.3  The effects of freezing and chilling

There are a few reports on the effects of freezing and chilling on the mobility of water-soluble toxins in tissues. Quayle (1969) reported an experiment where 32 lots of butter clams (*Saxidomus giganteus*) (mean toxicity 74 µg STX-equivalents/100 g tissue, range 34 to 256 µg STX-equivalents) were frozen for three months. At the end of that time mouse bioassays showed virtually no change in toxicity (mean 79 µg STX-equivalents/100 g, range 33 to 342 µg STX-equivalents).

Noguchi *et al.* (1984) examined the distribution of PSP toxicity (measured by the mouse bioassay) in highly toxic specimens of the clam *Patinopecten yessoensis* and the effect of freezing. In unfrozen clams containing very high concentrations of toxins (117 000 to 198 000 µg STX-equivalents/100 g digestive gland) the concentration in the adductor muscle was 54 to 234 µg STX-equivalents/100 g. In less toxic unfrozen clams containing 18 000 to 52 200 µg STX-equivalents/100 g digestive gland the adductor muscle, washed or unwashed, was not detectably toxic. These less toxic specimens were kept frozen (temperature not specified) for five months; when thawed by heating to 100°C for 5 min or by standing at 17° to 21°C for 4 h, the toxicity of the non-washed adductor muscle was <36 µg STX-equivalents/100 g but rose to between 54 and 162 µg STX-equivalents/100 g when allowed to thaw slowly at 5°C for 24 h. When the whole clams were subjected to three freeze–thaw cycles the toxicity of the adductor muscle rose to 972 µg saxitoxin equivalents/100 g, which indicated migration of toxins between tissues. Shumway (unpublished, cited in Shumway and Cembella, 1993) has obtained similar results.

Studies have been carried out on whole cooked Dungeness crab (*Cancer magister*) where domoic acid was confined mainly to the viscera; small amounts were also detectable in leg and body meat. After storage of cooked crabs for 90 days at −23°C slightly increased concentrations of domoic acid were found in the leg and body meat. In cooked crabs held at 1°C for one to six days there was evidence of diffusion of toxin from the viscera to the body meat (Hatfield *et al.*, 1995).

## 8.11 Monitoring and regulation

The first line of defence against phycotoxins endangering human health is the monitoring of toxin levels in seafoods and the implementation of legislation to prevent harvesting and marketing if toxin levels exceed the statutory limit.

Monitoring programmes exist on local, regional and national scales in countries where phycotoxins are a problem and detailed accounts of these have been published for the USA (Hungerford and Wekell, 1993), Canada (Cembella and Todd, 1993) and Europe (van Egmond et al., 1992, 1993; Shumway et al., 1995). The definitive reference work is that by Andersen (1996), which provides details for over 20 countries of national management plans, monitoring strategies, toxin tolerance limits, cost–benefit analyses, responsible authorities and many more useful facts.

In addition to causing public health problems, toxic phytoplankton can have a significant effect on the use of coastal waters for mariculture, commercial fisheries and recreation (Premazzi and Volterra, 1993; Andersen, 1996). Given the need to minimize economic losses and the potential risk to the public caused by these outbreaks, two monitoring strategies have been used: regular testing of seafoods and the screening of natural phytoplankton populations for the presence of harmful species

*8.11.1  Monitoring of shellfish tissues for toxicity.* When shellfish resources are well developed, intensive monitoring has proven cost-effective and has permitted flexible management so as to optimize the areas of shellfish open to harvesting. This strategy has been used in France (Berthomé and Lassus, 1986), Japan (Yamamoto and Yamasaki, 1996), New Zealand (Trusewich et al., 1996) and in Maine, USA (Shumway et al., 1988). In contrast, when shellfish resources are limited or under-exploited it may only be cost-effective to impose widespread closures in a region, with little or no monitoring being carried out, such as in California, USA where the harvesting of mussels is prohibited every year between April and October each year regardless of the level of toxicity (ICES, 1992, but see also Hungerford and Wekell, 1993). Examples of tolerance limits for PSP, DSP, NSP and ASP in various countries are given in Tables 8.5, 8.6 and 8.7.

*8.11.2  Phytoplankton monitoring*
Details of national strategies and methodologies adopted to monitor harmful algae have been discussed by Aune et al. (1995), Belin et al. (1995), Hallegraeff et al. (1995), Andersen (1996), Emsholm et al. (1996),

Table 8.5 PSP tolerance levels and official assay and/or analysis methods in various countries. Modified from Shumway (1995) and Andersen (1996)

| Country | Product | Toxin | Tolerable level (per 100 g soft tissue) | Method of assay or analysis |
|---|---|---|---|---|
| Australia | Shellfish | Saxitoxin | 80 µg | Mouse bioassay |
| Canada | Molluscs | PSP | <80 µg[a] | Mouse bioassay |
| European Union (EU)[b] | Bivalve molluscs | PSP | 80 µg | Mouse bioassay[c] |
| Guatemala | Molluscs | Saxitoxin | 400 MU[d] | Mouse bioassay |
| Hong Kong | Shellfish | PSP | 400 MU | Mouse bioassay |
| Japan | Bivalves | PSP | 400 MU | Mouse bioassay + HPLC |
| Korea | Bivalves | Gonyautoxins | 400 MU | Mouse bioassay + HPLC |
| New Zealand | Shellfish | PSP | 80 µg | Mouse bioassay |
| Norway | All types of mussels | PSP | 200 MU | Mouse bioassay |
| Panama | Bivalves | PSP | 400 MU | Mouse bioassay |
| Singapore | Bivalves | Saxitoxin | 80 µg | Mouse bioassay |
| Sweden | Molluscs | PSP | 80 µg | Mouse bioassay |
| USA | Bivalves | PSP | 80 µg | Mouse bioassay |

a In Canada products having levels between 80 and 160 µg /100 g prior to closure of fisheries may be canned.
b European Union countries include Belgium, France, Germany, Greece, Ireland, Italy, Luxembourg, The Netherlands, Portugal, Spain and UK.
c In the majority of countries within the EU, the mouse bioassay is used. However, The Netherlands uses HPLC alone and Denmark and the UK supplement the bioassay with HPLC.
d 1 mouse unit (MU) = approx. 0.18 µg saxitoxin (van Egmond et al. 1993).

**Table 8.6** DSP tolerance levels in shellfish and official assay and/or analysis methods in countries with monitoring programmes. Modified from Shumway (1995) and Andersen (1996)

| Country | Tolerable level (per 100 g tissue) | Method of assay or analysis |
|---|---|---|
| Canada | 20 µg | Mouse bioassay, HPLC, ELISA |
| Denmark | Presence (two out of three die within 24 h) | Mouse bioassay |
| France | Presence (two out of three die within 5 h) | Mouse bioassay |
| Italy | 5 h mouse test | Mouse bioassay |
| Ireland | Positive bioassay | Mouse bioassay + LC-MS |
| Japan | 5 MU[a] | Mouse bioassay |
| Korea | 5 MU | Mouse bioassay |
| The Netherlands | 20–40 µg (digestive gland) | Rat bioassay |
| Norway | 5–7 MU | Mouse bioassay |
| Portugal | Presence (20 µg) | Mouse bioassay |
| Spain | Presence | Mouse bioassay |
| Sweden | 40–60 µg | HLPC, mouse bioassay for confirmation |
| UK (including N. Ireland) | 200 µg | Rat bioassay |
| Uruguay | Mortality in 24 h | Mouse bioassay |

[a] 1 mouse unit (MU) = approx. 5 µg okadaic acid (van Egmond et al., 1993).

**Table 8.7** NSP and ASP (domoic acid) tolerance levels and official assay and/or analysis methods in countries with monitoring programmes. Modified from Shumway (1995) and Andersen (1996)

| Country | Product | Toxin | Tolerable level (per 100 mg soft tissue) | Method of analysis |
|---|---|---|---|---|
| Canada | Shellfish | Domoic acid | 2 mg | HPLC |
| Denmark | Bivalve shellfish | Domoic acid | 2 mg | HPLC |
| Italy | Shellfish | NSP | n.d.[a] | |
| | | Domoic acid | | Mouse bioassay |
| New Zealand | Shellfish | NSP | n.d. | Mouse bioassay |
| Portugal | Shellfish | Domoic acid | | Mouse bioassay |
| Spain | Shellfish | Domoic acid | 2 mg | Mouse bioassay and HPLC |
| USA | Bivalve shellfish | NSP[b] | n.d. | Mouse bioassay |
| | Bivalve shellfish | Domoic acid | 2 mg | HPLC |
| | Cooked crab viscera | Domoic acid | 3 mg | HPLC |

[a] n.d. = must not be detectable.
[b] NSP only tested for in certain states of the USA (Florida, North Carolina).

Trusewich *et al.* (1996) and Yamamoto and Yamasaki (1996). By itself, phytoplankton monitoring does not provide sufficient protection to public health but it is often used as an early warning system on which to base intensive sampling programmes of toxicity testing of shellfish (or finfish) tissue. Examples of some countries which monitor potentially toxic species and the concentrations of these that elicit further action are given in Table 8.8.

**Table 8.8** Examples of countries with toxic algal monitoring schemes and cell concentrations at which action is taken (this ranges from intensified monitoring to closure of fisheries). Modified from Shumway (1995) and Andersen (1996)

| Country | Algal species monitored | Cell concentration at which action is taken |
|---|---|---|
| Australia | *Alexandrium catanella* | $>5 \times 10^4$ cells $l^{-1}$ based on |
| | *Gymnodinium catenatum* | level of toxin |
| Canada | *Alexandrium* spp. | Presence |
| | *Pseudonitzschia multiseries* | $5 \times 10^4$ |
| | *Pseudonitzschia pseudodelicatissima* | $1 \times 10^5$ |
| | *Dinophysis* spp. | ?? |
| Denmark | *Alexandrium* spp. | 500 |
| | *Dinophysis* spp. | 500 |
| | *Prorocentrum lima* | 500 |
| | *Pseudo-nitzschia seriata* | $2 \times 10^5$ |
| | *Pseudo-nitzschia delicatissima* | $2 \times 10^5$ |
| | *Nodularia spumigena* | $1 \times 10^5 – 2 \times 10^5$ colonies $l^{-1}$ |
| Italy | *Dinophysis* spp. | $10^3$ and DSP in mussels |
| The Netherlands | *Alexandrium* spp. | $10^3 – 10^4$ |
| | *Dinophysis* spp. | 100 |
| | *Pseudo-nitzschia* spp. | $10^4 – 10^5$ |
| Norway | *Alexandrium* spp. | Presence in net hauls |
| | *Dinophysis* spp. | $500 – 1.2 \times 10^3$ |
| Philippines | *Pyrodinium bahamense* var. *compressum* | 200 cells $l^{-1}$ |
| Spain | | |
|   Valencia | *Alexandrium catanella* | $2 \times 10^7 – 5 \times 10^7$ |
|   Balearic Islands | *Alexandrium minutum* | $10^3$ |
|   Balearic Islands | *Alexandrium* spp. | $10^3$ |
|   Balearic Islands | *Dinophysis acuminata* | $10^3$ |
|   Valencia | *Dinophysis acuminata* | $2 \times 10^7 – 5 \times 10^7$ |
|   Andalusia | *Gymnodinium catenatum* | $>500$ |
|   Andalusia | *Prorocentrum lima* | ?? |
| UK | | |
|   Northern Islands | *Alexandrium tamarense* | Presence |
|   Scotland | *Dinophysis* spp. | $>100$ |
| | *Prorocentrum lima* | Presence |
| USA | | |
|   Florida | *Gymnodinium breve* (*Ptychodiscus brevis*) | $>5 \times 10^3$ |

## 8.12 Future prospects

The phycotoxins represent a particularly problematical group of compounds as regards detection and quantitation in food. The original algal toxins may undergo chemical or biological transformations in the vector organisms to other, often more toxic, derivatives and the lack of pure analytical standards makes it difficult to quantify many of these compounds. In addition, it is known that pharmacologically or chemically dissimilar phycotoxins may occur together, for example DTX-1 and YTX have been found together in mussels (Lee *et al.*, 1988), and PSP and DSP toxins have been found simultaneously in shellfish (Gago-Martinez *et al.*, 1996), making detection an even more complex task.

As analytical techniques become increasingly sophisticated so new toxic compounds, which may originate from microalgae, are constantly being discovered in shellfish. For example, various macrocyclic compounds, such as spirolide-B and spirolide-D, have been found in the digestive glands of mussels and scallops (Hu *et al.*, 1995c) and pinnatoxin-A has been found in the mollusc *Pinna muricata* (Chou *et al.*, 1996). In addition, there is evidence for the presence in shellfish of potential toxins that have yet to be characterized (Holmes, 1991; Luu *et al.*, 1993; Amzil *et al.*, 1996). The effect, if any, of many of these toxins on human health has yet to be established.

Detection and analysis of mixtures of existing, novel and unsuspected phycotoxins in seafoods will, therefore, continue to be a challenge both to analysts and to toxicologists for the forseeable future.

## 8.13 A note on the IOC harmful algal bloom programme

The Intergovernmental Oceanographic Commission (IOC) of UNESCO has long been aware of the detrimental effects that harmful algal blooms (HAB) can have on national economies and aims to support research to mitigate these effects on fisheries, aquaculture, human health, recreation areas and ecosystems (Kullenberg, 1995). To this end the IOC maintains a Science and Communication Centre on Harmful Algae, which serves as an important international channel of communication for information on many aspects of HAB. The Centre publishes a regular international newsletter, *Harmful Algal News* (also available at WWW site http://www.unesco.org/ioc/news/netslet/han.htm), a number of useful manuals on HAB (e.g. Hallegraeff *et al.*, 1995; Ravn, 1995) and other publications, including an international directory of experts (also available at WWW site http://www.unesco.org/ioc/isisdb/html/habd.htm), all available free or at nominal cost. These publications will be of particular interest to scientists in developing countries. Further information can be obtained from the IOC Centre on Harmful Algae, University of Copenhagen Botanical Institute, Øster Farimagsgade 2D, DK-1353 Copenhagen K, Denmark (e-mail: hab@bot.ku.dk).

## Acknowledgements

The authors thank the Intergovernmental Oceanographic Commission of UNESCO and Dr P. Andersen, Prof. D. Baden, Prof. G. Hallegraeff, Dr R. Lewis, Prof. Y. Oshima, Dr M. Quilliam, Dr S. Shumway, Dr V. Trainer and Dr J. Wright for permission to reproduce diagrams and/or parts of tables.

## References

Amzil, Z., Marcaillou-Le Baut, C. and Bohec, M. (1996) Unexplained toxicity in molluscs gathered during phytoplankton monitoring, in *Harmful and Toxic Algal Blooms*, Proceedings of the Seventh International Conference on Toxic Phytoplankton, 1995 (eds T. Yasumoto, Y. Oshima and Y. Fukuyo), Intergovernmental Oceanographic Commission of UNESCO, Paris, pp. 543-46.

Andersen, P. (1996) *Design and Implementation of some Harmful Algal Monitoring Systems*, Intergovernmental Oceanographic Commission Technical Series No. 44, UNESCO, Paris, 102 pp.

Anderson, D.M. (1994) Red tides. *Scientific American*, **271** (2) 52-58.

Aune, T., Yasumoto, T. and Engeland, E. (1991) Light and scanning electron microscopic studies on effects of marine algal toxins toward freshly prepared hepatocytes. *Journal of Toxicology and Environmental Health*, **34** 1-9.

Aune, T. and Yndestad, M. (1993) Diarrhetic shellfish poisoning, in *Algal Toxins in Seafood and Drinking Water* (ed. I.R. Falconer), Academic Press, London, pp. 87-104.

Aune, T., Dahl, E. and Tangen, K. (1995) Algal monitoring, a useful tool in early warning of shellfish toxicity?, in *Harmful Marine Algal Blooms*, Proceedings of the Sixth International Conference on Toxic Marine Phytoplankton, 1993 (eds P. Lassus, G. Arzul, E. Erard-Le Denn, P. Gentien and C. Marcaillou-Le Baut), Lavoisier, Paris, pp. 765-70.

Baden, D.G. and Trainer, V.J. (1993) Mode of action of toxins in seafood poisoning, in *Algal Toxins in Seafood and Drinking Water* (ed. I.R. Falconer), Academic Press, London, pp. 49-74.

Bagnis, R. (1993) Ciguatera fish poisoning, in *Algal Toxins in Seafood and Drinking Water* (ed. I.R. Falconer), Academic Press, London, pp. 105-15.

Bauder, A.G., Cembella, A.D. and Quilliam, M.A. (1996) Dynamics of diarrhetic shellfish toxins from the dinoflagellate, *Prorocentrum lima*, in the bay scallop, *Argopecten irradians*, in *Harmful and Toxic Algal Blooms*, Proceedings of the Seventh International Conference on Toxic Phytoplankton, 1995 (eds T. Yasumoto, Y. Oshima and Y. Fukuyo), Intergovernmental Oceanographic Commission of UNESCO, Paris, pp. 433-36.

Belin, C., Beliaeff, B., Raffin, B, Rabia, M. and Ibanez, F. (1995) Phytoplankton time-series data of the French phytoplankton monitoring network: Toxic and dominant species, in *Harmful Marine Algal Blooms*, Proceedings of the Sixth International Conference on Toxic Marine Phytoplankton, 1993 (eds P. Lassus, G. Arzul, E. Erard-Le Denn, P. Gentien and C. Marcaillou-Le Baut), Lavoisier, Paris, pp. 771-76.

Benoit, E., Juzans, P., Legrand, A.M. and Molgo, J. (1996) Nodal swelling produced by ciguatoxin-induced selective activation of sodium channels in myelinated nerve-fibers. *Neuroscience*, **71** (4) 1121-31.

Berenguer, J.A., Gonzalez, L., Jimenez, I., Legarda, T.M., Olmedo, J.B. and Burdaspal, P.A. (1993) The effect of commercial processing on the paralytic shellfish poison (PSP) content of naturally contaminated *Acanthocardia tuberculatum* L. *Food Additives and Contaminants*, **10** (2) 217-30.

Berthomé, J.P. and Lassus, P. (1986) French status of shellfish monitoring with regard to toxic dinoflagellates contamination, in *Quatrième colloque interdisciplinaire franco-japonais d'Océanographie. Les aménagements côtiers et la gestion du littoral*, Marseille, 16–21 September 1985 (eds H.J. Ceccaldi and G. Champalbert) fascicule **2** 37-50.

Blay, J. and Poon, A.S.L. (1995) Use of cultured permanent lines of intestinal epithelial cells for the assay of okadaic acid in mussel homogenates. *Toxicon,* **33** (6) 739-46.

Boney, A.D. (1989) *Phytoplankton*, 2nd edn, New Studies in Biology, Edward Arnold, London.

Bouaicha, N., Hennion, M.-C. and Sandra, P. (1997) Determination of okadaic acid by micellar electrokinetic chromatography with ultraviolet detection. *Toxicon*, **35** (2) 273-81.

Bravo, I., Cacho, E., Franco, J.M., Miguez, A., Reyero, M.I. and Martinez, A. (1996) Study of PSP toxicity in *Haliotis tuberculata* from the Galician coast, in *Harmful and Toxic Algal Blooms*, Proceedings of the Seventh International Conference on Toxic Phytoplankton, 1995 (eds T. Yasumoto, Y. Oshima and Y. Fukuyo), Intergovernmental Oceanographic Commission of UNESCO, Paris, pp. 421-24.

Bricelj, V.M. and Cembella, A.D. (1995) Fate of gonyautoxins accumulated in surfclams, *Spisula solidissima*, grazing upon toxigenic *Alexandrium*, in *Harmful Marine Algal Blooms*, Proceedings of the Sixth International Conference on Toxic Marine Phytoplankton, 1993 (eds P. Lassus, G. Arzul, E. Erard-Le Denn, P. Gentien and C. Marcaillou-Le Baut), Lavoisier, Paris, pp. 413-18.

Bricelj, V.M., Cembella, A.D., Laby, D., Shumway, S.E. and Cucci, T.L. (1996) Comparative physiological and behavioral responses to PSP toxins in two bivalve molluscs, the softshell clam, *Mya arenaria*, and surfclam, *Spisula solidissima*, in *Harmful and Toxic Algal Blooms*, Proceedings of the Seventh International Conference on Toxic Phytoplankton, 1995 (eds T. Yasumoto, Y. Oshima and Y. Fukuyo), Intergovernmental Oceanographic Commission of UNESCO, Paris, pp. 405-408.

Carmichael, W.W. and Falconer, I.R. (1993) Diseases related to freshwater blue–green algal toxins, and control measures, in *Algal Toxins in Seafood and Drinking Water* (ed. I.R. Falconer), Academic Press, London, pp. 187-209.

Carmody, E.P., James, K.J., Kelly, S.S. and Thomas, K. (1995) Complex diarrhetic shellfish toxin profiles in Irish mussels, in *Harmful Marine Algal Blooms*, Proceedings of the Sixth International Conference on Toxic Marine Phytoplankton, 1993 (eds P. Lassus, G. Arzul, E. Erard-Le Denn, P. Gentien and C. Marcaillou-Le Baut), Lavoisier, Paris, pp. 273-78.

Carmody, E.P., James, K.J. and Kelly, S.S. (1996) Dinophysistoxin-2: The predominant diarrhoetic shellfish toxin in Ireland. *Toxicon*, **34** (3) 351-59.

Cembella, A.D., Shumway, S.E. and Lewis, N.I. (1993) Anatomical distribution and spatio-temporal variation in paralytic shellfish toxin composition in two bivalve species from the Gulf of Maine. *Journal of Shellfish Research*, **12** (2) 389-403.

Cembella, A.D. and Todd, E. (1993) Seafood toxins of algal origin and their control in Canada, in *Algal Toxins in Seafood and Drinking Water* (ed. I.R. Falconer), Academic Press, London, pp. 129-44.

Cembella, A.D., Shumway, S.E. and Laroque, R. (1994) Sequestering and putative biotransformation of paralytic shellfish toxins by the sea scallop *Placopecten magellanicus*: seasonal and spatial scales in natural populations. *Journal of Experimental Marine Biology and Ecology*, **180** 1-22.

Cembella, A.D., Milenkovic, L., Doucette, G. and Fernandez, M. (1995) *In vitro* biochemical methods and mammalian bioassays for phycotoxins, in *Manual on Harmful Marine Microalgae* (eds G.M. Hallegraeff, D.M. Anderson and A.D. Cembella), Intergovernmental Oceanographic Commission Manuals and Guides No. 33, UNESCO, Paris, pp. 177-228.

Chen, D.Z.X., Boland, M.P., Smillie, M.A., Klix, H., Ptak, C., Andersen, R.J. and Holmes, C.F.B. (1993) Identification of protein phosphatase inhibitors of the microcystin class in the marine environment. *Toxicon*, **31** (11) 1407-14.

Chou, H.-N., Shimizu, Y., Van Duyne, G.D. and Clardy, J. (1985) Two new polyether toxins of *Gymnodinium breve* (= *Ptychodiscus brevis*), in *Toxic Dinoflagellates*, Proceedings of the Third International Conference on Toxic Dinoflagellates (eds D.M. Anderson, A.W. White and D.G. Baden), Elsevier, New York, pp. 305-308.

Chou, T., Kamo, O. and Uemura, D. (1996) Pinnatoxin-A, a potent shellfish poison from *Pinna muricata*. *Tetrahedron Letters*, **37** (23) 4023-26.

Ciminiello, P., Fattorusso, E., Forino, M., Magno, S., Poletti, R., Satake, M., Vivani, R. and Yasumoto, T. (1997) Yessotoxin in mussels of the northern Adriatic Sea. *Toxicon*, **35** (2) 177-83.

Codd, G.A. (1994) Blue–green algal toxins: water-borne hazards to health, in *Water and Public*

*Health* (eds A.M.B. Golding, N. Noah and R. Stanwell-Smith), Smith-Gordon, London, pp. 271-78.

Croci, L., Toti, L., De Medici, D. and Cozzi, L. (1994) Diarrhetic shellfish poison in mussels: Comparison of methods of detection and determination of the effectiveness of depuration. *International Journal of Food Microbiology*, **24** (1–2) 337-42.

Croci, L., Cozzi, L., Stacchini, A., DeMedici, D. and Toti, L. (1997) A rapid tissue culture assay for the detection of okadaic acid and related compounds in mussels. *Toxicon*, **35** (2) 223-30.

Dahl, E., Rogstad, A., Aune, T., Hormazabal, V. and Underdal, B. (1995) Toxicity of mussels related to the occurrence of *Dinophysis* species, in *Harmful Marine Algal Blooms*, Proceedings of the Sixth International Conference on Toxic Marine Phytoplankton, 1993 (eds P. Lassus, G. Arzul, E. Erard-Le Denn, P. Gentien and C. Marcaillou-Le Baut), Lavoisier, Paris, pp. 783-88.

Desbiens, M. and Cembella, A.D. (1995) Occurrence and elimination kinetics of PSP toxins in the American lobster (*Homarus americanus*), in *Harmful Marine Algal Blooms*, Proceedings of the Sixth International Conference on Toxic Marine Phytoplankton, 1993 (eds P. Lassus, G. Arzul, E. Erard-Le Denn, P. Gentien and C. Marcaillou-Le Baut), Lavoisier, Paris, pp. 433-38.

Draisci, R., Lucentini, L., Giannetti, L., Boria, P. and Poletti, R. (1996) First report of pectenotoxin-2 (PTX-2) in algae (*Dinophysis fortii*) related to seafood poisoning in Europe. *Toxicon*, **34** (8) 923-35.

Edebo, L., Lang, E.S., Li, X.P. and Mark, S.A. (1988) Toxic mussels and okadaic acid induce rapid hypersecretion in the rat small intestine. *Acta Pathologica, Microbiologica Scandinavia, Section C Immunology*, **96** (11) 1029-35.

Emsholm, H., Andersen, P. and Hald, B. (1996) Results of the Danish monitoring programme on toxic algae and algal toxins in relation to the mussel fisheries 1991–1994, in *Harmful and Toxic Algal Blooms*, Proceedings of the Seventh International Conference on Toxic Phytoplankton, 1995 (eds T. Yasumoto, Y. Oshima and Y. Fukuyo), Intergovernmental Oceanographic Commission of UNESCO, Paris, pp. 15-18

Eriksson, J.E., Meriluto, J.A.O. and Lindholm, T. (1989) Accumulation of a peptide toxin from the cyanobacterium *Oscillatoria agardhii* in the freshwater mussel *Anodonta cygnea*. *Hydrobiologia*, **183** 211-16.

Falconer, I.R. (1991) Tumour promotion and liver injury caused by oral consumption of cyanobacteria. *Environmental Toxicology and Water Quality*, **6** 177-84.

Falconer, I.R., Choice, A. and Hosja, W. (1992) Toxicity of the edible mussel (*Mytilus edulis*) growing naturally in an estuary during a water bloom of the blue–green alga *Nodularia spumigena*. *Environmental Toxicology and Water Quality*, **7** 119-23.

Falconer, I.R. (1993) Measurement of toxins from blue–green algae in water and foodstuffs, in *Algal Toxins in Seafood and Drinking Water* (ed. I.R. Falconer), Academic Press, London, pp. 165-75.

Falconer, I.R. (1996) Potential impact on human health of toxic cyanobacteria. *Phycologia*, **35** (suppl. 6) 6-11.

Falconer, I.R. and Humpage, A.R. (1996) Tumour promotion by cyanobacterial toxins. *Phycologia*, **35** (suppl. 6) 74-79.

Fleming, L.E., Bean, J.A. and Baden, D.G. (1995) Epidemiology and public health, in *Manual on Harmful Marine Microalgae* (eds G.M. Hallegraeff, D.M. Anderson and A.D. Cembella), Intergovernmental Oceanographic Commission Manuals and Guides No. 33, UNESCO, Paris, pp. 475-86.

Franca, S., Pinto, L., Alvito, P., Sousa, I., Vasconcelos, V. and Doucette, G.J. (1996) Studies on prokaryotes associated with PSP-producing dinoflagellates, in *Harmful and Toxic Algal Blooms*, Proceedings of the Seventh International Conference on Toxic Phytoplankton, 1995 (eds T. Yasumoto, Y. Oshima and Y. Fukuyo), International Oceanographic Commission of UNESCO, Paris, pp. 347-50.

Gago-Martinez, A., Rodriguez-Vazquez, J.A., Thibault, P. and Quilliam, M.A. (1996) Simultaneous occurrence of diarrhetic and paralytic shellfish poisoning toxins in Spanish mussels in 1993. *Natural Toxins*, **4** (2) 72-79.

Gallacher, S., Flynn, K.J., Leftley, J., Lewis, J., Munro, P.D. and Birkbeck, T.H. (1996) Bacterial production of sodium channel blocking toxins, in *Harmful and Toxic Algal Blooms*, Proceedings of the Seventh International Conference on Toxic Phytoplankton, 1995 (eds T. Yasumoto, Y. Oshima and Y. Fukuyo), Intergovernmental Oceanographic Commission of UNESCO, Paris, pp. 355-58.

Gallacher, S., Flynn, K.J., Franco, J.M., Brueggemann, E.E. and Hines, H.B. (1997) Evidence for production of paralytic shellfish toxins by bacteria associated with *Alexandrium* spp. (Dinophyta) in culture. *Applied and Environmental Microbiology*, **63** (1) 239-45.

Goldin, A.L., Snutch, T., Lubbert, H., Dowsett, A., Marshall, J., Auld, V., Downey, W., Fritz, L.C., Lester, H.A., Dunn, R., Catterall, W.A. and Davidson, N. (1986) Messenger RNA coding for only the alpha subunit of the rat brain Na channel is sufficient for expression of functional channels in *Xenopus* oocytes. *Proceedings of the National Academy of Sciences, USA (Neurobiology)*, **83** 7503-507.

Hallegraeff, G.M. (1995) Harmful algal blooms: a global overview, in *Manual on Harmful Marine Microalgae* (eds G.M. Hallegraeff, D.M. Anderson and A.D. Cembella), Intergovernmental Oceanographic Commission Manuals and Guides No. 33, UNESCO, Paris, pp. 1-22.

Hallegraeff, G.M., Anderson, D.M. and Cembella, A.D. (eds.) (1995) *Manual on Harmful Marine Microalgae*, Intergovernmental Oceanographic Commission Manuals and Guides No. 33, UNESCO, Paris, 551 pp.

Hatfield, C.L., Gauglitz, E.J., Barnett, H.J., Lund, J.A.K., Wekell, J.C. and Eklund, M. (1995) The fate of domoic acid in Dungeness crab (*Cancer magister*) as a function of processing. *Journal of Shellfish Research*, **14** (2) 359-63.

Haya, K., Young-Lai, W.W., Stewart, J.E. and Jellet, J.F. (1992) Uptake and excretion of paralytic shellfish toxins by lobster-fed scallop digestive glands, in *Proceedings of the Third Canadian Workshop on Harmful Marine Algae*, Maurice Lamontagne Institute, Mont-Joli, Quebec, May 12–14, 1992 (eds J.-C. Therriault and M. Levasseur), Canadian Technical Reports in Fisheries and Aquatic Sciences No. 1893, p. 38.

Holmes, C.F.B. (1991) Liquid chromatography-linked protein phosphatase bioassay: a highly sensitive marine bioscreen for okadaic acid and related diarrhetic shellfish toxins. *Toxicon*, **29** 469-77.

Holmes, M.J., Lewis, R.J., Jones, A. and Hoy, A.W.W. (1995) Cooliatoxin, the first toxin from *Coolia montis* (Dinophyceae). *Natural Toxins*, **3** (5) 355-62.

Honkanen, R.E., Mowdy, D.E. and Dickey, R.W. (1996a) Detection of DSP-toxins, okadaic acid and dinophysis toxin-1 in shellfish by the serine/threonine protein phosphatase assay. *Journal of AOAC International*, **79** (6) 1336-43.

Honkanen, R.E., Stapleton, J.D., Bryan, D.E. and Abercrombie, J. (1996b) Development of a protein phosphatase-based assay for the detection of phosphatase inhibitors in crude whole cell and animal extracts. *Toxicon*, **34** (11/12) 1385-92.

Hu, T.M., Curtis, J.M., Walter, J.A., McLachlan, J.L. and Wright, J.L.C. (1995a) Two new water-soluble DSP toxin derivatives from the dinoflagellate *Prorocentrum maculosum* — possible storage and excretion products. *Tetrahedron Letters*, **36** (51) 9273-76.

Hu, T.M., Curtis, J.M., Walter, J.A. and Wright, J.L.C. (1995b) Identification of DTX-4, a new water-soluble phosphatase inhibitor from the toxic dinoflagellate *Prorocentrum lima*. *Journal of the Chemical Society, Chemical Communications*, No. 5 597-99.

Hu, T.M., Curtis, J.M., Oshima, Y., Quilliam, M.A., Walter, J.A, Watson-Wright, W.M. and Wright, J.L.C. (1995c) Spirolide-B and spirolide-D, two novel macrocycles isolated from the digestive glands of shellfish. *Journal of the Chemical Society, Chemical Communications*, No. 20 2159-61.

Hu, T.M., De Freitas, S.W., Curtis, J.M., Oshima, Y., Walter, J.A. and Wright, J.L.C. (1996) Isolation and structure of prorocentrolide-B, a fast-acting toxin from *Prorocentrum maculosum*. *Journal of Natural Products*, **59** (11) 1010-14.

Hua, Y.S., Lu, W.Z., Henry, M.S., Pierce, R.H. and Cole, R.B. (1996) Online liquid- chromatography electrospray-ionization mass-spectrometry for determination of the brevetoxin profile in natural red tide algae blooms. *Journal of Chromatography A*, **750** (1–2) 115-25.

Hungerford, J.M. and Wekell, M.M. (1993) Control measures in shellfish and finfish industries in the USA, in *Algal Toxins in Seafood and Drinking Water* (ed. I.R. Falconer), Academic Press, London, pp. 117-28.

ICES (1992) *Effects of Harmful Algal Blooms on Mariculture and Marine Fisheries*, International Council for the Exploration of the Sea Co-operative Research Report, No. 181, p. 10.

Jasperse, J.A. (ed.) (1993) *Marine Toxins and New Zealand Shellfish*, Proceedings of a workshop on research issues, June 1993, The Royal Society of New Zealand, Miscellaneous Series, No. 24.

Kao, C.Y. (1993) Paralytic shellfish poisoning, in *Algal Toxins in Seafood and Drinking Water* (ed. I.R. Falconer), Academic Press, London, pp. 75-86.

Khan, S., Arakawa, O. and Onoue, Y. (1996) Neurotoxin production by a chloromonad *Fibrocapsa japonica* (Raphidophyceae). *Journal of the World Aquaculture Society*, **27** (3) 254-63.

Khan, S., Arakawa, O. and Onoue, Y. (1997) Neurotoxins in a toxic red tide of *Heterosigma akashiwo. Aquaculture Research*, **28** (1) 9-14.

Kullenberg, G. (1995) Preface, in *Manual on Harmful Marine Microalgae* (eds G.M. Hallegraeff, D.M. Anderson and A.D. Cembella), Intergovernmental Oceanographic Commission Manuals and Guides No. 33, UNESCO, Paris, p. i.

Lawrence, J.F., Maher, M. and Watson-Wright, W. (1994) Effect of cooking on the concentration of toxins associated with paralytic shellfish poison in lobster hepatopancreas. *Toxicon*, **32** (1) 57-64.

Laycock, M.V., Thibault, P., Ayer, S.W. and Walter, J.A. (1994) Isolation and purification procedures for the preparation of paralytic shellfish poisoning toxin standards. *Natural Toxins*, **2** (4) 175-83.

Lee, J.-S., Tangen, K., Dahl, E., Hovgaard, P. and Yasumoto, T. (1988) Diarrhetic shellfish toxins in Norwegian mussels. *Nippon Suisan Gakkaishi*, **54** (11) 1953-57.

Legrand, A.-M., Fukui, M., Cruchet, P., Ishibashi, Y. and Yasumoto, T. (1992) Characterization of ciguatoxins from different fish species and wild *Gambierdiscus toxicus*, in *Proceedings of the Third International Conference on Ciguatera Fish Poisoning*, Puerto Rico (ed. T.R. Tosteson), Polyscience Publications, Quebec, pp. 25-32.

Levasseur, M., Monfort, P., Doucette, G.J. and Michaud, S. (1996) Preliminary study of bacteria as PSP producers in the Gulf of St. Lawrence, Canada, in *Harmful and Toxic Algal Blooms*, Proceedings of the Seventh International Conference on Toxic Phytoplankton, 1995 (eds T. Yasumoto, Y. Oshima and Y. Fukuyo), Intergovernmental Oceanographic Commission of UNESCO, Paris, pp. 363-66.

Lewis, R.J., Sellin, M., Poli, M.A., Norton, R.S., MacLeod, J.K. and Sheil, M.M. (1991) Purification and characterization of ciguatoxins from moray eel (*Lycodontis javanicus*, Muraenidae). *Toxicon*, **29** (9) 1115-27.

Lewis, R.J. and Holmes, M.J. (1993) Origin and transfer of toxins involved in ciguatera. *Comparative Biochemistry and Physiology C – Pharmacology, Toxicology and Endocrinology*, **106** (3) 615-28.

Lewis, R.J., Holmes, M.J., Alewood, P.F. and Jones, A. (1994) Ionspray mass spectrometry of ciguatoxin-1, maitotoxin-2 and -3 and related marine polyether toxins. *Natural Toxins*, **2** (2) 56-63.

Lewis, R.J. (1995) Detection of ciguatoxins and related benthic dinoflagellate toxins: *in vivo* and *in vitro* methods, in *Manual on Harmful Marine Microalgae* (eds G.M. Hallegraeff, D.M. Anderson and A.D. Cembella), Intergovernmental Oceanographic Commission Manuals and Guides No. 33, UNESCO, Paris, pp. 135-61.

Lewis, R.J. and Jones, A. (1997) Characterization of ciguatoxins and ciguatoxin congeners present in ciguateric fish by gradient reverse-phase high-performance liquid chromatography mass spectrometry. *Toxicon*, **35** (2) 159-68.

Luu, H.A., Chen. D.Z.X., Magoon, J., Worms, J., Smith, J. and Holmes, C.F.B. (1993) Quantification of diarrhetic shellfish toxins and identification of novel protein phosphatase inhibitors in marine phytoplankton and mussels. *Toxicon*, **31** (1) 75-83.

Mackenzie, L., Haywood, A., Adamson, J., Truman, P., Till, D., Seki, T., Satake, M. and Yasumoto, T. (1996) Gymnodimine contamination of shellfish in New Zealand, in *Harmful and Toxic Algal Blooms*, Proceedings of the Seventh International Conference on Toxic Phytoplankton, 1995 (eds T. Yasumoto, Y. Oshima and Y. Fukuyo), Intergovernmental Oceanographic Commission of

UNESCO, Paris, pp. 97-100.

Manger, R.L., Leja, L.S., Lee, S.Y., Hungerford, J.M., Hokama, Y., Dickey, R.W., Granade, H.R., Lewis, R., Yasumoto, T. and Wekell, M.M. (1995) Detection of sodium channel toxins: directed cytotoxicity assay of purified ciguatoxins, brevetoxins, saxitoxins, and seafood extracts. *Journal of AOAC International,* **78** (2) 521-27.

Marcaillou-Le Baut, C., Bardin, B., Bardouil, M., Bohec, M., LeDean, L., Masselin, P. and Truquet, P. (1993) DSP depuration rates of mussels reared in a laboratory and in an aquaculture pond, in *Toxic Phytoplankton Blooms in the Sea,* Proceedings of the Fifth International Conference on Toxic Marine Phytoplankton, 1991 (eds T.J. Smayda and Y. Shimizu), Elsevier, Amsterdam, pp. 531-35.

Morris, P.D., Campbell, D.S., Taylor, T.J. and Freeman, J.I. (1991) Clinical and epidemiological features of neurotoxic shellfish poisoning in North Carolina. *American Journal of Public Health,* **81** 471-74.

Murata, M., Kumagai, M., Lee, J.-S. and Yasumoto, T. (1987) Isolation and structure of yessotoxin, a novel polyether compound implicated in diarrhetic shellfish poisoning. *Tetrahedron Letters,* **28** 5869-72.

Murata, M., Naoki, H., Matsunaga, S., Satake, M. and Yasumoto, T. (1994) Structure and partial stereochemical assignments for maitotoxin, the most toxic and largest natural non-biopolymer. *Journal of the American Chemical Society,* **116** (16) 7098-7107.

Nagashima, Y., Noguchi, T., Tanaka, M. and Hashimoto, K. (1991) Thermal degradation of paralytic shellfish poison. *Journal of Food Science,* **56** (6) 1572-75.

Negri, A.P. and Jones, G.J. (1995) Bioaccumulation of paralytic shellfish poisoning (PSP) toxins from the cyanobacterium *Anabaena circinalis* by the freshwater mussel *Alathyria condola. Toxicon,* **33** (5) 667-78.

Noguchi, T., Ueda, Y., Onoue, Y., Kono, M., Koyama, K., Hashimoto, K., Seno,Y. and Mishima, S. (1980a). Reduction in toxicity of PSP infested scallops during canning process. *Bulletin of the Japanese Society of Scientific Fisheries,* **46** (10) 1273-77.

Noguchi, T., Ueda, Y., Onoue, Y., Kono, M., Koyama, K., Hashimoto, K., Takeuchi, T., Seno, Y. and Mishima, S. (1980b) Reduction in toxicity of highly PSP-infested scallops during canning process and storage. *Bulletin of the Japanese Society of Scientific Fisheries,* **46** (11) 1339-44.

Noguchi, T., Nagashima, Y., Maruyama, J., Kamimura, S. and Hashimoto, K. (1984) Toxicity of the adductor muscle of markedly-infested scallop *Patinopecten yessoensis. Bulletin of the Japanese Society of Scientific Fisheries,* **50** (3) 517-20.

Nonomura, T., Sasaki, M., Matsumori, N., Murata, M., Tachibana, K. and Yasumoto, T. (1996) The complete structure of maitotoxin. 2. Configuration of the C135–C142 side-chain and absolute configuration of the entire molecule. *Angewandte Chemie – International Edition in English,* **35** (15) 1675-78.

Novaczek, I., Madhyastha, M.S., Ablett, R.F., Donald, A., Johnson, G., Nijjar, M.S. and Sims, D.E. (1992) Depuration of domoic acid from live blue mussels (*Mytilus edulis*). *Canadian Journal of Fisheries and Aquatic Sciences,* **49** (2) 312-18.

Nunez, P.E. and Scoging, A.C. (1997) Comparison of a protein phosphatase inhibition assay, HPLC assay and enzyme-linked immunosorbent assay with the mouse bioassay for the detection of diarrhetic shellfish poisoning toxins in European shellfish. *International Journal of Food Microbiology,* **36** (1) 39-48.

Ohta, T., Nomata, H., Takeda, T. and Kaneko, H. (1992) Studies on shellfish poison of scallop *Patinopecten yessoensis.* I. Reduction in toxicity of PSP infested scallops during extrusion processing. *Scientific Reports of the Hokkaido Fisheries Experimental Station,* **38** 23-30.

Oshima, Y. (1995a) Chemical and enzymatic transformations of paralytic shellfish toxins in marine organisms, in *Harmful Marine Algal Blooms,* Proceedings of the Sixth International Conference on Toxic Marine Phytoplankton, 1993 (eds P. Lassus, G. Arzul, E. Erard-Le Denn, P. Gentien and C. Marcaillou-Le Baut), Lavoisier, Paris, pp. 475-80.

Oshima, Y. (1995b) Post-column derivatization HPLC methods for paralytic shellfish poisons, in

*Manual on Harmful Marine Microalgae* (eds G.M. Hallegraeff, D.M. Anderson and A.D. Cembella), Intergovernmental Oceanographic Commission Manuals and Guides No. 33, UNESCO, Paris, pp. 81-94.

Poletti, R., Viviani, R., Casadei, C., Lucentini., L., Giannetti, L., Funari, E. and Draisci, R. (1996) Decontamination dynamics of mussels naturally contaminated with diarrhetic toxins relocated to a basin of the Adriatic Sea, in *Harmful and Toxic Algal Blooms*, Proceedings of the Seventh International Conference on Toxic Phytoplankton, 1995 (eds T. Yasumoto, Y. Oshima and Y. Fukuyo), Intergovernmental Oceanographic Commission of UNESCO, Paris, pp. 429-32.

Prakash, A., Medcof, J.C. and Tennant, A.D. (1971) Paralytic shellfish poisoning in eastern Canada. *Bulletin of the Fisheries Research Board of Canada*, **177** 1-87.

Premazzi, G. and Volterra, L. (1993) *Microphyte Toxins: A Manual for Toxin Detection, Environmental Monitoring and Therapies to Counteract Intoxications*, EUR 14854, Office for Official Publications of the European Communities, Luxembourg.

Quayle, D.B. (1969) Paralytic shellfish poisoning in British Columbia. *Bulletin of the Fisheries Research Board of Canada*, **168** 1-69.

Quilliam, M.A., Gilgan, M.W., Pleasance, S., De Freitas, A.S.W., Douglas, D., Fritz, L., Hu, T., Marr, J.C., Smyth, C. and Wright, J.L.C. (1993) Confirmation of an incident of diarrhetic shellfish poisoning in eastern Canada, in *Toxic Phytoplankton Blooms in the Sea*, Proceedings of the Fifth International Conference on Toxic Marine Phytoplankton, 1991 (eds T.J. Smayda and Y. Shimizu), Elsevier, Amsterdam, pp. 547-52.

Quilliam, M.A. and Wright, J.L.C. (1995) Methods for diarrhetic shellfish poisons, in *Manual on Harmful Marine Microalgae* (eds G.M. Hallegraeff, D.M. Anderson and A.D. Cembella), Intergovernmental Oceanographic Commission Manuals and Guides No. 33, UNESCO, Paris, pp. 95-111.

Quilliam, M.A. (1995) Seafood toxins. *Journal of AOAC International*, **78** (1) 144-48.

Quilliam, M.A., Hardstaff, W.R., Ishida, N., McLachlan, J.L., Reeves, A.R., Ross, N.W. and Windust, A.J. (1996) Production of diarrhetic shellfish poisoning (DSP) toxins by *Prorocentrum lima* in culture and development of analytical methods, in *Harmful and Toxic Algal Blooms*, Proceedings of the Seventh International Conference on Toxic Phytoplankton, 1995 (eds T. Yasumoto, Y. Oshima and Y. Fukuo), Intergovernmental Oceanographic Commission of UNESCO, Paris, pp. 289-92.

Quilliam, M.A. (1996) Seafood toxins. *Journal of AOAC International*, **79** (1) 209-14.

Quilliam, M.A. (1997) Phycotoxins. *Journal of AOAC International*, **80** (1) 131-36.

Ravn, H. (1995) *Amnesic Shellfish Poisoning (ASP)*. HAB Publication Series Volume 1, Intergovernmental Oceanographic Commission Manuals and Guides No. 31, Paris.

Ressom, R., Soong, F.S., Fitzgerald, J., Turcznowicz, L., Saadi, O.E., Roder, D., Maynard, T. and Falconer, I. (1994) *Health Effects of Toxic Cyanobacteria (Blue–Green Algae)*, National Health and Medical Research Council, The Australian Government Publishing Service, Canberra, Australia.

Satake, M., Terasawa, K., Kadowaki, Y. and Yasumoto, T. (1996) Relative configuration of yesso-toxin and isolation of two new analogs from toxic scallops. *Tetrahedron Letters*, **37** 5955-58.

Seki, T., Satake, M., Mackenzie, L., Kaspar, H.F. and Yasumoto, T. (1995) Gymnodimine, a new marine toxin of unprecedented structure isolated from New Zealand oysters and the dinoflagellate *Gymnodinium* sp. *Tetrahedron Letters*, **36** 7093-96.

Seki, T., Satake, M., Mackenzie, L., Kaspar, H.F. and Yasumoto, T. (1996) Gymnodimine, a novel toxic imine isolated from the Foveaux Strait oysters and *Gymnodinium* sp., in *Harmful and Toxic Algal Blooms*, Proceedings of the Seventh International Conference on Toxic Phytoplankton, 1995 (eds T. Yasumoto, Y. Oshima and Y. Fukuyo), Intergovernmental Oceanographic Commission of UNESCO, Paris, pp. 495-98.

Shea, D. (1997) Analysis of brevetoxins by micellar electrokinetic capillary chromatography and laser-induced fluorescence detection. *Electrophoresis*, **18** (2) 277-83.

Shimizu, Y. (1996) Microalgal metabolites: A new perspective. *Annual Review of Microbiology* **50**

431-65.

Shimizu, Y., Giorgio, C., Koerting-Walker, C. and Ogata, T. (1996) Nonconformity of bacterial production of paralytic shellfish poisons – neosaxitoxin production by a bacterium strain from *Alexandrium tamarense* Ipswich strain and its significance, in *Harmful and Toxic Algal Blooms*, Proceedings of the Seventh International Conference on Toxic Phytoplankton, 1995 (eds T. Yasumoto, Y. Oshima and Y. Fukuyo), Intergovernmental Oceanographic Commission of UNESCO, Paris, pp. 359-62.

Shumway, S.E., Sherman-Caswell, S. and Hurst, J.W. (1988) Paralytic shellfish poisoning in Maine: Monitoring a monster. *Journal of Shellfish Research,* **7** (4) 643-52.

Shumway, S.E. and Cembella, A.D. (1993) The impact of toxic algae on scallop culture and fisheries. *Reviews in Fisheries Science,* **1** (2) 121-50.

Shumway, S.E. (1995) Phycotoxin-related shellfish poisoning: Bivalve molluscs are not the only vectors. *Reviews in Fisheries Science,* **3** (1) 1-31.

Shumway, S.E., van Egmond, H.P., Hurst, J.W. and Bean, L.L. (1995) Management of shellfish resources, in *Manual on Harmful Marine Microalgae* (eds G.M. Hallegraeff, D.M. Anderson and A.D. Cembella), Intergovernmental Oceanographic Commission Manuals and Guides No. 33, UNESCO, Paris, pp. 433-61.

Silvert, W. and Rao, D.V.S. (1992) Dynamic-model of the flux of domoic acid, a neurotoxin, through a *Mytilus edulis* population. *Canadian Journal of Fisheries and Aquatic Sciences,* **49** (2) 400-405.

Steidinger, K.A. (1993) Some taxonomic and biologic aspects of toxic dinoflagellates, in *Algal Toxins in Seafood and Drinking Water* (ed. I.R. Falconer), Academic Press, London, pp. 1-28.

Sullivan, J.J. (1993) Methods of analysis for algal toxins: Dinoflagellate and diatom toxins, in *Algal Toxins in Seafood and Drinking Water* (ed. I.R. Falconer), Academic Press, London, pp. 29-48.

Takahashi, H., Kusumi, T., Kan, Y., Satake, M. and Yasumoto, T. (1996) Determination of the absolute configuration of yessotoxin, a polyether compound implicated in diarrhetic shellfish poisoning, by NMR spectroscopic method using a chiral anisotropic reagent, methoxy-(2-naphthyl)acetic acid. *Tetrahedron Letters,* **37** 7087-90.

Terao, K., Ito, E., Yasumoto, T. and Yamaguchi, K. (1990) Enterotoxic, hepatotoxic and immunotoxic effects of dinoflagellate toxins on mice, in *Toxic Marine Phytoplankton*, Proceedings of the Fourth International Conference on Toxic Marine Phytoplankton, 1989 (eds E. Granéli, B. Sundström, L. Edler and D.M. Anderson), Elsevier, New York, pp. 418-23.

Terao, K., Ito, E., Ohkusu, M. and Yasumoto, T. (1993) A comparative study of the effects of DSP-toxins on mice and rats, in *Toxic Phytoplankton Blooms in the Sea*, Proceedings of the Fifth International Conference on Toxic Marine Phytoplankton, 1991 (eds T.J. Smayda and Y. Shimizu), Elsevier, Amsterdam, pp. 581-86.

Todd, E.C.W. (1993) Domoic acid and amnesic shellfish poisoning – a review. *Journal of Food Protection,* **56** 69-83.

Torigoe, K., Murata, M., Yasumoto, T. and Iwashita, T. (1988) Prorocentrolide, a toxic nitrogenous macrocycle from a marine dinoflagellate, *Prorocentrum lima. Journal of the American Chemical Society,* **110** 7876-77.

Tripuraneni, J., Koutsouris, A., Pestic, L., deLanerolle, P. and Hecht, G. (1997) The toxin of diarrhetic shellfish poisoning, okadaic acid, increases intestinal epithelial paracellular permeability. *Gastroenterology,* **112** (1) 100-108.

Trusewich, B., Sim, J., Busby, P. and Hughes, C. (1996) Management of marine biotoxins in New Zealand, in *Harmful and Toxic Algal Blooms*, Proceedings of the Seventh International Conference on Toxic Phytoplankton, 1995 (eds T. Yasumoto, Y. Oshima and Y. Fukuyo), Intergovernmental Oceanographic Commission of UNESCO, Paris, pp. 27-30.

Usami, M., Satake, M., Ishida, S., Inoue, A., Kan, Y. and Yasumoto, T. (1995) Palytoxin analogs from the dinoflagellate *Ostreopsis siamenis. Journal of the American Chemical Society,* **117** (19) 5389-90.

van Egmond, H.P., Speijers, G.J.A. and van den Top, G.J.A. (1992) Current situation on worldwide regulation for marine phycotoxins. *Journal of Natural Toxins,* **1** (1) 67-85.

van Egmond, H.P., Aune, T., Lassus, P., Speijers, G.J.A. and Waldock, M. (1993) Paralytic and diar-rhoeic shellfish poisons: occurrence in Europe, toxicity, analysis and regulation. *Journal of Natural Toxins*, **2** (1) 41-83.

Vasconcelos, V.M. (1995) Uptake and depuration of the heptapeptide toxin microcystin-LR in *Mytilus galloprovincialis*. *Aquatic Toxicology*, **32** 227-37.

Vernoux, J.P and Lewis, R.J. (1997) Isolation and characterization of Caribbean ciguatoxins from the horse-eye jack (*Caranx latus*). *Toxicon*, **35** (6) 889-900.

Vernoux, J.P., Bansard, S., Simon, J.F., Nwal-Amang, D., Le-Baut, C., Gleizes, E., Fremy, J.M. and Lasne, M.C. (1994) Cooked mussels contaminated by *Dinophysis* sp.: a source of okadaic acid. *Natural Toxins*, **2** (4) 184-88.

Watson-Wright, W., Gillis, M., Smyth, C., Trueman, S., McGuire, A., Moore, W., McLachlan, D. and Sims, G. (1991) Monitoring of PSP in hepatopancreas of lobster from Atlantic Canada, in *Proceedings of the Second Canadian Workshop on Harmful Marine Algae*. Canadian Technical Reports on Fisheries and Aquatic Science No. 1799, pp. 27-28 (microfiche).

Wohlgeschaffen, G.D., Mann, K.H., Rao, D.V.S. and Pocklington, R. (1992) Dynamics of the phy-cotoxin domoic acid – Accumulation and excretion in two commercially important bivalves. *Journal of Applied Phycology*, **4** (4) 297-310.

Wright, J.L.C. (1995) Dealing with seafood toxins: present approaches and future options. *Food Research International*, **28** (4) 347-58.

Wright, J.L.C. and Quilliam, M.A. (1995) Methods for domoic acid, the amnesic shellfish poisons, in *Manual on Harmful Marine Microalgae* (eds G.M. Hallegraeff, D.M. Anderson and A.D. Cembella), Intergovernmental Oceanographic Commission Manuals and Guides No. 33, UNESCO, Paris, pp. 113-33.

Yamamoto, M. and Yamasaki, M. (1996) Japanese monitoring system on shellfish toxins, in *Harmful and Toxic Algal Blooms*, Proceedings of the Seventh International Conference on Toxic Phytoplankton, 1995 (eds T. Yasumoto, Y. Oshima and Y. Fukuyo), Intergovernmental Oceanographic Commission of UNESCO, Paris, pp. 19-22.

Yasumoto, T., Murata, M., Lee, J.-S. and Torigoe, K. (1989) Polyether toxins produced by dinoflagellates, in *Mycotoxins and Phycotoxins '88* (eds S. Natori, K. Hashimoto and T. Ueno), Elsevier, New York, pp. 375-82.

Yasumoto, T. (1990) Marine microorganisms toxins – An overview, in *Toxic Marine Phytoplankton*, Proceedings of the Fourth International Conference on Toxic Marine Phytoplankton, 1989 (eds E. Granéli, B. Sundström, L. Edler and D.M. Anderson), Elsevier, New York, pp. 3-8.

Yasumoto, T., Fukui, M., Sasaki, K. and Sugiyama, K. (1995) Determinations of marine toxins in foods. *Journal of AOAC International*, **78** (2) 574-82.

Yasumoto, T. and Satake, M. (1996) Chemistry, etiology and determination methods of ciguatera toxins. *Journal of Toxicology – Toxin Reviews*, **15** (2) 91-107.

Yu, S.-Z. (1994) Blue–green algae and liver cancer, in *Toxic Cyanobacteria, Current Status of Research and Management*, Proceedings of an International Workshop, Adelaide, Australia, 1994 (eds D.A. Steffenson and B.C. Nicholson), Australian Centre for Water Quality Research, Salisbury, Australia, pp. 75-85.

Zhao, J., Lembeye, J., Cenci, G., Wall, B. and Yasumoto, T. (1993) The determination of okadaic acid and dinophysistoxin-1 in mussels from Chile, Italy and Ireland, in *Toxic Phytoplankton Blooms in the Sea*, Proceedings of the Fifth International Conference on Toxic Marine Phytoplankton, 1991 (eds T.J. Smayda and Y. Shimizu), Elsevier, Amsterdam, pp. 587-92.

Zhao, J.-Y., Thibault, P. and Quilliam, M.A. (1997) Analysis of domoic acid and isomers in seafood by capillary electrophoresis. *Electrophoresis*, **18** (2) 268-76.

Zheng, W.J., Demattei, J.A., Wu, J.P., Duan, J.J.W., Cook, L.R., Oinuma, H. and Kishi, Y. (1996) Complete relative stereochemistry of maitotoxin. *Journal of the American Chemical Society*, **118** (34) 7946-68.

Zhou, Z.-H., Komiyama, M., Terao, K. and Shimada, Y. (1994) Effects of pectenotoxin-1 on liver cells *in vitro*. *Natural Toxins*, **2** (3) 132-35.

# Developing areas of work on natural toxicants in food

# 9 The control of natural toxicants

Andrew Moore

## 9.1 Introduction

The content of this chapter is the personal interpretation of the author and does not supplement the law in this area. The chapter, which was written in June 1977, does not constitute any form of legal guidance.

There are vast numbers of naturally occurring compounds in food reported to have toxic and beneficial effects. These can be broken down into a number of sub-groups:

- those that are present by infection or spoilage caused by bacteria or fungi;
- materials present in animal products (consumed by humans) that are derived from food eaten by the animal;
- substances formed as a result of the breakdown of constituent chemicals during storage, processing and preparation of foods;
- substances made by the natural biological processes within plants (used as food) themselves.

Why is there interest in naturally occurring compounds? Should there be a concern over any of these compounds? Many compounds naturally occurring in food are considered to be detrimental to human health but should it be necessary to regulate the levels of any of these compounds? To answer these questions, two of these groups of compounds—the mycotoxins and inherent natural toxicants—are discussed in this chapter. These two groups of compounds are of particular interest to farmers. By changing the circumstances of food production, the presence and level of these compounds can also be altered. Mycotoxins can increase due to adverse climate or storage conditions and inherent toxicants can increase by stressing the plant. Therefore, the need for regulations in this area and the difficulties encountered are of interest to farmers, as well as to consumers and others.

## 9.2 The regulation of aflatoxins in the UK

The regulation of mycotoxins has mainly concentrated on aflatoxins. In the UK, for example, the only specific regulations covering mycotoxins in food are the Aflatoxins in Nuts, Nut Products, Dried Figs and Dried Fig Products Regulations 1992 (SI 1992/3236).

In the 1980s concern was expressed at the continuing level of aflatoxins found in samples of nuts and nut products. The government's independent expert advisory Committee on Toxicity of Chemicals in Food, Consumer Products and the Environment (COT) recommended that levels of aflatoxins in food should be reduced to the lowest level 'that is technologically achievable'. As a consequence, regulations to control the levels of aflatoxins in selected foodstuffs were proposed in 1986. Between May 1982 and December 1988 control of aflatoxins was achieved by a voluntary code of practice applied by shippers and manufacturers. From 1988, Port Health Authorities applied a 10 µg/kg total aflatoxins guideline limit to imported nuts and dried figs. The limits for aflatoxins and the commodities to which they should apply were considered and amended for inclusion in the 1992 Regulations.

The Aflatoxins in Nuts, Nut Products, Dried Figs and Dried Fig Products Regulations 1992 were made under the Food Safety Act 1990. Under this Act, responsibility for enforcement lies with local authorities. The Port Health Authorities have a particularly significant role to play in relation to these Regulations as most of the commodities that they deal with are not grown within the UK and are therefore imported. SI 1992/3236 therefore has a number of specific references to Port Health Authorities. The Food Safety Act 1990 also established the basic principles that food should not be rendered injurious to health or unfit for human consumption or so contaminated that it would not be reasonably expected to be used for human consumption in that state. SI 1992/3236 sets out the parameters by which those principles can be defined in relation to aflatoxins.

The Regulations contain prescribed limits for the specified foodstuffs for retail sale and for imports of raw commodities that are to be further processed. The respective limits are 4 µg/kg for retail sales and 10 µg/kg for imports. It should be noted that because of the European Single Market legislation the limit on imports only applies to those directly from non-European Union (EU) countries through designated ports. The lists of designated ports for the importation of nuts, nut products, dried figs and dried fig products is contained in the London and Edinburgh Gazettes of 29 December 1992. Although Schedule 1 of the Regulations gives the full chemical names of aflatoxins $B_1$, $B_2$, $G_1$ and $G_2$, they do not contain specific limits for each individual aflatoxin. Both the 4 µg/kg and 10 µg/kg limits refer to total aflatoxin levels. A list of nuts to which the Regulations apply is contained in Schedule 2.

These Regulations are unusual among UK regulations on chemical contaminants in that Schedule 4 is entitled *Requirements for Sampling and Analysis of Aflatoxins in Nut, Nut Products, Dried Figs and Dried Fig Products*. This schedule contains guidance on sampling and analysis for use by enforcement authorities and others. The methods outlined in the schedule are not intended to be definitive. However, paragraph 5 states that any method may be used providing it meets the specified performance parameters and Regulation 11(4) refers back to Section 30 of the Food Safety Act 1990, which also deals with the analysis of samples.

SI 1992/3236 applies to Great Britain only. Similar but separate regulations apply in Northern Ireland. They were made under the Northern Ireland Food Safety Order 1991. The reasons for this are purely to do with the historical development of the government process in Northern Ireland. The operation of the Aflatoxins in Nuts, Nut Products, Dried Fig Products Regulations (Northern Ireland) 1993 (Statuary Rules of Northern Ireland) SR 93 No. 31 is exactly the same in Northern Ireland as SI 1992/3236 in Great Britain. The law relating to aflatoxins in nuts, nut products, dried figs and dried fig products is therefore the same throughout the UK.

Legislation also exists in the UK for the control of aflatoxin $B_1$ in animal feed. The most recent legislation is the Feeding Stuffs Regulations 1995 (SI 1995/1412). The level of aflatoxin $M_1$ in milk is thereby controlled by the restriction of aflatoxin $B_1$ in animal feed. The only other control on the levels of aflatoxins in food in the UK is a guideline or advisory level of 50 μg/kg total aflatoxins in chilli powder. This guideline cannot be regarded as legislation as it is not legally enforceable but it is used as an indication of good practice.

## 9.3   Other national and international control of aflatoxins

Over 40 other countries in all continents have some aflatoxins legislation although the coverage of foodstuffs and the limits set vary considerably. Most countries include nuts, especially peanuts, in their controls. However, some countries, including a number of EU Member States such as Austria, Denmark, Finland, France, Germany, Spain and Sweden, have limits for virtually all foodstuffs. Norway, Switzerland and Iceland have similar coverage. Denmark, however, requires compliance certificates only for nuts and figs. As far as limits are concerned, many Asian and American countries follow the US in setting limits, for example 20 μg/kg, although Brazil has a limit of 30 μg/kg and Malaysia has a limi of 35 μg/kg.

The EU is currently considering a draft proposal on mycotoxins. Originally this proposal included other mycotoxins such as ochratoxin A and patulin. The European Commission (EC) has since decided that before proceeding with legislation further scientific consideration is necessary on these mycotoxins and has referred them to the Scientific Committee for Food. Currently, therefore, the proposed regulation covers only aflatoxins.

Council Regulation (EEC) No. 315/93 of 8 February 1993 provides the framework legislation for contaminants in food. In Article 1.1 it defines a contaminant as 'any substance not intentionally added to food which is present in such food as a result of the production (including operations carried out in crop husbandry, animal husbandry and veterinary medicine), manufacture, processing, preparation, treatment, packing, packaging, transport or holding of such food, or as a result of environmental contamination'. Article 2.1 states that 'food containing a contaminant in an amount which is unacceptable from the public health viewpoint and in particular at a toxicological level should not be placed on the market' and article 2.2 continues 'Furthermore contaminant levels should be kept as low as can reasonably be achieved by following good practices at all stages referred to in Article 1' (1.1 as noted above). These general principles are similar to those contained in the Food Safety Act 1990 noted above.

Regulation 315/93 gives the EC powers to make legislation on individual contaminants. Such regulations are seen as harmonisation measures to complete the single market. Since many of the EU Member States have regulations on aflatoxins this is a reasonable contention. The proposals on aflatoxins currently being considered follow the UK principal of dual limits for groundnuts. A limit of 10 µg/kg is proposed where the consignments are intended for further processing, with a lower limit of 4 µg/kg when they are intended for direct human consumption. This is the same as the retail limit in SI 1992/3236. The EC proposal, however, covers many commodities not included in SI 1992/3236. All dried fruits in addition to figs are included, plus cereals and milk. All nuts other than groundnuts, dried fruits and cereals have a proposed limit of 4 µg/kg. The proposal also differs from SI 1992/3236 in that each commodity has a separate limit for aflatoxin $B_1$ of half the total limit for aflatoxins $B_1 + B_2 + G_1 + G_2$. This principle is already established in the current legislation of Austria, Denmark, France, Germany, The Netherlands and Sweden. The proposed limit for milk is 0.05 µg/kg, which is similar to the level in most countries that already have specific limits for aflatoxin $M_1$ in milk and/or milk products.

At present the EC proposal is still being considered by the Working Group on Agricultural Contaminants, which is a group of experts with representatives from the fifteen Member States. When this group has concluded its discussions the proposal will then be passed to the Standing Committee for Foodstuffs for consideration.

There is at present only one subsidiary regulation made under Council Regulation (EEC) No. 315/93. This is EC Regulation (EC) No. 194/97, of 31 January 1997, on nitrate in lettuce and spinach. The regulation on mycotoxins (aflatoxins) will be an amending regulation to 194/97.

Beyond the EU the main international forum for the discussion of the control of mycotoxins has been the Codex Committee on Food Additives and Contaminants (CCFAC) of the Codex Alimentarius Commission. This is the joint food standards programme of the Food and Agriculture Organisation (FAO) and the World Health Organisation (WHO). As a United

Nations organisation, Codex brings together member states from all continents. Once again work on aflatoxins is most advanced, in the CCFAC review of natural toxicants, and has been on the agenda of the CCFAC for a number of years. There is as yet no general agreement on maximum levels for aflatoxins within the CCFAC. At present the producers, led by the US, have suggested a limit of 15 µg/kg for unprocessed nuts, whereas the nut-importing nations, particularly those in Europe, currently have limits of 10 µg/kg and therefore are unlikely to agree to any change in their limits. The Codex Alimentarius Commission may at some time in the future set maximum levels and standards that will be used by the World Trade Organisation, the successor to the General Agreement on Tariffs and Trade, to harmonise international trade in many commodities. However, we are still currently some way from that scenario in the control of natural toxicants in global food supplies.

## 9.4   Control of other mycotoxins

The regulatory situation with regard to mycotoxins other than aflatoxins is much less well defined. The UK, for example, has an advisory level of 50 µg/kg for patulin in apple juice. This advisory level, like that on aflatoxins in chilli powder, does not have any legal status. The advisory level for patulin was recommended by the Ministry of Agriculture, Fisheries and Food's independent expert advisory committee, the Food Advisory Committee, following surveillance on apple juice carried out in 1992. Further work in 1993 and 1994 indicated that the problem was mainly concerned with directly pressed juices. Surveys carried out in 1995 and 1996 concentrated on this type of juice. The results of these surveys indicated that the problem had been significantly reduced among directly pressed juices. The Food Advisory Committee reaffirmed its advisory level for patulin in 1996.

Few countries exercise regulatory control on patulin. Sweden is about to introduce a limit of 50 µg/kg. Austria, Finland, France, Greece and Iceland have sought to control the problem through maximum guidance limits, like the UK, although in some cases other products are included. The EC had originally proposed a limit for patulin (50 µg/kg in fruit, fruit products, fruit juices and fermented ciders) but this has been deferred for further consideration by the EC's Scientific Committee for Food.

The CCFAC has also considered patulin. A paper prepared by the French delegation was presented to the 29th session in March 1997. No formal decision has been taken on maximum; and there is still much work to be done if harmonised international maximum levels for patulin are to be agreed.

The other mycotoxin that has been the subject of some regulation is ochratoxin A. Limits for this substance were originally proposed by the EC at a level of 4 µg/kg in cereals and coffee, but the regulation of ochratoxin A has been deferred for further consideration by the EC's Scientific Committee for Food. Denmark and, very recently, Sweden have introduced legislative controls on ochratoxin A. In Denmark the controls concentrate on pigs' kidneys. Sweden, however, is about to introduce a limit of 5 µg/kg in cereals and cereal products. Few other countries have proposed guidelines for the regulation of ochratoxin A. The CCFAC has also considered the subject but as with aflatoxins and patulin it has yet to come to a conclusion.

There are at present very few regulatory controls throughout the world on mycotoxins other than aflatoxins, patulin and ochratoxin A. The control of mycotoxins can therefore be seen as a hierarchical process with the most sophisticated and widespread controls being developed where there is the greatest need for the control of mycotoxins, i.e. on aflatoxins. This makes some sense since aflatoxins, in particular aflatoxin $B_1$, are seen to have the highest potential as a human carcinogen amongst mycotoxins.

## 9.5  Other natural toxicants

It is not possible to deal with all groups of compounds in the same way for legislative purposes. Mycotoxins are going down the regulatory route while in contrast toxicants that are inherent to food-producing plants (inherent natural toxicants) are virtually unregulated. Where a toxicological opinion indicates the necessity, it is prudent to control the level of exposure to such compounds. Mycotoxin production can be minimised with good agricultural practice. It is therefore possible to reduce mycotoxin contamination by making compliance with any set limit a practical possibility. In addition, modern processing techniques, including optical sorters, are capable of removing individual contaminated items in the case of aflatoxins.

Inherent natural toxicants present different problems. A common problem for inherent natural toxicants is that there are often insufficient toxicological data to set tolerable daily intakes for individual compounds. This makes it difficult to set acceptable levels for such compounds in food. The other problem is that it is not possible to bring down levels of inherent natural toxicants by a code of practice or through good agricultural practice.

To define the level of risk for inherent natural toxicants would require an exhaustive analysis and identification of all the individual potential toxins present, followed by the assessment of the toxicological properties of each in turn. With data on concentration and potential intakes, the possible health hazards to humans from these toxicants could then be estimated. This is the approach commonly used for many toxic contaminants and food additives. However, for natural constituents of plants there are difficulties with this approach. The problem breaks down into three component parts: the assessment of hazard, intake and risk. The problem for hazard assessment in this case is the shortage of toxicological data. It would be an overwhelming task to identify, isolate and test all the possible toxicants and, unlike trials carried out on additives and drugs, there is no commercial incentive for industry to fund such work. Further difficulties are that the degree of bioavailability in man of the toxicant from the food is vitally important in determining whether health effects will occur. Indeed there may be interactions with other constituents of the food that influence the effects of the toxicant in humans. Thus, data generated through the usual toxicological studies on an isolated substance may not be relevant.

In terms of intake assessment, there is the problem of the large variability usually found in the concentrations of natural toxicants in plant-based foods. In terms of risk assessment, it is particularly important to do a risk–benefit assessment of the potential toxic effects of a substance against the nutritional advantages of the food(s) involved. The lack of quantitative data and absence of a forum with the necessary expertise renders this extremely difficult.

## 9.6  Problems with legislation

When developing legislation the practicalities must be considered. Using mycotoxins as an example, the issues to be borne in mind can be identified. Limits cannot be introduced without consideration being given to the practicalities of enforcement. This is not always straightforward in the European context as the different Member States have very different systems of enforcement. In the UK, it is thought to be particularly important to ensure that it is practically possible to enforce the legislation and that it is not prohibitively expensive to do so. If a regulation is expensive and difficult to enforce, it is likely that less testing will be carried out thereby reducing the effectiveness of any regulation—the protection to the consumer will be reduced. The area of natural toxicants is different from many others, such as the control of pesticides, in that any legislation is enforced by trading standards officers. Unlike pesticides, where industry is required to partially fund the monitoring for enforcement purposes in the UK, there is no such requirement for natural toxicants. Local authorities are not given funding by industry to monitor and enforce any regulations on mycotoxins.

With aflatoxins, it is important to have an agreed sampling plan. However, the difficulty with aflatoxins, and probably other mycotoxins too, is the heterogeneous distribution of the mycotoxin in the food sample. This means that there has to be a requirement for a representative but practical sampling plan when considering legislation for mycotoxins. Due to the extreme heterogeneity of the mycotoxin and the existence of 'hot-spots', any sampling plan should be as representative as possible while remaining practical. It is also necessary to consider methods of analysis: it should be decided whether a particular method, or performance parameters, should be used.

## 9.7   UK regulations on inherent toxicants

There are no regulations for inherent toxicants other than the Erucic Acid in Food Regulations 1977 (SI 1977/691). Erucic acid is a normal constituent of some foods and levels are controlled in rapeseed due to its potential cardiotoxic effects.

## 9.8   Regulations on inherent toxicants in other countries

Few countries have regulations for inherent natural toxicants. Among EU Member States only Sweden has a limit for an inherent natural toxicant—for glycoalkaloids in potatoes. The total maximum level of solanidine glycosides in raw and unpeeled potatoes is set at 200 mg/kg. There are no limits for inherent natural toxicants in the USA.

## 9.9   Consequences of legislation

It is tempting to consider that when legislation has been introduced it will act to control the problem area but will not affect anything else. However, this is not necessarily the case.

### 9.9.1   Changes in practices
By changing practices in order to comply with any regulations, other parameters may also change. For example, pesticide usage has been decreased in a number of areas. There is a suggestion that this would lead to increased levels of mycotoxins, e.g. patulin. However, there is no evidence to show that this has happened. Although there was no particular effect in this case, the possibility of changes due to altered agricultural or processing practices is present.

### 9.9.2   Changes to the properties of foodstuffs
By changing the levels of natural toxicants in food, other properties of the food may be altered. For example, in the case of potatoes, when the level of glycoalkaloids was modified the flavour of the potato also changed. A further example is controlling the erucic acid level in rapeseed, which can result in technological effects. This makes it difficult to make a margarine from rapeseed oil—a grainy texture results because only C-18 fatty acids are present. Other oils need to be added to give a mixture of fatty acids and obtain the required texture.

It may be possible, by reducing the level of a particular natural toxicant, perhaps by regulation, that another constituent of the plant may be increased; this should be borne in mind when developing any legislation or guidelines.

## 9.10  The future of regulation in this area

Current discussions within the EC will result in regulation of aflatoxins. It is possible that this will be amended to include other mycotoxins, such as ochratoxin A, patulin and fumonisins, at a later date. In some places, there is a keenness to develop legislation for inherent toxicants. However, this has mostly been hampered by difficulties with risk assessment. While discussion of possible regulations has been mooted in a number of fora, little has actually taken place.

## 9.11  Conclusions

Issues regarding the regulation of the various groups of natural toxicants can be very different. Natural toxicants cannot be regarded as one group for such purposes. Before considering regulation in this area a number of points should be considered. It can be seen that in the case of mycotoxins there can be a demonstrated need (depending on the toxicological opinion) for limiting levels and this can be achieved by regulation. However, in the case of inherent natural toxicants, it is more difficult to carry out risk assessment. Therefore, it is suggested that it is far more difficult to consider regulation in this area and even if regulation is introduced this may only lead to the biochemical balance in the plant being disturbed, resulting in further problems. Whenever regulations are introduced, the consequences for other properties of the foodstuff should be borne in mind.

# 10   Quality assurance

Roger Wood

## 10.1   Introduction

It is now internationally recognised that for a laboratory to produce consistently reliable data it must implement an appropriate programme of quality assurance measures. This is particularly the case when trace constituents, such as natural toxicants, are to be determined. Among such measures is the need for the laboratory to demonstrate that the methods it uses are 'fit-for-purpose' and in statistical control, and to participate in proficiency testing schemes. This chapter surveys some of the essential elements that a laboratory has to consider when wishing to implement a programme of quality assurance measures.

While it is generally recognised that it is necessary for the above measures to be implemented, in the food sector control laboratories determining natural toxicants in the European Union (EU) are required to do so by legislative requirements. These are described below as they provide good guidance as to the quality assurance measures that all laboratories can follow to produce reliable data. Other international organisations, most notably the Codex Alimentarius Commission, are taking a similar approach to the EU. The Codex approach is therefore also described in this chapter.

### 10.1.1   European Union food control directives
Methods of analysis have been prescribed by legislation for a number of foodstuffs since the formation of the European Community, now the EU. However, the EU now recognises that the quality of results from a laboratory is equally as important as the method used to obtain the results. This is best illustrated by consideration of the Council Directive on the Official Control of Foodstuffs (OCF), which was adopted by the Community in June 1989 (EEC, 1989).

In Article 13 it is stated:

'In order to ensure that the application of this Directive is uniform throughout the Member States, the Commission shall, within one year of its adoption, make a report to the European Parliament and to the Council on the possibility of establishing Community quality standards for all laboratories involved in inspection and sampling under this Directive'.

The Commission, in September 1990, produced a report that recommended establishing Community quality standards for all laboratories involved in inspections and sampling under the OCF Directive. Proposals on this have now been adopted by the Community in the Directive on

Additional Measures Concerning the Food Control of Foodstuffs (AMFC) (EEC, 1993).

The relevant articles in the AMFC Directive are Article 3, which states:

'1. Member States shall take all measures necessary to ensure that the laboratories referred to in Article 7 of Directive 89/397/EEC comply with the general criteria for the operation of testing laboratories laid down in European Standard EN 45001 supplemented by Standard Operating Procedures and the random audit of their compliance by quality assurance personnel, in accordance with the OECD principles Nos. 2 and 7 of good laboratory practice as set out in Section II of Annex 2 of the Decision of the Council of the OECD of 12 May 1981 concerning the mutual acceptance of data in the assessment of chemicals.

2. In assessing the laboratories referred to in Article 7 of Directive 89/397/EEC Member States shall:

(a)     apply the criteria laid down in European Standard EN 45002; and

(b)     require the use of proficiency testing schemes as far as appropriate.

Laboratories meeting the assessment criteria shall be presumed to fulfil the criteria referred to in paragraph 1. Laboratories that do not meet the assessment criteria shall not be considered as laboratories referred to in Article 7 of the said Directive.

3. Member States shall designate bodies responsible for the assessment of laboratories as referred to in Article 7 of Directive 89/397/EEC. These bodies shall comply with the general criteria for laboratory accreditation bodies laid down in European Standard EN 45003.

4. The accreditation and assessment of testing laboratories referred to in this article may relate to individual tests or groups of tests. Any appropriate deviation in the way in which the standards referred to in paragraphs 1, 2 and 3 are applied shall be adopted in accordance with the procedure laid down in Article 8.'

and Article 4, which states:

'Member States shall ensure that the validation of methods of analysis used within the context of official control of foodstuffs by the laboratories referred to in Article 7 of Directive 89/397/EEC comply whenever possible with the provisions of paragraphs 1 and 2 of the Annex to Council Directive 85/591/EEC of 23 December 1985 concerning the introduction of Community methods of sampling and analysis for the monitoring of foodstuffs intended for human consumption.' (EEC, 1985).

As a result of the adoption of the above Directives, legislation is now in place to ensure that there is confidence in food analysis laboratories. The legislation requirements serve as a valid model for the quality assurance measures that laboratories analysing for natural toxicants should follow.

### 10.1.2  Codex Alimentarius Commission

The Codex Committee on Methods of Analysis and Sampling has also developed objective criteria for assessing the competence of testing laboratories involved in the official import and export control of foods. These were recommended by the Committee at its twenty-first Session (FAO, 1997) and mirror the EU recommendations for laboratory quality standards and methods of analysis.

The Codex recommendations are that laboratories:

- comply with the general criteria for testing laboratories laid down in ISO/IEC Guide 25:1990 General requirements for the competence of calibration and testing laboratories (ISO, 1993a);
- participate in appropriate proficiency testing schemes for food analysis that conform to the requirements laid down in the international harmonised protocol for the proficiency testing of (chemical) analytical laboratories (as adopted for Codex purposes by the Codex Alimentarius Commission at its 21st Session in July 1995) (Thompson and Wood, 1993);
- whenever available, use methods of analysis that have been validated according to the principles laid down by the Codex Alimentarius Commission (these are identical to the requirements laid down by the EU in the Methods of Analysis and Sampling Directive) (EEC, 1985);
- use internal quality control procedures, such as those described in the harmonised guidelines for internal quality control in analytical chemistry laboratories (Thompson and Wood, 1995).

The Committee noted that the compliance with the above criteria for laboratories involved in the official import and export control of foods needed to be assessed by suitable mechanisms. The bodies assessing the laboratories should comply with the general criteria for laboratory accreditation, such as those laid down in ISO/IEC Guide 58:1993, 'Calibration and testing laboratory accreditation systems—General requirements for operation and recognition' (ISO, 1993b).

The Codex requirements are becoming of increasing importance because of the acceptance of Codex Standards in World Trade Organisation agreements.

The effect of the Additional Measures Food Control (AMFC) Directive and the Codex requirements is that food control laboratories must consider the following aspects within the laboratory:

- the organisation of the laboratory;
- how well the laboratory actually carries out analyses; and
- the methods of analysis used in the laboratory.

All these aspects are interrelated, but in simple terms may be thought of as:

- becoming accredited to an internationally recognised standard (such accreditation is aided by the use of internal quality control procedures);
- participating in proficiency schemes; and
- using validated methods.

These considerations will be addressed in turn, as will other quality assurance measures that a laboratory should consider, for example, the use of recovery factors.

## 10.2  Accreditation

Although to be formally accredited is not a necessity to ensure that a laboratory will produce 'quality data', an accredited laboratory has to be able to state that it has been third party assessed, which does give additional assurance to its 'customers'.

The AMFC Directive requires that food control laboratories should be accredited to the EN 45000 series of standards supplemented by some of the OECD Good Laboratory Practice (GLP) principles. In the EU Member States' governments will nominate the accreditation service to carry out the required accreditation under the Directive. For example, in the UK the United Kingdom Accreditation Service (UKAS) will be nominated to carry out the accreditation of official food control laboratories for all the aspects prescribed in the Directive. However, as the accreditation agency will also be required to comply to EN 45003 Standard and to carry out assessments in accordance with the EN 45002 Standard, any other accreditation agencies that are members of the European Co-operation for Accreditation of Laboratories (EAL) may also be nominated to carry out the accreditation. Similar procedures will be followed in the other Member States, all having developed, or in the process of developing, equivalent organisations to UKAS. The EN 45001 Standard adopted by the EU is related to the ISO Guide 25. Laboratories carrying out official control analyses in the natural toxicants area will have to be accredited. Other laboratories may wish to be seen to be of the same standard in order that confidence can be placed in their work.

In the UK it has been the normal practice for UKAS to accredit the scope of laboratories on a method-by-method basis. However, in the case of official food control laboratories undertaking non-routine or investigative chemical analysis, it is accepted that it is not practical to use an accredited fully documented method in the conventional sense, i.e. to specify each sample type and analyte. Such laboratories must have a protocol defining the approach to be adopted, including requirements for validation of methods and internal quality control. Full details of procedures used, including instrumental parameters, must be recorded at the time of each analysis in order to enable the procedure to be repeated in the same manner at a later date. Thus, for official food control laboratories undertaking analysis, appropriate methods may be accredited on a generic basis with such generic accreditation being underpinned where necessary by specific method accreditation. This approach will be particularly appropriate to laboratories carrying out natural toxicants work where the methodology may be continuously developed and where a laboratory may wish for any 'research' activities to be regarded as being accredited, as well as its defined methods being used on a routine basis.

## 10.3   Internal quality control: harmonised guidelines for internal quality control in analytical chemistry laboratories

An integral part of the accreditation process is the introduction of acceptable internal quality control (IQC) procedures. IQC is one of a number of concerted measures that analytical chemists can take to ensure that the data produced in the laboratory are of known quality and uncertainty. In practice this is determined by comparing the results achieved in the laboratory at a given time with a standard. IQC therefore comprises the routine practical procedures that enable the analyst to accept a result or group of results, or reject the results and repeat the analysis. IQC is undertaken by the inclusion of particular reference materials, 'control materials', into the analytical sequence and by duplicate analysis.

ISO, IUPAC and AOAC INTERNATIONAL (AOACI) have co-operated to produce agreed protocols on the design, conduct and interpretation of collaborative studies (Horwitz, 1988) and on the proficiency testing of (chemical) analytical laboratories (Thompson and Wood, 1993). The Working Group that produced these protocols has prepared a further protocol on the internal quality control of data produced in analytical laboratories. The document was finalised in 1994 and published in 1995 as the 'Harmonised guidelines for internal quality control in analytical chemistry laboratories' (Thompson and Wood, 1995). The use of the procedures outlined in the protocol should aid compliance with the accreditation requirements above.

### 10.3.1   Basic concepts

The protocol sets out guidelines for the implementation of IQC in analytical laboratories. IQC is one of a number of concerted measures that analytical chemists can take to ensure that the data produced in the laboratory are fit for their intended purpose. In practice, fitness for purpose is determined by a comparison of the accuracy achieved in a laboratory at a given time with a required level of accuracy. IQC therefore comprises the routine practical procedures that enable the analytical chemist to accept a result or group of results as fit for purpose, or reject the results and repeat the analysis. As such, IQC is an important determinant of the quality of analytical data and is recognised as such by accreditation agencies.

IQC is undertaken by the inclusion of particular reference materials, called 'control materials', into the analytical sequence and by duplicate analysis. The control materials should, wherever possible, be representative of the test materials under consideration in respect of matrix composition, the state of physical preparation and the concentration range of the analyte. As the control materials are treated in exactly the same way as the test materials, they are regarded as surrogates that can be used to characterise the performance of the analytical system, both at a specific time and over longer intervals. IQC is a final check of the correct execution of all of the procedures (including calibration) that are prescribed in the analytical protocol and all of the other quality assurance measures that underlie good analytical practice. IQC is therefore necessarily retrospective. It is also required to be as far as possible independent of the analytical protocol, especially the calibration, that it is designed to test.

Ideally both the control materials and those used to create the calibration should be traceable to appropriate certified reference materials or a recognised empirical reference method. When this is not possible, control materials should be traceable at least to a material of guaranteed purity or other well-characterised material. However, the two paths of traceability must not become coincident at too late a stage in the analytical process. For instance, if control materials and calibration standards were prepared from a single stock solution of analyte, IQC would not detect any inaccuracy stemming from the incorrect preparation of the stock solution.

In a typical analytical situation several, or perhaps many, similar test materials will be analysed together and control materials will be included in the group. Often determinations will be duplicated by the analysis of separate test portions of the same material. Such a group of materials is referred to as an analytical 'run'. (The words 'set', 'series' and 'batch' have also been used as synonyms for 'run'.) Runs are regarded as being analysed under effectively constant conditions. The batches of reagents, the instrument settings, the analyst and the laboratory environment will, under ideal conditions, remain unchanged during analysis of a run. Systematic errors should therefore remain constant during a run, as should the values of the parameters that describe random errors. As the monitoring of these errors is of concern, the run is the basic operational unit of IQC.

A run is therefore regarded as being carried out under repeatability conditions, i.e. the random measurement errors are of a magnitude that would be encountered in a 'short' period of time. In practice the analysis of a run may occupy sufficient time for small systematic changes to occur. For example, reagents may degrade, instruments may drift, minor adjustments to instrumental settings may be called for or the laboratory temperature may rise. However, these systematic effects are, for the purposes of IQC, subsumed into the repeatability variations. Sorting the materials making up a run into a randomised order converts the effects of drift into random errors.

### 10.3.2 Scope of the guidelines
The guidelines are a harmonisation of IQC procedures that have evolved in various fields of analysis, notably clinical biochemistry, geochemistry, environmental studies, occupational hygiene and food analysis. There is much common ground in the procedures from these various fields. However, analytical chemistry comprises an even wider range of activities, and the basic

principles of IQC should be able to encompass all of these. The guidelines will be applicable in the great majority of instances although there are a number of IQC practices that are restricted to individual sectors of the analytical community and so not included in the guidelines.

In order to achieve harmonisation and provide basic guidance on IQC, some types of analytical activity have been excluded from the guidelines. Issues specifically excluded are as follows:

(i) *Quality control of sampling.* While it is recognised that the quality of the analytical result can be no better than that of the sample, quality control of sampling is a separate subject and in many areas is not yet fully developed. Moreover, in many instances analytical laboratories have no control over sampling practice and quality.

(ii) *In-line analysis and continuous monitoring.* In this style of analysis there is no possibility of repeating the measurement, so the concept of IQC as used in the guidelines is inapplicable.

(iii) *Multivariate IQC.* Multivariate methods in IQC are still the subject of research and cannot be regarded as sufficiently established for inclusion in the guidelines. The current document regards multianalyte data as requiring a series of univariate IQC tests. Caution is necessary in the interpretation of this type of data to avoid inappropriately frequent rejection of data.

(iv) *Statutory and contractual requirements.*

(v) *Quality assurance measures.* Quality assurance measures such as pre-analytical checks on instrumental stability, wavelength calibration, balance calibration, tests on resolution of chromatography columns and problem diagnostics are not included. They are regarded as part of the analytical protocol and IQC tests their effectiveness together with the other aspects of the methodology.

### 10.3.3  Internal Quality Control and uncertainty

A prerequisite of analytical chemistry is the recognition of 'fitness for purpose', the standard of accuracy that is required for an effective use of the analytical data. This standard is arrived at by consideration of the intended uses of the data, although it is seldom possible to foresee all of the potential future applications of analytical results. For this reason, in order to prevent inappropriate interpretation, it is important that a statement of the uncertainty should accompany analytical results or be readily available to those who wish to use the data.

Strictly speaking, an analytical result cannot be interpreted unless it is accompanied by knowledge of its associated uncertainty at a stated level of confidence. A simple example demonstrates this principle. Suppose that there is a statutory requirement that a foodstuff must not contain more than 10 mg/kg of a particular constituent. A manufacturer analyses a batch and obtains a result of 9 mg/kg for that constituent. If the uncertainty on the result expressed as a half range (assuming no sampling error) is 0.1 mg/kg (i.e. the true result falls, with a high probability, within the range 8.9–9.1), then it may be assumed that the legal limit is not exceeded. If, in contrast, the uncertainty is 2 mg/kg then there is no such assurance. The interpretation and use that may be made of the measurement thus depends on the uncertainty associated with it.

Analytical results should therefore have an associated uncertainty if any definite meaning is to be attached to them or an informed interpretation made. If this requirement cannot be fulfilled, the use to which the data can be put is limited. Moreover, the achievement of the required measurement uncertainty must be tested as a routine procedure, because the quality of data can vary, both in time within a single laboratory and between different laboratories. IQC comprises the process of checking that the required uncertainty is achieved in a run.

### 10.3.4 Recommendations in the guidelines

The following recommendations represent integrated approaches to IQC that are suitable for many types of analysis and application areas. Managers of laboratory quality systems will have to adapt the recommendations to the demands of their own particular requirements. Such adoption could be implemented, for example, by adjusting the number of duplicates and control material inserted into a run or by the inclusion of any additional measures favoured in the particular application area. The procedure finally chosen and its accompanying decision rules must be codified in an IQC protocol that is separate from the analytical system protocol.

The practical approach to quality control is determined by the frequency with which the measurement is carried out and the size and nature of each run. The following recommendations are therefore made. (The use of control charts and decision rules are covered in Appendix 1 to the guidelines.) In all of the following the order in the run in which the various materials are analysed should be randomised if possible. A failure to randomise may result in an underestimation of various components of error.

(i) *Short (e.g. n <20) frequent runs of similar materials.* Here the concentration range of the analyte in the run is relatively small, so a common value of standard deviation can be assumed.

   Insert a control material at least once per run. Plot either the individual values obtained or the mean value on an appropriate control chart. Analyse in duplicate at least half of the test materials, selected at random. Insert at least one blank determination.

(ii) *Longer (e.g. n >20) frequent runs of similar materials.* Again a common level of standard deviation is assumed.

Insert the control material at an approximate frequency of one per ten test materials. If the run size will vary from run to run it is easier to standardise on a fixed number of insertions per run and plot the mean value on a control chart of means. Otherwise plot individual values. Analyse in duplicate a minimum of five test materials chosen at random. Insert one blank determination per ten test materials.

(iii) *Frequent runs containing similar materials but with a wide range of analyte concentration.* Here we cannot assume that a single value of standard deviation is applicable.

Insert control materials in total numbers approximately as recommended above. However, there should be at least two levels of analyte represented, one close to the median level of typical test materials and the other approximately at the upper or lower decile as appropriate. Enter values for the two control materials on separate control charts. Duplicate a minimum of five test materials and insert one procedural blank per ten test materials.

(iv) *Ad hoc analysis.* Here the concept of statistical control is not applicable. It is assumed, that the materials in the run are of a single type.

Carry out duplicate analysis on all of the test materials. Carry out spiking or recovery tests or use a formulated control material, with an appropriate number of insertions (see above) and with different concentrations of analyte if appropriate. Carry out blank determinations. As no control limits are available, compare the bias and precision with fitness-for-purpose limits or other established criteria.

By following the above recommendations laboratories introduce IQC measures, which are an essential aspect of ensuring that data released from a laboratory are fit for purpose. If properly executed, quality control methods can monitor the various aspects of data quality on a run-by-run basis. In runs where performance falls outside acceptable limits, the data produced can be rejected and, after remedial action on the analytical system, the analysis can be repeated.

The guidelines stress, however, that internal quality control is not foolproof even when properly executed. Obviously it is subject to 'errors of both kinds', i.e. runs that are in control will occasionally be rejected and runs that are out of control occasionally accepted. Of more importance, IQC cannot usually identify sporadic gross errors or short-term disturbances in the analytical system that affect the results for individual test materials. Moreover, inferences based on IQC results are applicable only to test materials that fall within the scope of the analytical method validation. Despite these limitations, which professional experience and diligence can alleviate to a degree, IQC is the principal recourse available for ensuring that only data of appropriate quality are released from a laboratory. When properly executed it is very successful.

The guidelines also stress that the perfunctory execution of any quality system will not guarantee the production of data of adequate quality. The correct procedures for feedback, remedial action and staff motivation must also be documented and acted upon. In other words, there must be a genuine commitment to quality within a laboratory for an IQC programme to succeed, i.e. the IQC must be part of a complete quality management system.

## 10.4   Proficiency testing

The need for laboratories carrying out analytical determinations to demonstrate to their customers that they are doing so competently has become paramount. Thus laboratories are required to become accredited, to use fully validated methods and to participate successfully in proficiency testing schemes. Proficiency testing has assumed a far greater importance than previously and, during negotiation on the AMFC Directive, it was agreed that proficiency testing schemes will comply with the requirements of the ISO/IUPAC/AOACI harmonised protocol for proficiency testing of (chemical) analytical laboratories (Thompson and Wood, 1993), thus eliminating the potential for different interpretations of the requirement for proficiency testing under the EN 45,000 Standards.

The essential elements of proficiency testing have now been accepted within the EU. Laboratories carrying out natural toxicants work must regard these as an integral part of their quality assurance activities. For that reason proficiency testing is described in detail below:

### 10.4.1   What is proficiency testing?
A proficiency testing scheme is defined as a system for objectively checking laboratory results by an external agency. It includes comparison of a laboratory's results at intervals with those of other laboratories, the main object being the establishment of trueness.

Proficiency testing schemes are based on the regular circulation of homogeneous samples by a co-ordinator, analysis of samples (normally by the laboratory's method of choice) and an assessment of the results. However, although many organisations carry out such schemes, it is only recently that the international protocol has been agreed and then used by many proficiency testing scheme organisers.

### 10.4.2   Why proficiency testing is important
Participation in proficiency testing schemes provides laboratories with a means of objectively assessing, and demonstrating, the reliability of the data they produce. Although there are several types of schemes, they all share a common feature of comparing test results obtained by one testing laboratory with those obtained by other testing laboratories. Schemes may be 'open' to

any laboratory or participation may be invited. Schemes may set out to assess the competence of laboratories undertaking a very specific analysis (e.g. lead in blood) or more general analysis (e.g. food analysis). Although accreditation and proficiency testing are separate exercises, accreditation assessments will increasingly use proficiency testing data. It is now recommended by ISO Guide 25 (ISO, 1993a), the prime standard to which accreditation agencies operate, that such agencies require laboratories seeking accreditation to participate in an appropriate proficiency testing scheme before accreditation is gained.

### 10.4.3 ISO/IUPAC/AOACI harmonised protocol for proficiency testing of (chemical) analytical laboratories

The International Standardising Organisations, AOACI, ISO and IUPAC, have co-operated to produce an agreed international harmonised protocol for proficiency testing of (chemical) analytical laboratories (Thompson and Wood, 1993). This protocol is recognised within the food sector of the EU and also by the Codex Alimentarius Commission. The protocol makes the following recommendations about proficiency testing, all of which are important to laboratories carrying out analysis for natural toxicants.

*Framework.* Samples must be distributed regularly to participants who are to return results within a given time. The results will be statistically analysed by the organiser and participants will be notified of their performance. Advice will be available to poor performers and participants will be kept fully informed of the scheme's progress. Participants will be identified by code only, to preserve confidentiality.

The scheme's structure for any one analyte or round in a series should be:

- samples prepared;
- samples distributed regularly;
- participants analyse samples and report results;
- results analysed and performance assessed;
- participants notified of their performance;
- advice available for poor performers, on request;
- co-ordinator reviews performance of scheme; and
- next round commences.

*Organisation.* The running of the scheme will be the responsibility of a co-ordinating laboratory or organisation. Sample preparation will either be contracted out or undertaken in-house. The co-ordinating laboratory must be of high reputation in the type of analysis being tested. Overall management of the scheme should be in the hands of a small steering committee (Advisory Panel) having representatives from the co-ordinating laboratory (who should be practising laboratory scientists), contract laboratories (if any), appropriate professional bodies and ordinary participants.

*Samples.* The samples to be distributed must be generally similar in matrix to the unknown samples that are routinely analysed (in respect of matrix composition and analyte concentration range). It is essential they are of acceptable homogeneity and stability. The bulk material prepared must be effectively homogeneous so that all laboratories will receive samples that do not differ significantly in analyte concentration.

The procedure to be followed to test for sample heterogeneity is:

- prepare whole of bulk material in a satisfactory form;
- divide the material into the containers;
- select between 10 and 20 containers randomly;
- homogenise contents of each selected container;
- from each take two test portions;
- analyse portions in random order as one batch;
- estimate sampling variance (one-way variance analysis, without exclusion of outliers);
- assign $\sigma$ as a precision standard at mean analyte value (i.e. the target value for the standard deviation for the proficiency test at the analyte concentration of interest);
- for effective homogeneity the square root of the sampling variance divided by $\sigma$ must be less than 0.3.

The co-ordinating laboratory should also show that the bulk sample is sufficiently stable throughout the duration of the proficiency test. Thus, prior to sample distribution, the stability of the sample matrix and of the analyte must be assessed after appropriate storage. Ideally the quality checks on prepared samples should be performed by a second laboratory although it is recognised that this would probably cause considerable difficulty to the co-ordinating laboratory. The number of samples to be distributed per round for each analyte should not be more than five.

*Frequency of sample distribution.* Ideally sample distribution frequency in any one series should not be more than every two weeks and not less then every four months. A frequency greater than once every two weeks could lead to problems in turn-round of samples and results. If the period between distributions extends much beyond four months, there will be unacceptable delays in identifying analytical problems and the impact of the scheme on participants will be small. The frequency also relates to the field of application and the amount of internal quality control that is required for that field. Thus, although the frequency range stated above should be adhered to, there may be circumstances where it is acceptable for a longer time-scale between sample distributions, e.g. if sample throughput per annum is very low. Advice on this respect would be a function of the Advisory Panel.

*Estimating the assigned value (the 'true' result).* There are a number of possible approaches to determining the nominally 'true' result for a sample but only three are normally considered:

- the result may be established from the amount of analyte added to the samples by the laboratory preparing the sample;
- a 'reference' laboratory (or group of such expert laboratories) may be asked to measure the concentration of the analyte using definitive methods;
- the results obtained by the participating laboratories (or a substantial sub-group of these) may be used as the basis for the nominal 'true' result.

The organisers of the scheme should provide the participants with a clear statement giving the basis for the assignment of reference values, which should take into account the views of the Advisory Panel.

*Choice of analytical method.* Participants can use the analytical method of their choice except when instructed to adopt a specified method. It is recommended that all methods should be properly validated before use. In situations where the analytical result is method-dependent, the true value will be assessed using those results obtained using a defined procedure. If participants use a method that is not 'equivalent' to the defining method, then an automatic bias in result will occur when their performance is assessed.

*Performance criteria.* For each analyte in a round a criterion for the performance score may be set, against which the score obtained by a laboratory can be judged. A 'running score' could be calculated to give an assessment of performance spread over a longer period of time.

*Reporting results.* Reports issued to participants should include data on the results from all laboratories together with the participant's own performance score. The original results should be presented to enable participants to check correct data entry. Reports should be made available before the next sample distribution.

Although all results should be reported, it may not be possible to do this in extensive schemes (e.g. 700 participants determining 20 analytes in a round). Participants should, therefore, receive at least a clear report with the results of all laboratories in histogram form.

*Liaison with participants.* Participants should be provided with a detailed information pack on joining the scheme. Communication with participants should be by newsletter or annual report together with a periodic open meeting; participants should be advised of changes in scheme design. Advice should be available to poor performers. Feedback from laboratories should be encouraged so that participants contribute to the scheme's development. Participants should view it as *their* scheme rather than one imposed by a distant bureaucracy.

*Collusion and falsification of results.* Collusion might take place between laboratories so that independent data are not submitted. Proficiency testing schemes should be designed to ensure that there is as little collusion and falsification as possible. For example, alternative samples could be distributed within a round. In addition, instructions should make it clear that collusion is contrary to professional scientific conduct and serves only to nullify the benefits of proficiency testing.

*Statistical procedure for the analysis of results.* The first stage in producing a score from a result $x$ (a single measurement of analyte concentration in a test material) is to obtain an estimate of the bias, thus:

$$\text{bias} = x - X$$

where $X$ is the true concentration or amount of analyte.

The efficacy of any proficiency test depends on using a reliable value for $X$. Several methods are available for establishing a working estimate of $\hat{X}$ (i.e. the assigned value, outlined above).

*Formation of a z score.* Most proficiency testing schemes compare bias with a standard error. An obvious approach is to form the $z$ score given by:

$$z = (x - \hat{X})/\sigma$$

where $\sigma$ is a standard deviation. $\sigma$ is either an estimate of the actual variation encountered in a particular round ($\hat{s}$) estimated from the laboratories' results after outlier elimination or a target representing the maximum allowed variation consistent with valid data. This is the procedure recommended in the International Protocol and hence that to be followed in the EU.

A fixed target value for $\sigma$ is preferable and can be arrived at in several ways: it could be fixed arbitrarily, with a value based on a perception of how laboratories should perform, it could be an estimate of the precision required for a specific task of data interpretation, or it could be derived from a model of precision, such as the Horwitz curve (Horwitz, 1982). However, while this model provides a general picture of reproducibility, substantial deviation

from it may be experienced for particular methods. In the case of natural toxicants data on the target deviations will have been drawn from both collaborative trials and from predictions using the Horwitz curve.

*Interpretation of z-scores.* If $\hat{X}$ and $\sigma$ are good estimates of the population
mean and standard deviation then $z$ will be approximately normally distributed with a mean of zero and unit standard deviation. An analytical result is
described as 'well behaved' when it complies with this condition.

An absolute value of $z$ ($|z|$) greater than 3 suggests poor performance
in terms of accuracy. This judgement depends on the assumption of the normal distribution, which, outliers apart, seems to be justified in practice.

As $z$ is standardised, it is comparable for all analytes and methods. Thus
values of $z$ can be combined to give a composite score for a laboratory in
one round of a proficiency test.

The $z$ scores can be interpreted as follows:

| | |
|---|---|
| $|z| < 2$ | 'satisfactory': will occur in 95% cases produced by 'well-behaved' results |
| $2 < |z| < 3$ | 'questionable': will occur in $\approx$ 5% of cases produced by 'well-behaved' results |
| $|z| > 3$ | 'unsatisfactory': will only occur in $\approx$ 0.1% of cases produced by 'well-behaved' results |

*National proficiency schemes.* Because of the EU requirements a number of
Member States have introduced proficiency testing schemes in the food
area. Most operate according to the harmonised protocol and thus conform
to the requirements internationally accepted for the operation of proficiency
testing schemes in the food sector. For example, in the UK the Ministry of
Agriculture, Fisheries and Food has developed a proficiency testing scheme
for food analysis laboratories (The Food Analysis Performance Assessment
Scheme, FAPAS). The scheme complies with the requirements of the harmonised protocol referred to above and thus may be regarded as a practical
demonstration of the effectiveness of the protocol. It covers some analytes
of concern in the natural toxicants field.

## 10.5  Methods of analysis

Methods of analysis are a vital part of the quality assurance measures that a
laboratory carrying out the analysis of natural toxicants must consider. This
is best achieved by a laboratory referring to the statutory requirements for
methods of analysis in the food sector in both the EU and Codex. In addition,
the requirements (see section 10.5.1 below) of the Association of Official
Analytical Chemists International (AOACI) and the European Committee for
Standardization are important sources of validated methods of analysis in the
natural toxicants area.

### 10.5.1  AOAC International

This organisation has required for many years that all of its methods, which are quoted worldwide, be collaboratively tested before being accepted for publication. The procedure for carrying out the necessary collaborative trials is well defined and has formed part of the internal requirements of the organisation for many years. In addition, methods are adopted by the organisation on a preliminary/tentative basis (as 'Official First Action Methods') before being adopted as 'Official Final Action Methods' by the organisation after at least two years in use by analysts on a routine basis. This procedure ensures that the methods are satisfactory on a day-to-day basis before being finally accepted by the AOACI.

The AOACI has also developed two other procedures for 'method validation', which, though not dealing directly with the production of methods of analysis that have been validated by collaborative trial, do result in some validation. These are:

- peer validated methods in which a method of analysis is assessed in a very limited number of laboratories (usually three) and an assessment made of its performance characteristics; and
- methods assessed by the AOAC Research Institute, which are normally proprietary products (e.g. 'test kits') for which a 'certificate' of conformance with specification is issued by the Research Institute.

### 10.5.2  The European Union

The EU is attempting to harmonise sampling and analysis procedures in order to meet the current demands of the national and international enforcement agencies and the likely increased problems that the open market will bring. To aid this the EU issued a Directive on Sampling and Methods of Analysis (EEC, 1985). The Directive contains a technical annex in which the need to carry out a collaborative trial before a method in the food sector can be adopted by the EU is emphasised and which contains important information for all food analysis laboratories.

The criteria to which EU methods of analysis for foodstuffs should now conform are as stringent as those recommended by any international organisation following adoption of the Directive. The annex states:

'1. Methods of analysis which are to be considered for adoption under the provisions of the Directive shall be examined with respect to the following criteria:

    (i)    specificity
    (ii)   accuracy
    (iii)  precision: repeatability intra-laboratory (within laboratory), reproducibility inter-laboratory (within laboratory and between laboratories)
    (iv)  limit of detection
    (v)   sensitivity

    (vi)     practicability and applicability under normal laboratory conditions

    (vii)    other criteria which may be selected as required.

2.   The precision values referred to in 1(iii) shall be obtained from a collaborative trial which has been conducted in accordance with an internationally recognised protocol on collaborative trials (e.g. International Organisation for Standardization Precision of Test Methods (ISO 5725/1981) (ISO, 1981)). The repeatability and reproducibility values shall be expressed in an internationally recognised form (e.g. the 95% confidence intervals as defined by ISO 5725/1981). The results from the collaborative trial shall be published or be freely available.

3.   Methods of analysis which are applicable uniformly to various groups of commodities should be given preference over methods which apply to individual commodities.

4.   Methods of analysis adopted under this Directive should be edited in the standard layout for methods of analysis recommended by the International Organisations for Standardization.'

### 10.5.3  The Codex Alimentarius Commission

This was the first international organisation working at the government level in the food sector that laid down principles for the establishment of its methods. That it was necessary for such guidelines and principles to be laid down reflects the confused and unsatisfactory situation in the development of legislative methods of analysis that existed until the early 1980s in the food sector. The principles for the establishment of Codex methods of analysis are given below; other organisations which subsequently laid down procedures for the development of methods of analysis in their particular sector followed these principles to a significant degree.

*Principles for the establishment of Codex methods of analysis*

*Purpose of Codex methods of analysis.* The methods are primarily intended as international methods for the verification of provisions in Codex standards. They should be used for reference, in calibration of methods in use or introduced for routine examination and control purposes.

*Methods of analysis*

  *(A) Definition of types of methods of analysis*

  (a) Defining methods (type I)

     Definition: a method that determines a value that can only be arrived at in terms of the method *per se* and serves by definition as the only method for establishing the accepted value of the item measure.

     Examples: Howard Mould Count, Reichert-Meissl value, loss on drying, salt in brine by density.

(b) Reference methods (type II)

Definition: a type II method is the one designated 'reference method' where type I methods do not apply. It should be selected from type III methods (as defined below). It should be recommended for use in cases of dispute and for calibration purposes.

Example: Potentiometric method for halides.

(c) Alternative approved methods (type III)

Definition: a type III method is one that meets the criteria required by the Codex Committee on Methods of Analysis and Sampling for methods that may be used for control, inspection or regulatory purposes.

Example: Volhard method or Mohr method for chlorides.

(d) Tentative method (type IV)

Definition: a type IV method is a method that has been used traditionally or else has been recently introduced but for which the criteria required for acceptance by the Codex Committee on Methods of Analysis and Sampling have not yet been determined.

Examples: chlorine by X-ray fluorescence, estimation of synthetic colours in foods.

*(B) General criteria for the selection of methods of analysis*

(a) Official methods of analysis elaborated by international organisations occupying themselves with a food or group of foods should be preferred.
(b) Preference should be given to methods of analysis the reliability of which have been established in respect of the following criteria, selected as appropriate:

- specificity
- accuracy
- precision: repeatability intra-laboratory (within laboratory), reproducibility inter-laboratory (within laboratory and between laboratories)
- limit of detection
- sensitivity
- practicability and applicability under normal laboratory conditions
- other criteria which may be selected as required

(c) The method selected should be chosen on the basis of practicability and preference should be given to methods that have applicability for routine use.

(d) All proposed methods of analysis must have direct pertinence to the Codex Standard to which they are directed.

(e) Methods of analysis that are applicable uniformly to various groups of commodities should be given preference over methods that apply only to individual commodities.

### 10.5.4 European Committee for Standardization (CEN)

In Europe the international organisation that is now developing most standardised methods of analysis in the food additive and contaminant area is the European Committee for Standardization (CEN). Although CEN methods are not prescribed by legislation, the European Commission does place considerable importance on the work that CEN carries out in the development of specific methods in the food sector. CEN has been given direct mandates by the Commission to publish particular methods, e.g. those for the detection of food irradiation. Because of this some of the methods in the food sector being developed by CEN are described below. CEN, like the other organisations described above, has adopted a set of guidelines to which its Methods Technical Committees should conform when developing a method of analysis. The guidelines are:

'Details of the interlaboratory test on the precision of the method are to be summarised in an annex to the method. It is to be stated that the values derived from the interlaboratory test may not be applicable to analyte concentration ranges and matrices other than given in the annex.

The precision clauses shall be worded as follows:

*Repeatability:* "The absolute difference between two single test results found on identical test materials by one operator using the same apparatus within the shortest feasible time interval will exceed the repeatability value $r$ in not more than 5% of cases.

The value(s) is (are): ..."

*Reproducibility:* "The absolute difference between two single test results on identical test material reported by two laboratories will exceed the reproducibility value $R$ in not more than 5% of cases.

The value(s) is (are): ..."

There shall be minimum requirements regarding the information to be given in an Informative Annex, this being:

- year of interlaboratory test and reference to the test report (if available)
- number of samples
- number of laboratories retained after eliminating outliers
- number of outliers (laboratories)
- number of accepted results
- mean value (with the respective unit)
- repeatability standard deviation ($s_r$) (with the respective unit)
- repeatability relative standard deviation ($RSD_r$) (%)
- repeatability limit ($r$)w (with the respective units)
- reproducibility relative standard deviation ($s_R$) (with the respective unit)
- reproducibility relative standard deviation ($RSD_R$) (%)

- reproducibility limit ($R$) (with the respective unit)
- sample types clearly described
- notes if further information is to be given'.

In addition, CEN publishes its methods as either finalised standards or as preliminary standards, which are required to be reviewed after two years and then either withdrawn or converted to a full standard. Thus, CEN follows the same procedure as the AOACI in this regard.

### 10.5.5 Requirements of official bodies for methods of analysis

Consideration of the above requirements means that all methods of analysis used in the food area, and hence for natural toxicants in food, must be fully validated, i.e. they have been subjected to a collaborative trial conforming to an internationally recognised protocol. It is important that this is fully recognised as it sets the quality standard for the methods of analysis aspects of quality assurance considerations. Because of this users of analytical methods must be fully appreciative of the requirements being imposed and have good reasons for not following them, e.g. the non-availability of suitably validated procedures in a particular determination.

The concept of the valid analytical method in the food sector and some of its requirements are described below.

*Accuracy.* Accuracy is defined as the closeness of the agreement between the result of a measurement and a true value of the measurand (ISO, 1993c). It may be assessed by the use of reference materials. However, in food analysis, there is a particular problem. In many instances, though not normally for food additives and contaminants, the numerical value of a characteristic (or criterion) in a standard is dependent on the procedures used to ascertain its value. This illustrates the need for the (sampling and) analysis provisions in a standard to be developed at the same time as the numerical value of the characteristics in the standard are negotiated to ensure that the characteristics are related to the methodological procedures prescribed.

*Precision.* Precision is defined as the closeness of agreement between independent test results obtained under prescribed conditions (ISO, 1992).

In a standard method the precision characteristics are obtained from a properly organised collaborative trial, i.e. a trial conforming to the requirements of an international standard (the AOAC/ISO/IUPAC harmonised protocol or the ISO 5725 standard). Because of the importance of collaborative trials, the fact that EU methods must have been subjected to a collaborative trial before acceptance and the resource that is now being devoted to the assessment of precision characteristics of analytical methods, collaborative trials are described in detail here.

### 10.5.6 Collaborative trials

As seen above, all 'official' methods of analysis are required to include precision data; such data can only be obtained through a collaborative trial and hence the stress that is given to collaboratively tested and validated methods in the food sector.

*What is a collaborative trial?* A collaborative trial is a procedure whereby the precision of a method of analysis may be assessed and quantified. The precision of a method is usually expressed in terms of repeatability and reproducibility values. Accuracy is not the objective.

*IUPAC/ISO/AOACI harmonisation protocol.* Recently there has been progress towards a universal acceptance of collaboratively tested methods and collaborative trial results and methods, no matter by whom these trials are organised. This has been aided by the publication of the IUPAC/ISO/AOACI harmonisation protocol on collaborative studies (Horwitz, 1988). This protocol was developed under the auspices of the International Union of Pure and Applied Chemists (IUPAC) aided by representatives from the major organisations interested in conducting collaborative studies. In particular, from the food sector, AOACI, the International Organisation for Standardisation (ISO), the International Dairy Federation (IDF), the Collaborative International Analytical Council for Pesticides (CIPAC), the Nordic Analytical Committee (NMKL), the Codex Committee on Methods of Analysis and Sampling and the International Office of Cocoa and Chocolate were involved.

The protocol gives a series of recommendations, the most important of which are described below:

*The components that make up a collaborative trial*
(i) *Participants*
It is of paramount importance that all the participants taking part in the trial are competent, i.e. they are fully conversant and experienced in the techniques used in the particular trial, and they can be relied upon to act responsibly in following the method/protocol. It is the precision of the method that is being assessed, not the performance of the trial participants.

The number of participants must be at least eight. However, to use only laboratories who are 'experts' in the use of the method in question but will not ultimately be involved in the routine use of the method could give an exaggerated precision performance for the method.

(ii) *Sample type*
Samples should, if possible, be normal materials containing the required levels of analyte. If this is not possible, then alternative laboratory-prepared

samples must be used. These have the obvious disadvantage of a different analyte/sample matrix from that of the normal materials. The types of samples used should cover as wide an area as possible of sample types for which the method is to be used. Ideally for collaborative trial purposes the individual sample/sample types should be identical in appearance so as to preserve sample anonymity.

## (iii) *Sample homogeneity*
The bulk sample, from which all sub-samples that form the collaborative trial samples are taken, should be homogenous and the sub-sampling procedure such that the resulting sub-samples have an equivalent composition to that of the original bulk sample. Tests should also be carried out to determine the stability of the sample over the intended time period of the trial. The precision of the method can only be as good as the homogeneity of the samples allows it to be. There must be little or no variability due to sample heterogeneity.

## (iv) *Sample plan*
For the study of method performance at least five samples, covering a range of analyte concentrations representative of the commodity, should be used. These samples should be duplicated, making a minimum of ten samples in all. The samples should be visually identical and given individual sample codes to preserve sample anonymity as far as possible.

However, in the case of blind duplicates it may be possible to link the pairs together. This possibility may be reduced by the use of *split-level samples*, where the samples differ only slightly in concentration of analyte. Any artificial attempt to draw these 'duplicate' samples closer together will in fact give decreased precision as it is the difference *between* the split-level samples that is involved in the calculation of the precision parameter and this will be a quantifiable amount.

Sometimes it is not feasible to have blind duplicates or split-level samples and laboratories are requested to analyse samples as known duplicates. This is the least favoured option.

*The method(s) to be tested.* The method(s) to be tested should have been tested for robustness (i.e. how susceptible the procedure is to small variations in method protocol/instructions) and optimised before circulation to participants. A thorough evaluation of the method at this stage can often eliminate the need for a retrial at a later stage.

*Pilot study/pre-trial.* These are invaluable exercises if resources permit. A pilot study involves at least three laboratories testing the method, checking the written version, highlighting any hidden problems that may be encountered during the study and giving an initial estimation of the precision of the method. A pre-trial can be used in place of or to supplement the pilot study. It is particularly useful where a new method or technique is to be used. Participants are sent one or two reference samples with which to familiarise themselves with the method before starting the trial proper. A successful pre-trial is usually a prerequisite to starting the trial proper and can be used to rectify any individual problems that the laboratories are having with the method.

*The trial proper.* Participants should be given clear instructions on the protocol of the trial, the time limit for return of results, the number of determinations to be carried out per sample and how to report results (to how many decimal places, as received or on a dry matter basis, corrected or uncorrected for recovery, etc.).

*Statistical analysis.* It is important to appreciate that the statistical significance of the results is wholly dependent on the quality of the data obtained from the trial. Data which contain obvious gross errors should be removed prior to statistical analysis. It is essential that participants inform the trial co-ordinator of any gross error that they know has occurred during the analysis and also if any deviation from the method as written has taken place. The statistical parameters calculated and the outlier tests performed are those used in the internationally agreed protocol for the design, conduct and interpretation of collaborative studies (Horwitz, 1988).

*Analysis of data for outliers.* More time has been devoted to the procedures to be used for the removal of outliers than is warranted. However, the procedure prescribed in the harmonised protocol is now accepted within the food sector.

*Precision parameters.* The most commonly quoted precision parameters are repeatability and reproducibility. Typical definitions of these are:

$r$      repeatability, the value below which the absolute difference between two single test results obtained under repeatability conditions (i.e. same sample, same operator, same apparatus, same laboratory and short interval of time) may be expected to lie within a specific probability (typically 95%), hence $r = 2.8 \times s_r$

$s_r$      standard deviation, calculated from results generated under repeatability conditions

$RSD_r$      relative standard deviation, calculated from results generated under repeatability conditions [$(s_r / \bar{x}) \times 100$], where $\bar{x}$ is the average of results over all laboratories and samples

$R$      reproducibility, the value below which the absolute difference between single test results obtained under reproducibility conditions (i.e. on identical material

obtained by operators in different laboratories, using the standardised test method)
may be expected to lie within a certain probability (typically 95%), $R = 2.8 \times s_R$.

$s_R$      standard deviation, calculated from results under reproducibility conditions

$RSD_R$    relative standard deviation, calculated from results generated under reproducibility conditions [$(s_R / \bar{x}) \times 100$].

### 10.5.7 Assessment of the acceptability of the precision characteristics of a method of analysis

The calculated repeatability and reproducibility values of a method can be compared with existing methods and a comparison made. If these are satisfactory then the method can used as a validated method. If there is no method with which to compare the precision parameters then theoretical repeatability and reproducibility values can be calculated from the Horwitz equation (Horwitz, 1982):

$$RSD_R = 2^{(1-0.5\log C)}$$

Values for this equation are given in Table 10.1.

**Table 10.1**

| Concentration ratio | $RSD_R$ |
|---|---|
| 1 (100%) | 2 |
| $10^{-1}$ | 2.8 |
| $10^{-2}$ (1%) | 4 |
| $10^{-3}$ | 5.6 |
| $10^{-4}$ | 8 |
| $10^{-5}$ | 11 |
| $10^{-6}$ (ppm) | 16 |
| $10^{-7}$ | 23 |
| $10^{-8}$ | 32 |
| $10^{-9}$ (ppb) | 45 |

Horwitz derived the equation after studying the results from many (~3000) collaborative trials. Although it represents the average $RSD_R$ values and is an approximation of the possible precision that can be achieved, the data points from 'acceptable' collaborative trials lie within a range plus and minus twice the values derived from the equation. This idealised smoothed curve is found to be independent of the nature of the analyte or of the analytical technique that was used to make the measurement. In general the values taken from this curve are indicative of the precision that is achievable and acceptable for an analytical method by different laboratories. Its use provides a satisfactory and simple means of assessing method precision acceptability.

*10.5.8  Summary of requirements for a collaborative trial*
For a method to be considered fully validated it must have been subjected to
a collaborative trial that conforms to the following critical characteristics:

- the minimum number of laboratories should be eight (i.e. there
  should be eight sets of valid data available for the calculation of precision characteristics);
- the minimum number of samples should be five;
- samples should not be sent to participants for analysis as known
  duplicates, except as a last resort; and
- all the original data obtained in the trial should be reproduced in the
  final report on the trial. A number of outlier identification procedures
  are given in the recommendations. Although it is desirable that they
  should be used in the statistical analysis of the trial results it is not
  essential provided the raw collaborative trial data are available, thus
  enabling other organisations to re-calculate if they so desire.

## 10.6  Recovery factors: development of an internationally agreed protocol for the use of recovery factors

*10.6.1  Introduction*
The estimation and use of recovery is an area where practice differs among
analytical chemists. The variations in practice are most obvious in the determination of analytes such as veterinary drug residues and pesticide residues
in complex matrices, such as foodstuffs. The same considerations apply in
the determination of natural toxicants. Typically, methods of analysis for the
determination of these analytes rely on transferring the analyte from the
complex matrix into a much simpler solution that is used to present the analyte for instrumental determination. However, the transfer procedure results
in loss of analyte. Quite commonly in such procedures a substantial proportion of the analyte remains in the matrix after extraction so that the transfer
is incomplete and the subsequent measurement is lower than the true concentration in the original test material. If no compensation for these losses
is made, then markedly discrepant results may be obtained by different laboratories. Even greater discrepancies arise if some laboratories compensate
for losses and others do not.

Recovery studies are clearly an essential component of the validation
and use of analytical methods. It is important that all concerned with the
production and interpretation of analytical results are aware of the problems
and the basis on which the result is being reported. At present, however,
there is no single well-defined approach to estimating, expressing and applying recovery information.

The most important inconsistency in analytical practice concerns the correction of a raw measurement, which can (in principle) eliminate the low bias due to loss of analyte. The difficulties involved in reliably estimating the correction factor deter practitioners in some sectors of analysis from applying such corrections.

In the absence of consistent strategies for the estimation and use of recovery it is difficult to make valid comparisons between results produced in different laboratories or to verify the suitability of data for the intended purpose. This lack of transparency can have important consequences in the interpretation of data. For example, in the context of enforcement analysis, the difference between applying or not applying a correction factor to ana-lytical data can mean, respectively, that a legislative limit is exceeded or that a result is in compliance with the limit. Thus, where an estimate of the *true concentration* is required, there is a compelling case for compensation for losses in the calculation of a reported analytical result.

Examples of the difference in approach towards the use of recovery fac-tors come from the US FDA, where the adjustment of data in the food sec-tor for recovery factors is not encouraged, and the UK, where for all surveillance data in the food sector it is required that laboratories adhere to the following instructions:

'*Correcting for analytical recovery*
The Steering Group has promulgated advice on correcting for analytical recovery. It con-cluded that corrected values give a more accurate reflection of the true concentration of the analyte and facilitate interpretation of data and made the following recommendations:

1. Unless there are overriding reasons for not doing so, results should be corrected for recovery.
2. Recovery values should always be reported, whether or not results are corrected, so that measured values can be converted to corrected values and vice versa.
3. Where there is a wide variation around the mean recovery value, correcting for recovery can give misleading results and therefore the standard deviation should also be reported.
4. Each Working Party should establish upper and lower limits for acceptable recov-ery and for variability of recovery. Samples giving recovery values outside the range should be re-analysed or results reported as semi-quantitative.
5. It is important to report analytical data in a way that ensures that their significance is fully understood. It is particularly important, especially where results are close to legal or advisory limits, to explain those factors, such as sampling and analyti-cal errors and corrections for recovery, which are sources of uncertainties. Both enforcement authorities and working parties need to consider the most appropri-ate way to present results.'

As a result of such discrepancies in approach, guidelines are being pre-pared that will provide a conceptual framework for consistent decisions on the estimation and use of recovery information in various sectors of analyt-ical science.

*10.6.2  Sources of error in analytical chemistry*
The guidelines are being developed in the light of the sources of error that may occur in an analytical process, as given in Table 10.2, and the sources of uncertainty in recovery estimation, which are given in Table 10.3.

**Table 10.2**  Sources of error that may occur in an analytical process

1.  Incomplete definition of the measurand (for example, failing to specify the exact form of the analyte being determined)
2.  Sampling: the sample measured may not represent the defined measurand
3.  Incomplete extraction and/or pre-concentration of the measurand, contamination of the measurement sample, interferences and matrix effects
4.  Inadequate knowledge of the effects of environmental conditions on the measurement procedure or imperfect measurement of environmental conditions
5.  Cross-contamination or contamination of reagents or blanks
6.  Personal bias in reading analogue instruments
7.  Uncertainty of weights and volumetric equipment
8.  Instrument resolution or discrimination threshold
9.  Values assigned to measurement standards and reference materials
10. Values of constants and other parameters obtained from external sources and used in the data reduction algorithm
11. Approximations and assumptions incorporated in the measurement method and procedure
12. Variations in repeated observations of the measurand under apparently identical conditions

**Table 10.3**  Sources of uncertainty in recovery estimation

1.  Repeatability of the recovery experiment
2.  Uncertainties in reference material values
3.  Uncertainties in added spike quantity
4.  Poor representation of native analyte by the added spike
5.  Poor or restricted match between experimental matrix and the full range of sample matrices encountered
6.  Effect of analyte/spike level on recovery and imperfect match of spike or reference material analyte level and analyte level in samples

*10.6.3  International guidelines*
ISO, IUPAC and AOACI have co-operated to produce agreed protocols or guidelines on the design, conduct and interpretation of collaborative studies, on the proficiency testing of (chemical) analytical laboratories and on internal quality control for analytical laboratories. These organisations are preparing guidelines on the use of recovery information in analytical measurement.

### 10.6.4 Recommendations

The following recommendations are made regarding the use of recovery information in the latest draft of the guidelines.

1. Results should be corrected for recovery, unless there are overriding reasons for not doing so. Such reasons would include the situation where a limit (statutory or contractual) has been established using uncorrected data or where recoveries are close to unity.

2. Recovery values should always be established as part of method validation, whether or not recoveries are reported or results are corrected, so that measured values can be converted to corrected values and vice versa.

3. IQC control charts for recovery should be established during method validation and used in all routine analysis. Runs giving recovery values outside the control range should be considered for re-analysis in the context of acceptable variation or the results reported as semi-quantitative.

It is important for the determination of natural toxicants that due consideration is given to these guidelines as they provide information and justification for selecting the approach to be taken towards the use of recovery factors, an important aspect of the quality assurance of the laboratory.

## 10.7  Conclusions

The need for a laboratory to demonstrate that it is producing reliable and acceptable results has become of major importance. The quality assurance measures adopted by the laboratory must be such that this is achieved. This demonstration is aided by the introduction of the following:

1. The achievement of formal laboratory accreditation by the laboratory. However, even if this is not deemed to be necessary in the light of the individual circumstance of the laboratory, it is important that the requirements of accreditation are recognised and followed by the laboratory in its internal procedures.

2. Participation in proficiency testing schemes.

3. Use of validated methods.

4. Introduction of appropriate IQC procedures.

All the above are essential aspects of ensuring that data released from a laboratory are fit for purpose. The last three aspects have now been described in appropriate international protocols and Guidelines, and due note should be taken of these if appropriate quality assurance measures are to be followed.

# References

EEC (1985) Council Directive 85/591/EEC concerning the introduction of community methods of sampling and analysis for the monitoring of foodstuffs intended for human consumption, O.J. L372 of 31.12.1985.

EEC (1989) Council Directive 89/397/EEC on the official control of foodstuffs, O.J. L186 of 30.6.1989.

EEC (1993) Council Directive 93/99/EEC on the subject of additional measures concerning the official control of foodstuffs, O.J. L290 of 24.11.1993.

FAO (1997) *Report of the Twenty-First Session of the Codex Committee on Methods of Analysis and Sampling*, ALINORM 97/23A, FAO, Rome.

Horwitz, W. (1982) Evaluation of analytical methods for regulation of foods and drugs. *Analytical Chemistry*, **54** 67A-76A

Horwitz, W. (1988) Protocol for the design, conduct and interpretation of method performance studies. *Pure and Applied Chemistry*, **60** 855-64 (now revised).

ISO (1981) *Precision of Test Methods*, ISO, Geneva (revised 1986 with further revision in preparation).

ISO (1992) *Terms and Definitions used in Connection with Reference Materials*, ISO Guide 30, ISO, Geneva.

ISO (1993a) *General Requirements for the Competence of Calibration and Testing Laboratories*, ISO Guide 25, 2nd edn, ISO, Geneva.

ISO (1993b) *Calibration and Testing Laboratory Accreditation Systems—General Requirements for Operation and Recognition*, ISO/IEC Guide 58, ISO, Geneva.

ISO (1993c) *International Vocabulary for Basic and General Terms in Metrology*, 2nd edn, ISO, Geneva.

Thompson, M. and Wood, R. (1993) The international harmonised protocol for the proficiency testing of (chemical) analytical laboratories. *Pure and Applied Chemistry*, **65**, 2123-44 (also published in *JAOAC International*, 1993, **76** 926).

Thompson, M. and Wood, R. (1995) Harmonized guidelines for internal quality control in analytical chemistry laboratories. *Pure and Applied Chemistry*, **67**, 649-66.

# 11 Quantifying exposure to natural toxicants in food

David Tennant

## 11.1 Introduction

Other chapters in this book have shown that many foods can contain natural chemicals that could present a toxic hazard to consumers. Whether natural toxicants actually cause any harm depends on two factors: the potency and the dose. The potency of any toxic substance is the amount that is required to cause a given toxicological response. This can be measured by either the severity of effect or the proportion of the exposed population who are affected. This chapter is about methods that can be used to estimate the dose or exposure to natural toxicants via food.

There are two main situations where it is necessary to estimate exposures to natural toxicants: when carrying out a risk assessment and in epidemiological studies. The approaches taken to estimate exposure differ according to the situation.

## 11.2 Risk assessment

Risk assessment is the process of estimating the likelihood that a particular adverse effect will occur in a population following exposure to a hazard. In this case the hazards are natural toxicants and the potential adverse effects range from the relatively trivial, such as nausea or skin rashes, to the very severe, such as death from liver disease or cancer. Risk assessment can be carried out prospectively or retrospectively. Prospective risk assessment is used when it is necessary to predict the consequences of a change to the food supply, such as the introduction of a novel food. Retrospective risk assessment is used when it is necessary to discover whether a substance already in the food supply is likely to be having any effect on health, for example to investigate whether aflatoxins are likely to contribute significantly to the incidence of liver cancer in a given population. The process of risk assessment can be conveniently described by the flow-chart in Figure 11.1 (based on Tennant, 1997), which identifies the main steps involved.

*Hazard identification* is the first step of the risk assessment process. Hazards may sometimes be identified as a result of the chemical analysis of foodstuffs. In other cases, poisoning of either people or animals may alert toxicologists to a potential hazard. The introduction of a novel or genetically modified food may also present the possibility of altering exposure to natural toxicant hazards. When a potential hazard has been identified the risk assessment process divides into two paths: exposure analysis and hazard characterisation.

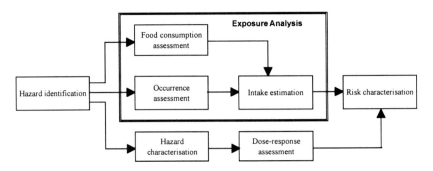

**Figure 11.1**   Flow chart for chemical risk assessment

*Exposure analysis* combines data on the levels and incidences of substances found in food with information about people's food consumption habits, to generate an estimate of intake.

*Food consumption assessments* are usually based on the results of dietary surveys. Such surveys may be carried out for a variety of reasons, such as nutritional analysis or economic studies. This means that they are seldom tailored to the particular data requirements of chemical risk assessment. Therefore ingenuity is often required in adapting dietary survey data for chemical intake estimations (Douglass and Tennant, 1997). One particular problem is that many surveys are conducted at the household level. A consequence of this is that it is difficult to estimate the range of individual exposure to a substance found in food. It is sometimes only possible to estimate the average intake of a population and this figure is not necessarily relevant to risk assessment. A more detailed discussion of dietary survey data is provided later in this chapter.

*Occurrence assessment* provides information about the levels and incidences of a substance in foods. The concentration of a particular substance may vary according to plant variety or degree of ripeness and may be affected by storage or spoilage. Not all varieties of a particular food may contain a particular substance and the incidence may also be related to the country of origin and be affected by the storage conditions. For example, aflatoxins tend to be present only in certain food products that have been grown or stored in the warm, humid conditions found near the tropics. It is also vital to understand the statistical distribution of concentrations if relevant estimates of intake are to be created. If a potential toxicant is a normal physiological constituent of a plant then its levels may be biologically regulated so that concentrations fall into a very narrow range. If this is the case then it is usually only necessary to use the mean to represent the concentration. However, it is often the case that natural toxicants arise as fungal contaminants or as a consequence of unusual circumstances, such as plant disease or other stresses. In these cases concentrations are unlikely to be normally distributed about the mean. Log-normal and bimodal distributions can frequently be expected. The arithmetic mean may still be a suitable measure of the concentration to which a population is exposed in this situation. However, this will depend on the toxicological characteristics of the substance, the distribution of the food supply and patterns of eating habits. It should never be assumed that the arithmetic mean is always relevant. At least the minimum and maximum levels should always be quoted along with the mean. Ideally the whole distribution should be described.

*Intake estimation* combines data about the levels and occurrence of a substance in particular foods with information about the amounts of those foods consumed. Thus:

$$\text{intake (mg/day)} = \text{occurrence (mg/kg)} \times \text{consumption (kg/day)}$$

Intakes are frequently expressed per unit bodyweight of a consumer (mg/kg bw/day). This is to allow comparison with the toxicologically determined acceptable daily intake (ADI) or tolerable daily intake (TDI), which are expressed in these units.

While data on average intakes by populations are useful and sometimes relevant to risk assessment, it is often necessary to consider intakes of people who are relatively high level consumers of foods in which a natural toxicant occurs. If detailed data on individual intakes are available it is sometimes possible to estimate intakes at the 90th, 95th or even 97.5th percentile. If intake data are log-normally distributed it is not unusual to find that high-level intakes are more than three times those at the arithmetic mean. It is also necessary to consider the time period over which intake estimates are averaged. The relevant time period will be determined by the toxicological characteristics of the particular substance. In the extreme case, for something that is acutely toxic such as botulinum toxin, it is the amount eaten on one occasion which is important. At the other extreme, such as for genotoxic carcinogens, it is the total intake averaged over the entire lifetime which is relevant. For most substances the relevant period will fall somewhere between these acute and chronic extremes. However, this is vital information for intake estimation. In situations where the substance of concern is present in foods at a constant level and those foods are eaten in steady amounts throughout life, the difference between acute and chronic intakes will be minimal. However, if the substance has very variable concentrations or is present in foods that are infrequently consumed, then the difference between chronic and acute intakes can be considerable.

*Hazard characterisation* aims to identify the toxicological characteristics associated with a particular substance. All relevant human, animal and *in vitro* data are assessed in order to identify the toxicologically relevant end-point likely to be associated with potential exposure. Sometimes the end-point is specific, such as carcinoma of a particular organ or tissue. In other cases the end-point is vague and related to non-specific effects like weight loss or failure to thrive. In all cases it is necessary to consider whether the end-point is an immediate (acute) or long-term (chronic) effect and to identify the time period over which intakes should be estimated. Hazard characterisation must also consider whether any particularly vulnerable groups should be the focus of the risk assessment. Such groups could include infants and children, pregnant women (to protect the foetus) or people suffering from chronic illnesses such as diabetes.

*Dose–response assessment* determines the relationship between the amount of a substance ingested and the expression of adverse effects. In some cases the expression of effect can relate to the severity of illness and in other cases to the proportion of the population affected. There are two principal types of dose–response relationship: those with thresholds (thresholded effects) and those without (non-thresholded effects).

For thresholded effects there comes a point where, as the dose increases, the body's protective mechanisms are overcome. Up to this point—the 'no observable adverse effect level' (NOAEL)—no harmful effects are seen. Above the NOAEL increasing severity of adverse effects is observed as the dose increases. Because of variability in individuals' no-effect levels, the incidence of harmful effects will also increase around the NOAEL. For human risk assessments the NOAEL is usually based on animal studies. Safety factors to allow for inter-species extrapolation and inter-individual variation are applied to determine the ADI for an additive or TDI for contaminants (Rubery *et al.*, 1990). The ADI or TDI is the amount of a substance that can be ingested daily over an entire lifetime without harmful effect. Sometimes a provisional tolerable weekly intake (PTWI) has been used instead of a TDI for contaminants. Non-thresholded toxicants do not have a NOAEL. Even the smallest dose can have a correspondingly small effect. The effect of increasing the dose is not usually an increase in severity of the effect but an increase in the incidence of that effect in a population. For example, increasing the levels of a genotoxic carcinogen in the food supply would result in greater numbers of deaths from certain types of cancer. It would not affect the severity of the cancer in any particular individual. Mathematical models have been developed that are aimed at indicating the level of risk associated with a given exposure to a genotoxic carcinogen. There is considerable debate about the reliability of these methods.

*Risk characterisation* compares the intake estimate with the result of the dose–response assessment. For thresholded toxicants it is necessary to compare the ADI or TDI with the estimate of intake. If intakes appear to exceed the ADI or TDI then some kind of risk management activity is required. For non-thresholded toxicants the intake estimate is compared with the dose–response curve. The threshold of concern is usually some risk level that is considered to be so low as to be insignificant—the acceptable risk level. What is an acceptable risk is a political rather than a scientific question. However, in many situations an arbitrary 'one death per one million lifetimes' is used. Risk characterisation should not be seen as a simple arithmetic operation. Care must be taken to ensure that when chronic or acute hazards have been identified then appropriate intake estimates are used. It is also necessary to consider how risks vary between different population groups, particularly those identified as being especially vulnerable in the hazard characterisation. The accuracy of any estimate of intake and its relevance to the toxicological characteristics of the substance should always be considered and made explicit to others who may interpret the results.

## 11.3  Epidemiological studies

Diet has long been implicated as a potential source of human cancers and epidemiological assessments have been used to investigate the evidence (Armstrong and Doll, 1975). Like risk assessment, epidemiological studies can be retrospective or prospective. In both cases, studies rely on comparing data on the incidences of particular diseases in specified populations with environmental, dietary or other factors. In retrospective epidemiological dietary studies, records of morbidity and mortality are examined and compared with evidence of dietary patterns. Prospective studies can be more specifically related to individuals. For example, the dietary habits of the study population can be compared with records of their subsequent ill-health or cause of death.

Both retrospective and prospective epidemiological studies require information about the food consumed by the study population. Retrospective studies can sometimes be an insensitive tool because it is not possible to determine the specific dietary patterns of those individuals who succumbed to the disease of concern. In general only the average consumption of certain foods can be compared between populations living in different locations or differing in some other unique way. While the average consumption might be the relevant parameter, there may be cases where it is not. In some circumstances it may be the proportion of the population that consumes above a given threshold level that is paramount. In other cases it may be exposure during a particular phase of life that is important.

Prospective studies can be planned to gather data that may be more relevant to the particular toxicological characteristics of the substance being studied or the disease end-point of concern. For example, it may be sufficient to obtain qualitative information only, such as 'does the individual's diet contain a particular food like cassava?' In other cases food frequency questionnaire data may be adequate, such as 'how often do you eat brassicas?' Generally speaking portion sizes of vegetables are relatively constant compared to the variability in the frequency of consumption. Alternatively fully quantitative data may be required, such as 'how much wine do you consume?' Most people drink wine from time to time but the amount consumed can vary considerably from individual to individual.

## 11.4   Novel foods and novel food ingredients

Regulation (EC) No. 258/97 concerning novel foods and novel food products provides an example of where intakes of natural toxicants may need to be considered. The role of some natural toxicants in plants is believed to be as 'natural pesticides'. Their toxicity to insect pests protects plants from attack, but some observers believe that these natural compounds could be at least as harmful as synthetic plant protection products (Gold *et al.*, 1997). If a plant has been modified so that it is more resistant to attack by pests this may be as a result of increased levels of these natural toxicants. It may therefore be necessary to carry out a risk assessment of the substance to confirm that public health is not at risk.

Draft European Union (EU) Guidelines, which are intended to accompany the above Regulation, are based on establishing the principal of 'substantial equivalence'. The Guidelines state that 'If a new food or new food component is found to be substantially equivalent to an existing food or food component then it can be treated in the same manner with regard to safety.' If substantial equivalence cannot be demonstrated then it becomes necessary to take account of the chemical composition of the new food and to estimate potential intakes. The greater the predicted intake, the greater the need for toxicological testing. Intake estimates must take account of not just normal levels but also maximum levels of consumption. The Regulations may therefore require reliable estimates of intakes of natural toxicants or other chemicals associated with food.

## 11.5   Using food consumption data to estimate intakes

Food consumption data are collected for a variety of purposes. The aims of the study normally determine the form of the survey required. Food consumption surveys vary considerably in levels of detail. This means that estimates of food consumption and natural toxicant intake can range from the very crude to the highly sophisticated.

It is not always necessary to use highly sophisticated methods to get a useful answer, however. Crude methods, provided that they are conservative (i.e. they do not significantly underestimate the true situation), can often provide useful screening tools. If intakes appear to be well below the TDI using a conservative screen then there may be no need to do any further analyses. Care must be taken in using such screens to ensure that they really are conservative for all population groups in all circumstances. For example, there is no justification for using population per capita intakes as a screening tool if the population of concern is children with a high consumption of certain foods, such as soya milk.

### 11.5.1 Disappearance data

Very often it is possible to calculate the amount of a food produced and, together with import and export figures, estimate the amount that 'disappears':

disappearance = total production + imports − exports.

If the average concentration of a natural toxicant in particular foods is known and the disappearance rate is available, then the amount of that natural toxicant entering the food chain can be calculated:

$$\text{natural toxicant in food chain (mg)} = \text{disappearance of foods (kg)} \times \text{concentration (mg/kg)}$$

It is then a small step to divide the amount in the food chain by the population to obtain an estimate of intake:

$$\text{per capita intake (mg/person)} = \frac{\text{natural toxicant in food chain (mg)}}{\text{population}}$$

Per capita intakes should not be discounted just because they are simple. They may be of relevance in some circumstances such as when a population is exposed to a genotoxic carcinogen and the risk to the *population*, rather than to the *individual*, is required. Such estimates are therefore sometimes useful in epidemiological studies where different populations in different locations are being compared. However, if risks to individuals with high level intakes within a population are required, then per capita intakes are of very limited value.

### 11.5.2 Market basket studies

Data are sometimes available on the amounts of foods purchased by a sample population. For example, in household budget surveys householders may be asked to keep a record of all their purchases for a week. The amount spent on each food is then converted back to the amount of food by using the price of each item purchased. This kind of survey is often used for economic or nutritional analyses.

Household budget surveys provide more reliable data than per capita estimates, but their value is still limited. While food consumption can be related to separate households it is still very difficult to use these kinds of data to estimate individual food consumption or natural toxicant intake.

Because household budget surveys are routinely conducted in many countries (Table 11.1), they can serve a useful purpose in risk assessment. They are frequently employed in total diet studies. Data from the household budget survey are used to purchase representative samples of foods from retail outlets. Samples are combined in the proportions found in the household budget survey to create composite samples representing several food groups. The composite samples may then be analysed for contaminants, natural toxicants or any other chemical. This is the total diet study approach. It is, however, of limited value for risk assessment. It has proved to be of great value in monitoring annual trends or when making international comparisons.

**Table 11.1**   Household level surveys completed in European countries[a]

| Country | Date | Type of survey | Methodology |
|---------|------|----------------|-------------|
| Belgium | 1987–88 | Household budgets | Purchase records |
|  | 1972–91 | Purchase records | Diary |
| Denmark | 1981 | Food purchases | Purchase records |
|  | 1987 | Food consumption | Purchase records |
| France | 1963–91 | Purchases + gifts | 7-day purchase records |
|  | Continuous | Purchases + gifts | 52, 7-day purchase records. (single households interviewed only) |
| Greece | 1981/82 | Purchases | 7-day purchase records |
|  | 1987/88 | Purchases | 7-day purchase records |
|  | 1994 | Purchases | 7-day purchase records |
| Italy | 1980 | Food consumption | Inventory |
| Spain | 1989–93 | Foods consumed | Purchase records |
|  | 1991 | Foods consumed | Inventory weighing |
| UK | 1981/82 | Foods purchased | 7-day diary |
| Europe-wide | Continuous | Household budgets | Purchase records (EUROSTAT survey) |

[a] Based on personal communication from A. Møller, quoted in Douglass and Tennant (1997).

### 11.5.3   Food consumption surveys of individuals
Several countries gather data on the food consumption of individuals (Table 11.2). In such surveys individuals are asked to record the quantities of every food or drink item that they consume for periods ranging from two to seven days. Subjects are normally provided with scales so that they can weigh the food and any wastage or left-overs. In theory, weighed diary methods should provide very accurate data but unfortunately the task of recording everything eaten or drunk during the survey can prove onerous. People may sometimes either fail to record properly or alter their diet to make the survey easier. Some individuals may also wish to conceal how much they eat

(too much or too little) out of feelings of guilt. Weighed diaries are notoriously poor measures of alcohol consumption and weak at indicating calorie intakes. Nevertheless, even with their shortcomings individual survey databases are valuable tools for risk assessment and currently are the best generally available method for generating reliable estimates of dietary intake. Data are usually assembled in such a way that each individual has a record of the quantity of each food eaten on every eating occasion, on every day of the survey. Data on age, sex, bodyweight and other social and biological factors are often included. This means that statistical distributions of food consumption patterns can be investigated so that high end consumers of particular foods are identified and their consumption quantified. Intakes can be corrected for bodyweight on an individual basis. Age, sex and other characteristics of high- or low-level consumers can sometimes be defined.

**Table 11.2**    Some examples of surveys of food consumption of individuals

---

*UK*

Survey data are published by the Ministry of Agriculture, Fisheries and Food.

1.  *Food and Nutritional Survey of British Adults*: October 1986 to August 1987; 2197 adults aged 16 to 64; based on 7-day weighed food consumption records (Gregory *et al.*, 1990)
2.  *Food and Nutrient Intakes of British Infants Aged 6 to 12 Months*: 1986; 488 infants; based on 7-day weighed food consumption records
3.  *National Diet and Nutrition Survey: Children Aged 1¹/₂ to 4¹/₂ Years*: July 1992 and June 1993; 1675 children; based on 4-day food consumption records (Gregory *et al.*, 1995)
4.  *The Diets of British Schoolchildren*: 1983; 3581 children ages 10 to 11 and 14 to 15; based on 7-day food consumption records (Department of Health, 1989)

*Germany*

*National Consumption Study* (*NVS*): former West Germany only; October 1985 to January 1989; over 25 000 individuals aged over 4 years; 6000 food codes; 7-day weighed food consumption records (unpublished)

*USA*

*Continuing Surveys of Food Consumption by Individuals* (*CSFII*): 1989–90, 1990–91 and 1991–92; over 11 000 individuals; 3-day food consumption record (USDA, 1991, 1992, 1993)

---

It is also possible to use food consumption databases to estimate chemical intakes for individuals. For example, if the concentrations of a given natural toxicant are known in a number of foods then the data on levels found could be combined with food consumption values for every individual in the survey to calculate the intake of the toxicant at each eating occasion. These intake estimates can then be summed for each individual to provide an estimate of intake of that contaminant for any time period, from one eating occasion to the duration of the survey. The statistical distribution of intake values would also be available so high end intakes at the 95th or 97.5th percentile could be calculated.

### 11.5.4  Monte Carlo analysis

The estimates based on individual food consumption described above suffer from one principal drawback: it is only possible to consider one level of natural toxicant in each food at a time. This means that a single value must be selected to represent the entire statistical distribution. If the mean or median is chosen, this might provide a reasonable estimate over the long term, if the physical distribution of foods is such that all individuals face the same probability of consuming a given concentration of the toxicant.

For short-term intakes the problem is more difficult. Concentration levels at the maximum could be used but this becomes unrealistic if the natural toxicant is present in several different foods. This is especially pronounced if the statistical distribution of natural toxicant levels is highly skewed. It is very unlikely that an individual would consume the maximum concentration from all foods at any given time. Nevertheless, it is not impossible. Monte Carlo and other distributional analysis techniques allow the exposure expert to determine the probability that intakes will occur at a given level.

Monte Carlo techniques allow two or more statistical distributions to be combined to create a new distribution (Figure 11.2). For natural toxicants the frequency distribution of food consumption for each food can be combined (by multiplication) with the distribution of concentrations of the natural toxicant in the foods to generate an intake frequency distribution. This can be done for each food source and the resulting distributions combined (by addition) to produce a total intake distribution.

There are two main approaches in use for combining distributions. Put simply, one way combines the actual food consumption and concentration data by selecting values at random from each distribution to gradually build up the new distribution. The quality of the final distribution will depend on the number of sampling rounds. An alternative approach is to estimate the parameters (e.g. mean, median, maximum, minimum and skew) of each distribution to create hypothetical distributions that represent the original data. The two distributions can then be combined mathematically.

It is usually better to use real data rather than a hypothetical model. This is particularly true in cases where bimodal or other non-parametric distributions can be expected. A good example of this is mycotoxins, for which distributions in food are rarely normal.

If enough sampling cycles are included then the output distribution will include the worst possible case, where the highest value has been selected from all of the contributing distributions. A probability value will also be produced, which will indicate how frequently this worst-case scenario is likely to arise. At this point a decision must be made as to the acceptability of that probability and of all other points on the distribution. However, this is a risk management decision that needs input on social and economic factors beyond the bounds of science.

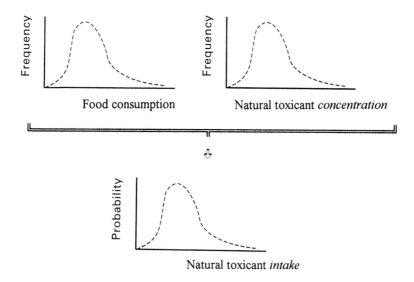

**Figure 11.2**   Probabilistic approaches to natural toxicant intake estimation

### 11.5.5   Food frequency questionnaires

Food frequency questionnaires provide a relatively simple and sometimes effective method for gathering data on food consumption. Respondents are interviewed about their food consumption habits in terms of 'how often do you eat a certain food?' They may also be invited to suggest a typical portion size for when they eat that food.

Responses are usually quantitative so that respondents may be asked to tick one box from several, for example:

| | | | |
|---|---|---|---|
| Every mealtime | | Every other week | |
| More than once a day | | Monthly | |
| Every day | | More than once a year | |
| Every other day | | Less than once a year | |
| Every week | | Never | |

The specific frequencies can be tailored to the needs of the survey.

The amount of a respondent's time is less than required by other surveys and this allows more respondents to be accommodated within a given budget. This means that while the quality of information obtained from each respondent may sometimes be poorer, by including more respondents the overall accuracy and precision can be increased.

The main advantage of food frequency questionnaires is that they are capable of capturing data that go beyond the time limits of conventional dietary surveys. These can be combined with distributional data on portion sizes by using Monte Carlo techniques to generate food consumption distributions. This means that it is possible to estimate food consumption or natural toxicant intakes over time intervals ranging from one meal to a year, or possibly even longer.

### 11.5.6  Duplicate diet studies

Long regarded as the best method for obtaining data about chemical intakes, duplicate diet studies are also the least frequently employed because of the expense. Subjects are invited to purchase and prepare double the normal amounts of food they would need for themselves. A separate portion of the meal is then saved and taken for analysis. Duplicate diet studies provide excellent information about individuals' intakes (provided that these individuals are honest about their normal diet), but because meals tend to be composited before analysis, they give less information about the food sources of a particular chemical.

## 11.6   Some case studies

### 11.6.1  Aflatoxin and patulin intakes in Australia

The Australia/New Zealand Food Authority (ANZFA) has carried out studies to estimate intakes of aflatoxins and patulin in the Australian population (ANZFA, 1996). Aflatoxins are considered to be potential human carcinogens and no ADI has been established because this is a non-thresholded effect. In contrast, patulin is believed to be associated with short-term gastro-intestinal effects and the Joint FAO/WHO Expert Committee on Food Additives has set a PTWI of 7 µg/kg bw (WHO, 1990).

In the ANZFA work, aflatoxins were found only in peanut butter and patulin found only in apple juice (Table 11.3). Estimates of consumption of peanut butter and apple juice were based on Australian National Dietary Surveys conducted between 1983 and 1985 (Table 11.4). Consumption at the 95th percentile level was estimated using the ratio between energy intake at the mean and 95th percentile levels. This ratio was applied to mean food consumption levels to estimate consumption at the 95th percentile level. Using this method, means and 95th consumption figures will relate to the entire population over the long term rather than to consumers only or actual daily consumption.

Table 11.3    Occurrence of aflatoxins and patulin in Australia

| Mycotoxin | Food | Mycotoxin levels found (mg/kg) | | |
| | | Minimum | Average | Maximum |
| --- | --- | --- | --- | --- |
| Aflatoxins | Almonds | n.d. | n.d. | n.d. |
| | Milk, whole | n.d. | n.d. | n.d. |
| | Peanut butter | n.d. | 0.002 | n.d. |
| | Sunflower seeds | n.d. | n.d. | n.d. |
| Patulin | Apple juice | n.d. | 0.0117 | 0.05 |
| | Fruit sticks | n.d. | n.d. | n.d. |

n.d. = not detected.

Mean and 95th percentile intakes of aflatoxins calculated by ANZFA fell into the range 0.0001 to 0.0005 µg/kg bw/day (Table 11.5). Since these are per capita long-term consumption figures, this intake range probably represents a reasonable representation of lifetime intakes of aflatoxins by the Australian population.

Since patulin is associated with an acute end-point, high-level intakes by individuals over the short term are critical. The highest intake reported in the ANZFA study is 0.137 µg/kg bw/day by toddlers aged two (Table 11.5). This reflects a 95th percentile apple juice consumption of 144.7 g/day, which is approximately the volume of a small cup. With a PTWI of 7 µg/kg bw (equivalent to 1 µg/kg bw/day), this estimate of intake appears to provide a large margin of safety. However, if a 13 kg two-year-old consumed two cups of apple juice (total 289.4 g of apple juice) every day for one week and the concentration was at the maximum found in the survey (0.05 mg/kg), then the child would have an average intake of 1.1 µg/kg bw/day for that week. This is not a realistic scenario, and exceeding the PTWI by such a small margin as 0.7 µg/kg bw is unlikely to be significant. Nevertheless this example shows how varying the underlying assumptions used in intake estimation significantly effects the outcome of the risk assessment.

### 11.6.2    Agaratine intakes from mushrooms
Agaratine is a hydrazine derivative found in mushrooms. Agaratine is believed to be a potential carcinogen but this is unconfirmed (Ministry of Agriculture, Fisheries and Food, 1996). Levels in mushrooms vary, for example decreasing with age. Storage and processing may also affect agaratine concentrations. Levels in fresh raw mushrooms have been found to be between 80 and 250 mg/kg. Processed mushroom products usually contain from less than 5 mg/kg to 33 mg/kg, while dried mushrooms contain over 7000 mg/kg (Ministry of Agriculture, Fisheries and Food, 1996).

**Table 11.4** Consumption of peanut butter and apple juice in Australia (g/day)

| Food | Men Mean | Men 95th percentile | Women Mean | Women 95th percentile | Boys Mean | Boys 95th percentile | Girls Mean | Girls 95th percentile | Toddlers Mean | Toddlers 95th percentile | Infants Mean | Infants 95th percentile |
|---|---|---|---|---|---|---|---|---|---|---|---|---|
| Peanut butter | 5.3 | 8.6 | 4.2 | 7 | 5.9 | 9.3 | 2.6 | 3.7 | 1.3 | 1.5 | 0[a] | 0[a] |
| Apple juice | 59.4 | 96.1 | 47.7 | 79.2 | 71.9 | 113.4 | 76.9 | 111.5 | 123.9 | 144.7 | 32 | 37.9 |

[a] No consumers.

**Table 11.5:** Estimated intakes of aflatoxins and patulin in Australia ($\upsilon$g/kg bw/day).

| Mycotoxin | Men Mean | Men 95th percentile | Women Mean | Women 95th percentile | Boys Mean | Boys 95th percentile | Girls Mean | Girls 95th percentile | Toddlers Mean | Toddlers 95th percentile | Infants Mean | Infants 95th percentile |
|---|---|---|---|---|---|---|---|---|---|---|---|---|
| Aflatoxins | 0.0002 | 0.0002 | 2E-04 | 0.0003 | 0.0003 | 0.0005 | 0.0001 | 0.0002 | 0.0002 | 0.0003 | 0[a] | 0[a] |
| Patulin | 0.009 | 0.015 | 0.009 | 0.016 | 0.021 | 0.033 | 0.022 | 0.031 | 0.117 | 0.137 | 0.041 | 0.048 |

[a] No consumers.

The Ministry of Agriculture, Fisheries and Food used consumption of mushrooms by pre-school children, schoolchildren and adults, averaged over one week, to calculate intakes of agaratine. Their calculations were based on data only from those individuals who reported consuming mushrooms during the one-week survey (Table 11.6). However, even if reported consumption of mushrooms by adults from all sources is considered, only 6% reported consumption. This is unlikely to be a true representation of long-term mushroom consumption since most people consume mushrooms from time to time if not every week. If the reported consumption could be taken to be typical of consumption by all individuals in these age groups over an extended period of time, then population average (per capita) consumption might provide a better representation of real consumption patterns (Table 11.7). This produces much lower estimates of mushroom consumption, which are probably more relevant for carcinogenic risk assessment; for populations if not individuals. In reality, consumption by individuals in these age groups is probably somewhere between these extremes. Unfortunately data do not exist to provide more accurate estimates of consumption.

In order to be compatible with the potential carcinogenic effect of agaratine, intake estimates should ideally be based on lifetime exposure. Crude estimates of lifetime mushroom consumption can be generated by integrating intake for those age groups where we have data and extrapolating to estimate the others. Before this can be done it is necessary to correct for bodyweights (Table 11.8). For such calculations bodyweights were assumed to be 60 kg, 15 kg and 7.5 kg for adults, schoolchildren and pre-schoolchildren, respectively (Rees and Harris, 1995). Lifetime per capita consumption of mushrooms is probably the most relevant parameter on which to base calculations of intake for dietary risk assessment of agaratine:

Per capita 'lifetime' consumption* = 0.021 mg/kg bw/day = 0.995 mg/person*/day

(*average lifetime bodyweight estimated to be 47.4 kg)

This works out to be very close to 1 g of mushrooms per person per day, which is close to adults' mean consumption. Relatively high consumption of mushrooms during childhood (on a bodyweight basis) is therefore probably of limited relevance to lifetime risk. Providing estimates of intakes for consumers only, over one week (Table 11.6), could in this example lead to overestimates of the true level of risk.

**Table 11.6** Consumption of mushrooms: consumers only (g/person/day)

| Type of mushroom | Adults | | Schoolchildren | | Pre-school children | |
|---|---|---|---|---|---|---|
| | % consumers | Mean consumption | % consumers | Mean consumption | % consumers | Mean consumption |
| Canned | 0.8 | 10 | 0.0 | 0 | 0.1 | 8 |
| Dried | 0.0 | 0 | 0.0 | 0 | 0.0 | 0 |
| Raw | 3.3 | 6 | 0.7 | 4 | 1.2 | 4 |
| Canned soup | 2.0 | 39 | 1.4 | 32 | 0.7 | 39 |
| All sources | 6.0 | 18 | 2.1 | 23 | 2.1 | 16 |

**Table 11.7** Mean consumption of mushrooms: population average (g/person/day)

| Type of mushroom | Adults | Schoolchildren | Pre-school children |
|---|---|---|---|
| Canned | 0.1 | 0.0 | 0.0 |
| Dried | 0.0 | 0.0 | 0.0 |
| Raw | 0.2 | 0.0 | 0.0 |
| Canned soup | 0.8 | 0.4 | 0.3 |
| All sources | 1.1 | 0.5 | 0.3 |

**Table 11.8** Consumption of mushrooms: bodyweight corrected (g/kg bw/day)

| Type of mushroom | Adults | | Schoolchildren | | Pre-school children | |
|---|---|---|---|---|---|---|
| | Per capita | Consumers | Per capita | Consumers | Per capita | Consumers |
| Canned | 0.001 | 0.167 | 0.000 | 0.000 | 0.001 | 1.067 |
| Dried | 0.000 | 0.000 | 0.000 | 0.000 | 0.000 | 0.000 |
| Raw | 0.003 | 0.100 | 0.002 | 0.267 | 0.006 | 0.533 |
| Canned soup | 0.013 | 0.650 | 0.030 | 2.133 | 0.036 | 5.200 |
| All sources | 0.018 | 0.300 | 0.032 | 1.533 | 0.045 | 2.133 |

## 11.7  Conclusions

Data on food consumption and the methods available to estimate chemical intakes are many and varied. Very often the type of intake analysis that can be undertaken is limited by the amount and quality of data. However, a very critical look should be taken at any estimates of intake to ensure that they are not providing misleading information. At the most basic level it is vital to know whether population mean intakes are relevant or whether it is necessary to consider intakes at the individual level.

It is critically important that any estimate of intake should correspond to the toxicological characteristics of the natural toxicant being studied. In particular it is vital to know not only whether the toxicological end-point is an acute or chronic effect but also the specific time interval over which it is appropriate to average intakes. For some natural toxicants in food this will make only a relatively minor difference but for those toxicants that occur in infrequently consumed foods the difference can be orders of magnitude.

It is also important to be aware of any particular sub-populations that may be more susceptible. If, for example, a substance is thought to be foetotoxic then it is necessary to consider potential maternal intakes during the critical period of development. Other substances may be more likely to affect people with inherent defects of metabolism. It is now routine practice to consider children separately because their low bodyweight often means that they are automatically the greatest consumers on a bodyweight basis. Nevertheless, children's intakes may not necessarily be relevant to a particular risk assessment. There may be other sub-populations such as vegetarians and cultural groups whose food consumption habits put them at particular risk. For example, the Japanese have a particular fondness for young bracken fern stems which may contain natural toxicants.

Estimates of intake should never be assumed to be accurate. In fact it is more reliable to assume that they are *in*accurate. The question that must be asked is: does the estimate overestimate or underestimate intake and, if so, by how much?

Decisions about risks from natural toxicants in the diet can be made only when one understands the essential uncertainties involved in the risk assessment process. Only then can realistic conclusions be reached.

## References

ANZFA (1996) *The 1994 Australian Market Basket Survey*, Australia/New Zealand Food Authority, Canberra.

Armstrong, B. and Doll, R. (1975) Environmental factors and cancer incidence and mortality in different countries, with special reference to dietary practices. *International Journal of Cancer*, **15** 617-31.

Department of Health (1989) The diets of British schoolchildren, Report on Health and Social Subjects No. 36, HMSO, London.

Douglass, J.S. and Tennant, D.R. (1997) Estimations of dietary intake of food chemicals, in *Food Chemical Risk Analysis* (ed. D.R. Tennant), Blackie Academic & Professional, Chapman & Hall, London, pp. 195-216.

Gold, L., Slone, T.H. and Ames, B.N. (1997) Prioritization of possible carcinogenic hazards in food, in *Food Chemical Risk Analysis* (ed. D.R. Tennant), Blackie Academic & Professional, Chapman & Hall, London, pp. 267-89.

Gregory, J., Tyler, H. and Wiseman, M. (1990) *The Dietary and Nutritional Survey of British Adults*, HMSO, London.

Gregory, J., Collins, D., Davies, P., Hughes, J. and Clarke, P. (1995) *National Diet and Nutrition Survey: Children aged 1¹/₂ to 4¹/₂ years*, HMSO, London.

Ministry of Agriculture, Fisheries and Food (1996) Inherent natural toxicants in food, Food Surveillance Paper No. 51, HMSO, London.

Rees, N.R. and Harris, C.A. (1995) *UK Methods for the Estimation of Dietary Intakes of Pesticide Residues*, Pesticides Safety Directorate, Ministry of Agriculture, Fisheries and Food, HMSO, London.

Rubery, E.D., Barlow, S.M. and Steadman, J.H. (1990) Criteria for setting quantitative estimates of acceptable intakes of chemicals in food in the UK. *Food Additives and Contaminants*, **7** 287-302.

Tennant, D.R. (1997) Food, chemicals and risk analysis, in *Food Chemical Risk Analysis* (ed. D.R. Tennant), Blackie Academic & Professional, Chapman & Hall, London, pp. 1-18.

USDA (1991, 1992, 1993) *Continuing Surveys of Food Consumption by Individuals, 1989–90, 1990–91 and 1991–92*, United States Department of Agriculture, Washington DC.

WHO (1990) *Toxicological Evaluation of Certain Food Additives and Contaminants, No. 26*, International Programme on Chemical Safety, World Health Organisation, Geneva.

# 12  The chemical detoxification of aflatoxin-contaminated animal feed

Raymond D. Coker

## 12.1  Introduction

The mycotoxin problem may be conceptualised (Coker, 1997) as the result of interacting spoilage, mycotoxin, socio-economic and control 'systems', where a 'system' may be viewed as a set of interacting components in which the interactions are just as important as the components themselves (after Open University Business School, 1987).

The mycotoxin control system, illustrated in Figure 12.1, describes the three main types of intervention that are likely to be employed to alleviate the impact of mycotoxins: (a) prevention of contamination, (b) identification and segregation of contaminated material and (c) detoxification. The control of mycotoxins in animal feeds, by means of chemical detoxification procedures, will be discussed in considerable detail in this chapter.

## 12.2  Chemical detoxification

It has been estimated that annual losses in the USA and Canada arising from the impact of mycotoxins on the feed and livestock industries are of the order of $5 billion (Miller, personal communication). Consequently, it is essential that a strategy is developed for the utilisation of feeds in those instances where mycotoxin contamination cannot be prevented.

Numerous oxidising agents, aldehydes, acids and bases (inorganic and organic) have been investigated as potential chemical detoxification agents (Park *et al.*, 1988). Patented procedures exist that utilise ammonia, calcium hydroxide, hydrogen peroxide, methylamine and a mixture of calcium hydroxide and methylamine. Commodities that have been experimentally treated in this way include groundnut meal (with ammonia, hydrogen peroxide, formaldehyde, calcium hydroxide plus methylamine, sodium hydroxide), cottonseed meal (ammonia, sodium hydroxide, calcium hydroxide), corn (ammonia, sodium bisulphite, calcium hydoxide), copra (calcium hydroxide) and poultry feed (sodium hydroxide). Detoxification equipment has included large plastic silage bags (ammonia/corn,cottonseed), pelleters (sodium hydroxide/poultry feed; calcium hydroxide/copra), pressurised reaction vessels (ammonia/groundnut and cottonseed meal), unpressurised reaction vessels (calcium hydroxide plus formaldehyde/groundnut cake) and screw press extruders (calcium hydroxide plus methylamine/groundnut meal).

## 12.3   Ammonia detoxification

The chemical detoxification reagent that has attracted the widest interest is ammonia, as both an anhydrous vapour and an aqueous solution. Consequently, many studies have been performed, within the European Union and on other continents, on the efficiency of ammonia detoxification and on the nutritional and toxicological properties of ammoniated feeds.

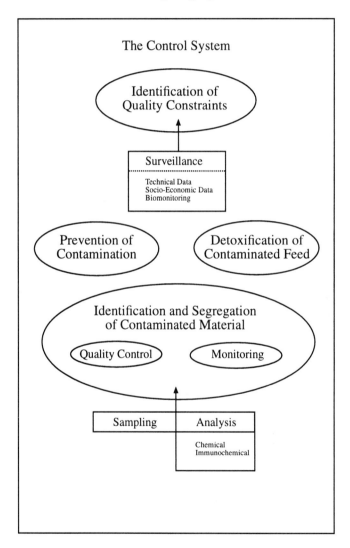

**Figure 12.1**   The mycotoxin control system

Ammonia was first used for the detoxification of aflatoxin-contaminated cottonseed meal, in the USA, in the late 1960s (Park *et al.*, 1988). Food and Drug Administraton (FDA) approval was obtained, temporarily, for utilising ammoniated cottonseed meal in feedstuffs for non-lactating ruminants and laying hens. However, although numerous nutritional and toxicological studies have since been performed, under the auspices of the National Cottonseed Growers' Association, formal approval of the ammoniation process, by the FDA, is still awaited.

In the USA, Arizona, California and Texas permit the 'ammoniation' of cottonseed products and the states of Texas, North Carolina, Georgia and Alabama allow the ammoniation of contaminated corn.

In Arizona, for example, procedures operating either at atmospheric pressure/ambient temperature (APAT) or at elevated temperature and pressure have been used successfully for the decontamination of whole cottonseed and cottonseed meal for ten years and have played a key role in controlling the occurrence of aflatoxin $M_1$ in milk produced by cows fed cottonseed products (Park, 1993). During 1978, for example, some 400 tonnes of milk were destroyed, with contamination levels of up to $10\,\mu g/kg$ aflatoxin $M_1$. Since the ammoniation of cottonseed was instituted by statute in 1980, the destruction of milk has only been ordered on one occasion (when cottonseed awaiting ammoniation was fed to cows in error).

The APAT procedure involves the spraying of cottonseed with aqueous ammonia and storage for approximately two weeks in large white silage bags. The elevated temperature/pressure procedure utilises a large, rotating pressure vessel. Ammonia (4% w/w) and steam are added to the cottonseed to afford a pressure of 40 pounds per square inch (psi) and a temperature of 100°C. A dwell time of 30 min is employed. Although the APAT process has not been approved by the Californian authorities, a high temperature/pressure treatment is utilised involving 1.5% ammonia, 14% moisture and a pressure of 30 psi.

A procedure used for the detoxification of corn includes the successive addition of water (to 17.5% moisture) and ammonia to 29 tonne batches of corn held in special bins (Coker *et al.*, 1985). A mixture of ammonia and air is recycled through the corn for 48 h, after which the treated material is held at a mean temperature of approximately 36°C for a further 11 days. The ammoniated corn is then transferred to a drying bin where it is deodorised and dried, to a moisture content of about 10%, using hot air.

### 12.3.1 Large-scale ammoniation

Currently, groundnut products are subjected to commercial-scale ammoniation in Senegal, France and the UK. Typically, commercially operated ammoniation processes employ an anhydrous ammonia concentration of 1 to 4% (w/w), a moisture level of 12 to 17%, a pressure of approximately 30 psi and a temperature of at least 80°C. Dwell times are normally of the order of 30 min to 1 h.

The Senegalese process, for example, is performed in a large, stirred reaction vessel and is reported to involve the addition of gaseous ammonia, at 2 bars, to groundnut meal at 5 to 15% moisture content, which has been heated to 80°C; 0.3 to 0.6% formaldehyde is also added as an anti-caking agent (Pemberton and Simpson, 1991). In 1984, the total throughput of ammoniated groundnut cake was approaching 600 000 tonnes a year.

The operation of an elevated temperature/pressure ammoniation process may be further illustrated by outlining the main features of an experimental low pressure process developed at the Natural Resources Institute (Coker *et al.*, 1985). Briefly, the process involves the addition of the aflatoxin-contaminated commodity to a steam-jacketed, stirred reaction vessel, followed by the sequential injection of steam and ammonia gas. After a dwell period of 30 min, or less, the excess ammonia is removed by drawing air through the ammoniated product. Additional purging by steam may be performed if necessary. Typical operating conditions are shown in Table 12.1. The quantity of animal feed treated varied from 200 to 300 kg, and the maximum pressure and temperature attained within the reaction vessel were 17 psi and 124°C respectively (during the treatment of comminuted groundnut cake). Mean flow rates for the addition of steam and ammonia were of the order of 1.4 and 0.2 kg per minute, respectively, and the temperature of the feeds at the beginning of the steam and ammonia treatments were, typically, about 70 and 115°C, respectively. For groundnut meal, groundnut cake and corn, high rates of detoxification were obtained using only 1% (w/w) ammonia, or less, and high levels of aflatoxin contamination.

Groundnut cake was also pelleted immediately after treatment. Ammoniated cake (10.8% moisture) was successfully pelleted, without preconditioning, using a 4.8 mm die and a throughput of 207 kg per hour. The temperatures of the groundnut cake immediately before and after pelleting were 69 and 80°C respectively and the moisture content of the pellets, after cooling, was 9.3%.

## 12.3.2 Ammoniation in the developing world

The presence of aflatoxin in livestock feed may result in reduced feed efficiency, poor growth rates, decreased disease resistance, increased vaccination failure and increased mortality. The perceived financial consequences of these manifestations of aflatoxicosis will determine the premium that end-users (e.g feed manufacturers and livestock farmers) are prepared to pay for feeds with acceptably low levels of aflatoxin.

The cost of ammonia detoxification will vary with the location of the ammoniation plant. A rapid appraisal performed in India, in 1990 (Coker *et al.*, 1991) evaluated the costs associated with four possible types of location

Table 12.1 A low-pressure ammoniation process

| Commodity | Weight (kg) | Moisture (%, w/w) Before[a] | Moisture (%, w/w) After[b] | Ammonia (%, w/w) | Maximum pressure (psi) | Maximum temperature (°C) | Aflatoxin content (mg/kg) Before[a] | Aflatoxin content (mg/kg) After[b] | Detoxification % |
|---|---|---|---|---|---|---|---|---|---|
| Groundnut meal (ground) | 250 | 9.1 | ND[c] | 0.94 | 17 | 122 | 2220 | 58 | 97 |
| Groundnut meal (not ground) | 218 | 9.0 | 10.8 | 0.92 | 17 | 117 | 1871 | 33 | 98 |
| Groundnut cake (ground) | 238 | 8.2 | 10.8 | 1.00 | 17 | 124 | 1242 | 58 | 95 |
| Corn (ground) | 300 | 8.7 | 11.9 | 0.80 | 14 | 107 | 1939 | 45 | 98 |
| Cottonseed meal | 250 | 8.5 | 9.5 | 2.0 | 14 | 122 | 1220 | 45 | 96 |

[a] Before = before ammoniation.
[b] After = after ammoniation, purging and drying.
[c] ND = not determined.

for a plant: (a) as an integral component of a feed manufacturing plant, (b) at an export port, (c) attached to an oil extraction plant and (d) a stand-alone, centrally operated facility. The estimated cost for the ammoniation of groundnut and cottonseed cakes, as a percentage of the value of the commodity, is shown in Table 12.2 for models of each of the four locations. Costs are given for operational capacities of 25 and 100%, assuming that 100% capacity is equivalent to 300 days per year.

It is evident that, for both commodities, the least costly location is model (c), where the ammoniation plant is attached to an oil extraction facility, and that the most costly location is model (b), where the plant is located at an export port. When operating at 100% capacity it was estimated that the costs of ammoniating groundnut and cottonseed cakes at an oil extraction facility were equivalent to 5.3 and 7.5% of the commodity value, respectively.

**Table 12.2** Ammoniation cost as a percentage of the commodity value

| Commodity | Capacity (%) | Percentage detoxification | | | |
|---|---|---|---|---|---|
| | | Model (a) | Model (b) | Model (c) | Model (d) |
| Groundnut cake | 100 | 7.2 | 8.7 | 5.3 | 6.7 |
| | 25 | 12.7 | 14.4 | 7.9 | 9.2 |
| Cottonseed cake | 100 | 11.0 | 12.5 | 7.5 | 9.6 |
| | 25 | 18.1 | 20.5 | 11.0 | 13.0 |

Model (a): as an integral component of a feed manufacturing plant.
Model (b): at an export port.
Model (c): attached to an oil extraction plant.
Model (d): a stand-alone, centrally operated facility.

### 12.3.3 Ammoniation and the nutritional quality of feed

Ammoniation produces changes in protein patterns with an accompanied reduction in, for example, the levels of cystine, methionine and available lysine. The nitrogen solubility index is also reduced (Park *et al.,* 1988), indicating that some degree of thermal/chemical denaturation of protein has occurred. Residual ammonia, of course, increases the level of non-protein nitrogen in ammoniated feeds. Although small increases of this nature can be accommodated by ruminants, excessive residual ammonia is highly undesirable in monogastric feeds. No significant changes have been reported in the levels of starch and lipid components (Peplinski *et al.,* 1983).

Following *in vitro* studies, ammoniation has been reported to increase amino acid digestibility (Adrian, 1976) and amyloglucosidase activity (Brekke *et al.,* 1978). In general, ruminants demonstrated improvements in weight gain and feed efficiency when fed ammoniated diets. Non-ruminants either showed no effect or suffered a decrease in these parameters.

## 12.4  Ammoniation and feed toxicity

The interaction of ammonia both with the aflatoxin and with the constituents of the feed will produce a complex mixture of reaction products, the metabolic fate of which will determine the toxicological properties of the treated commodity.

### 12.4.1  Animal feeding trials

Very extensive feeding trials, using ammoniated feeds, have been performed with a variety of animals including trout, rats, poultry, swine, and beef and dairy cattle. The effect of ammoniation on the toxicity of aflatoxin-contaminated feeds has been determined by monitoring animal growth and organ weights, together with haematological, histopathological and biochemical parameters.

A 90-day feeding trial, using weaning male and female Fischer 344 rats, was performed using low-pressure, ammoniated (1.5% ammonia, 10 psi, 90°C) groundnut cake (Manson and Neal, 1987). Four diets were prepared, each containing 75% groundnut cake and 25% powdered rat diet. Two diets (at 600 ppb) contained naturally aflatoxin-contaminated groundnut cake, while the remaining diets were uncontaminated (the contaminated diet contained 40 ppb aflatoxin after ammoniation).

The hepatotoxic and potential hepatocarcinogenic effects of the diets were assessed by assaying the activity of gamma-glutamyl transferase (GGT) in the rats' livers. The results indicated that ammoniation of the aflatoxin-contaminated cake eliminated the development of focal GGT positive (preneoplastic) lesions in both male and female animals. However, in the female rat, histochemical GGT staining of periportal hepatocytes was increased by all the experimental diets (including the ammoniated, uncontaminated diet), compared with the untreated, uncontaminated diet. Ammoniated diets also produced decreased bodyweight gains.

The toxicity of low-pressure ammoniated groundnut cake was also assessed by feeding ducklings five diets for 22 days (Coker *et al.*, 1983). The diets consisted of a control (zero aflatoxin) and feeds containing 5 and 25% ammoniated or untreated aflatoxin-contaminated cake. The group of ducklings that received the diet (300 ppb total aflatoxin) containing 25% untreated cake showed very low growth rates; all birds in this group had died by the 14th day of the trial. No significant difference in growth was apparent between those ducklings receiving a control diet (<2.0 ppb aflatoxin) and a diet containing 5% ammoniated cake (5 ppb). The performance of those birds fed diets containing 5% untreated cake (50 ppb) and 25% ammoniated cake (15 ppb) were slightly reduced compared to the other groups. (The high natural biological variation within each group of ducklings made an accurate assessment of the significance of small differences in performance extremely difficult.)

A microscopic examination of the livers of all the birds included in the trial demonstrated the absence of any abnormal lesions from the livers of the ducklings that had received a diet containing 5% ammoniated groundnut cake. Five out of the nine livers from ducklings fed on the diet that contained 25% ammoniated groundnut cake showed slight centriacinar bile duct proliferation; one liver also showed evidence of single cell necrosis. All of the nine birds receiving a diet containing 25% untreated cake afforded livers with marked bile duct proliferation, with five of the livers also showing single cell necrosis. Eight of the nine ducklings with 5% untreated cake in their diet produced livers showing slight bile duct proliferation; the liver of the remaining group member showed a marked proliferation of the bile duct. None of the livers from ducklings that had received diets containing ammoniated groundnut cake showed any evidence of centriacinar fibrosis.

Rat feeding trials have also been performed over a two-year period (Park *et al.,* 1988). Diets containing uncontaminated or aflatoxin-contaminated cottonseed meal, either ammoniated or untreated, at 20% inclusion rates were utilised. None of the male rats on untreated contaminated diets survived the trial. The number of female survivors was also significantly reduced compared to those fed an uncontaminated diet. All ammoniated diets led to similar organ weights among male rats, which were significantly lower than those obtained for animals fed uncontaminated feed. Rats receiving either uncontaminated or ammoniated diets did not exhibit liver neoplasms.

The safety of meat and eggs produced by animals receiving diets containing ammoniated feeds has been evaluated by the US Department of Agriculture (USDA) and FDA (Park *et al.,* 1988). Diets containing uncontaminated or aflatoxin-contaminated corn (either ammoniated or untreated) were fed to poultry, pigs and beef cattle. Meat and eggs from these animals were then fed to rats (as 20% of the diets) for a 15- to 18-month period. No toxic or carcinogenic effects were reported. (A reduction in the survival of male rats receiving eggs was attributed to nutritional deficiencies in the diet.) Multigeneration studies on rats have been performed by the USDA using poultry and beef tissue derived from animals fed ammoniated, aflatoxin-contaminated corn (Food and Drug Administration, 1982). A teratological evaluation indicated that foetal development was not affected by the consumption of tissue (as 20% of the diet), for periods of 15 to 18 months, derived from poultry and cattle fed ammoniated corn.

The toxicity of milk derived from dairy cattle fed ammoniated cottonseed meal has been evaluated using rainbow trout (Sinnhuber *et al.,* unpublished work). The aflatoxin content of contaminated cottonseed meal (c. 4000 ppb, total) was reduced to <5.0 ppb aflatoxin by ammoniation. Ingestion of the treated meal (c. 3.6 kg/cow/day) afforded milk with no detectable aflatoxin $M_1$. The freeze-dried milk was fed to rainbow trout, as 25% of the diet, for 12 months. The low incidence of observed hepatomas was similar to that induced by low dietary levels of aflatoxin.

Ammoniated corn has been directly fed to trout, as 25% of the diet (Brekke *et al.*, 1977). There was no significant difference in the incidence of hepatomas between those fish fed uncontaminated corn and those receiving the ammoniated diet.

The effect of ammoniated feeds on the productivity, disease resistance and biochemical parameters in poultry has been examined. Feeding trials, with day-old ducklings, using ammoniated groundnut cake produced using a low-pressure ammoniation process are described above. Studies with day-old chicks have also been reported (Delort-Laval *et al.*, 1980). Diets containing ammoniated groundnut cake did not affect the feed intake although a slight reduction in weight gain and feed conversion efficiency was observed. These reductions however, could be reversed by adding methionine to the diet.

The effect of ammoniation on the effectiveness of vaccination against Newcastle disease has been evaluated by feeding white leghorn layer-breeders with ammoniated corn (Boulton *et al.*, 1981). No reduction in haemagglutination-inhibition (HI) titres, after vaccination, were observed for birds receiving either ammoniated/contaminated or ammoniated/uncontaminated corn. A significant reduction in HI titres was exhibited by those birds receiving untreated diets contaminated with 500 ppb aflatoxin.

The effect of feeding ammoniated diets on egg production and quality has also been studied in white leghorn layer-breeders (Hughes and Jones, 1979; Hughes *et al.*, 1979). Ammoniation had no effect on egg production, egg weight, fertility or hatchability. However, reductions in feed consumption and weight gain were reported for those birds fed ammoniated diets.

Ammoniated corn has been fed to weanling pigs (Keyl and Norred, 1978). No reductions in weight gain or feed efficiency were observed after a period of 120 days.

The effect of ammoniated feeds on dairy cattle and on the concentration of aflatoxin $M_1$ in milk has been extensively studied (Park *et al.*, 1988). Three feeding trials using ammoniated groundnut cake and ammoniated cottonseed meal serve to illustrate the type of results typically observed. Ammoniated cottonseed meal and whole cottonseed was fed to lactating Holstein cows for 14 days. No aflatoxin $M_1$ could be detected in the milk compared to the 3–5 ng/l aflatoxin $M_1$ that was detected after feeding untreated contaminated feed, equivalent to a daily intake of approximately 6.0 (cottonseed) and 1.0 µg (meal) aflatoxin $B_1$ (McKinney *et al.*, 1973). The effect of feeding ammoniated groundnut cake, at 5–17 ppb aflatoxin $B_1$ to Holstein Friesian cows, over a 16-month period, has also been investigated (Fremy *et al.*, 1987). No aflatoxin $M_1$ levels in excess of 0.01 µg/l were observed. The contaminated untreated diet, containing 20% contaminated groundnut cake, contained approximately 220 ppb aflatoxin $B_1$.

The effect of ammoniation at low and medium pressure on the carry-over of residual aflatoxin $B_1$ into milk has also been studied (Coker *et al.*, 1995). Six groups of 10 Holstein cows were fed the diets containing groundnut cake described in Table 12.3. Statistically, there was no evidence of significant differences between diets B, C and D, and it was concluded that the incorporation of ammonia-detoxified groundnut meal into dairy feed did not lead to an enhancement of the carry-over of aflatoxin from feed to the milk

### 12.4.2 The chemistry of ammoniation

The nature of the reaction products produced by the ammoniation of aflatoxin is still poorly defined. Most studies have focused on the reaction products of aflatoxin $B_1$ produced under a variety of conditions including the treatment (a) *in vitro*, of pure toxin, (b) of pure toxin on an inert carrier, (c) of feedstuffs spiked with pure toxin and (d) of naturally contaminated feedstuffs.

**Table 12.3**  The percentage carry-over of aflatoxin $B_1$ into milk as aflatoxin $M_1$

| Diet | Aflatoxin $B_1$ in Feed ($\mu g/kg$) | Treatment | Percentage carry-over |
|------|------|------|------|
| A | 42.5 | Untreated groundnut meal (GNM) at 615 $\mu g/kg$ | 0.86 |
| B | 4.1 | Low-pressure detoxified GNM at 43 $\mu g/kg$ | 1.20 |
| C | 3.4 | Medium-pressure detoxified GNM at 21 $\mu g/kg$ | 1.72 |
| D | 3.0 | Uncontaminated GNM + GNM at 615 $\mu g/kg$ | 1.59 |

Ammoniation, *in vitro*, of pure aflatoxin $B_1$ has afforded four compounds of molecular weights (MW) 286, 256, 236 and 206, together with many unidentified compounds of MW less than 200. The compound of MW 286 has been characterised as the decarboxylated derivative (aflatoxin $D_1$) of aflatoxin $B_1$, whereas the compound of MW 206 lacks the cyclopentenone ring of aflatoxin $D_1$. The loss of the methoxy group from aflatoxin $D_1$ affords the compound with MW 256. The reaction product of molecular weight 236 has still to be identified (Figure 12.2).

When aflatoxin $B_1$ was treated with ammonium hydroxide at 100°C, approximately 30% of the crude reaction product was attributed to aflatoxin $D_1$ (Lee *et al.*, 1974). In a similar experiment, the reaction product contained between 3 and 26% of compound MW 206, depending on the duration of the reaction. An increase in the concentration of compound MW 206 was accompanied by a decrease in the concentration of aflatoxin $D_1$ (Cucullu *et al.*, 1976)

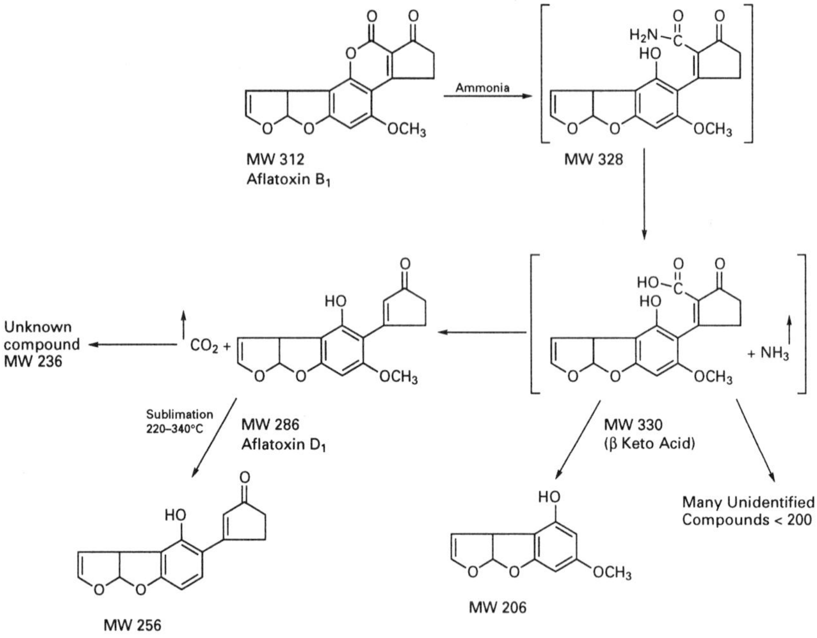

**Figure 12.2**   The *in vitro* ammoniation of aflatoxin $B_1$ from Park *et al.*, 1998

When pure radiolabelled aflatoxin $B_1$, on an inert carrier, was treated with ammonia at 40 psi and 100°C, 20% of the label was lost as volatile compounds while less than 1% remained as unreacted aflatoxin $B_1$. Although the reaction product of MW 206 was identified, no aflatoxin $D_1$ was detected (Lee *et al.*, 1984).

Further studies were performed using groundnut meal spiked with labelled aflatoxin $B_1$. Treatment at 75°C afforded an ammoniated product which contained only 45–50% of the label. Unreacted aflatoxin $B_1$ and aflatoxin $D_1$ accounted for only 0.3 and 0.2% of the reaction product, respectively. Some activity was also detected in the volatile fraction (Lee *et al.*, 1979).

Similar larger scale studies have involved the ammoniation of a 28 kg batch of naturally contaminated cottonseed meal, additionally spiked with labelled aflatoxin $B_1$. Treatment at 40 psi and 100°C produced an ammoniated product, which accounted for about 86% of the radioactivity. Subsequent mass spectral analysis of the ammoniated product confirmed the absence of *both* aflatoxin $D_1$ and compound MW 206 (Lee *et al.*, 1985). However, aflatoxin $D_1$ was detected, by tandem mass spectrometry, in very heavily aflatoxin-contaminated corn (175 ppm) after ammoniation at 37°C for 21 days. The yield of aflatoxin $D_1$ was estimated as substantially less than 10% (Grove *et al.*, 1984). 37% of the activity remained in the meal after solvent extraction and chemical and enzymic treatments (Park *et al.*, 1984). The final distribution of the radiolabel among the various fractions is summarised in Figure 12.3. When the mutagenicity of the fractions was determined using the Ames test, a methylene chloride extract of the final residue, shown in Figure 12.3, was the only extract that produced a positive response.

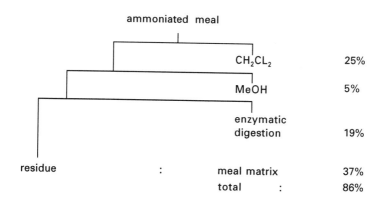

**Figure 12.3**     The distribution of radiolabel after ammoniation of cottonseed meal spiked with [14]C-labelled aflatoxin $B_1$. After Pemberton and Simpson (1991).

The apparent affinity of ammoniated aflatoxin for the feed matrix was further demonstrated when Norred (1981) fed rats with [14]C-labelled aflatoxin $B_1$ in corn. The radiolabel was excreted faster when the corn was ammoniated than when the rats were fed with untreated corn. Similarly, Beckwith and co-workers (1975) have reported that radiolabelled aflatoxin $B_1$ binds covalently to corn flour after ammoniation. Since the covalent binding did not change the spectral properties of the aflatoxin $B_1$ chromophore, it was surmised that the binding occurred via the bisdihydrofuran system.

### 12.4.3  The toxicity of ammoniation reaction products

The toxicity of the reaction product, aflatoxin $D_1$, has been compared to that of aflatoxin $B_1$ using (a) the Ames test (*Salmonella* mutagenicity), (b) the DNA covalent binding index (CBI) and (c) the chick embryo bioassay as indicators of toxicity. Aflatoxin $D_1$ was reported as representing a 450-fold decrease in mutagenic potential, a 300-fold decrease, at least, in the DNA CBI and a 20-fold decrease in toxicity to the chick embryo (Lee *et al.*, 1981). The reaction product, MW 206, was over 600 times less mutagenic than aflatoxin $B_1$ (Haworth *et al.*, 1989).

## 12.5  Conclusions

The presence of aflatoxin in feedstuff is producing severe economic losses and threatening human health throughout the world. Furthermore, the imposition of legislation, by importing countries within the developed world, is serving to heighten the aflatoxin problem within the exporting countries in the Third World.

Chemical detoxification of contaminated feeds has a major role to play in the prevention of economic loss and human disease. Although the use of ammonia as a detoxification reagent has been very widely investigated and commercially exploited, the use of ammoniated commodities as animal feeds has not been widely accepted. This acceptance will not be forthcoming until general agreement has been reached on the toxicological implications of ammoniation. The US FDA's Center for Veterinary Medicine has established a Public Master File as a repository of information on the toxicology of ammoniated feeds so that accumulated data on this matter can be effectively reviewed.

### Acknowledgements

The author acknowledges that this chapter contains material previously published in Coker, R.D. (1997) Mycotoxins and their Control: Constraints and Opportunities, NRI Bulletin 73, Chatham.

### References

Adrian, J. (1976) Evolution de la lysine, methionine et cystine dans le touteau d'arachide traite a l'ammoniac. *Revue Française Corps Gras*, **23** 209-12.
Beckwith, A.C., Vesonder, R.F. and Ciegler, A (1975) Action of weak bases upon aflatoxin $B_1$ in contact with macromolecular reactants. *Journal of Agricultural and Food Chemistry*, **23** 582.
Boulton, S.L., Dick, J.N. and Hughes, B.L. (1981) Effects of dietary aflatoxin and ammonia-inactivated aflatoxin on Newcastle disease antibody titers in layer-breeders. *Avian Diseases*, **26** 1-6.

Brekke, O.L., Sinnhuber, R.O., Peplinski, A.J., Wales, H.H., Putnam, G.B., Lee, D.J. and Ciegler, A. (1977) Aflatoxin in corn: ammonia inactivation and bioassay with rainbow trout. *Applied Environmental Microbiology,* **34** 34-37.

Brekke, O.L., Stringfellow, A.C. and Peplinski, A.J. (1978) Aflatoxin inactivation in corn by ammonia gas: laboratory trials. *Journal of Agricultural and Food Chemistry,* **26** 1383-89.

Coker, R.D., Jewers, K., Jones, N.R., Nabney, J. and Watson, D.H. (1983) Decontaminating aflatoxin-containing agricultural products, British Patent 2108365, London, 4 pp.

Coker, R.D., Jewers, K. and Jones, B.D. (1985) The destruction of aflatoxin by ammonia: practical possibilities, *Tropical Science,* **25** 139-54.

Coker, R.D., Hawkes, A.J., Watson, I.G. and Bennett, C.J. (1991) The control of mycotoxins in poultry feeds in India. *NRI Visit Report* R1820 (R).

Coker, R.D., Nagler, M.J., Neal, G.E. and Mansbridge, R. (1995) Project CSO 103: bovine feeding studies using ammonia detoxified groundnut derivative. *MAFF Report.*

Coker, R.D. (1997) Mycotoxins and their control: constraints and opportunities, *NRI Bulletin* 73, Natural Resources Institute: Chatham, UK.

Cucullu, A.F., Lee, L.S., Pons, P.A. and Stanley, I.B. (1976) Ammoniation of aflatoxin $B_1$: isolation and characterization of a product with molecular weight 206. *Journal of Agricultural and Food Chemistry,* **24** 408-10.

DeLort-Laval, J., Viroben, G. and Borgida, L.P. (1980) Efficacité biologique pour le poulet de chair du tourteau d'arachide traite a l'ammoniac ou a la monomethylamine en vue de l'inactivation des aflatoxines. *Annales de Zootechnie,* **29** 387-400.

Food and Drug Administration (1982) *NCTR Evaluation of Rat Fetuses from the USDA Aflatoxin Multigeneration Studies,* National Center for Toxicological Research Technical Report for Experiment 944/945, NCTR, Jefferson.

Fremy, J.M., Gautier, J.P., Herry, M.P., Terrier, C. and Calet, C. (1987) Effects of ammoniation on the 'carry-over' of aflatoxins into bovine milk. *Food Additives and Contaminants,* **5** 39-44.

Grove, M.D., Plattner, R.D. and Peterson, R.E. (1984) Detection of aflatoxin $D_1$ in ammoniated corn by mass spectrometry. *Applied Environmental Microbiology,* **48** 887-89.

Haworth, S.R., Lawlor, T.E., Zeiger, E., Lee, L.S. and Park, D.L. (1989) Mutagenic potential of ammonia-related aflatoxin reaction products in model systems. *Journal of the American Oil Chemists' Society,* **66** 102-104.

Hughes, B.L. and Jones, I.E. (1979) Hematology of single comb white leghorn pullets fed aflatoxin-contaminated and ammonia-treated corn. *Poultry Science,* **58** 981-82.

Hughes, B.L., Barnett, B.D., Jones, J.E., Dick, J.W. and Norred, W.P. (1979) Safety of feeding aflatoxin-inactivated corn to white leghorn layer breeders. *Poultry Science,* **58** 1202-1209.

Keyl, A.C. and Norred, W.P. (1978) Utilization of aflatoxin contaminated feed. *American Dairy Science Association/American Society for the Administration Science Meeting,* July, East Lansing, MI.

Lee, L.S., Stanley, J.B., Cucullu, A.F. and Pons, W.A. (1974) Ammoniation of aflatoxin $B_1$: isolation and identification of the major reaction product. *Journal of the Association of Analytical Chemists,* **57** 626-31.

Lee, L.S., Conkerton, E.J., Ory, R.L. and Bennett, J.W. (1979) [${}^{14}$C]-aflatoxin $B_1$ as an indicator of toxin destruction during ammoniation of contaminated peanut meal. *Journal of Agricultural and Food Chemistry,* **27** 598-602.

Lee, L.S., Dunn, J.J., DeLucca, A.J. and Ciegler, A. (1981) Role of lactone ring of aflatoxin $B_1$ in toxicity and mutagenicity. *Experientia,* **37** 16-17.

Lee, L.S., Koltun, S.P. and Stanley, I.B. (1984) Ammoniation of aflatoxin $B_1$ in a pressure chamber used to decontaminate toxin-containing cottonseed meal. *Journal of the American Oil Chemists' Society,* **61** 1607-1608.

Lee, L.S., Legendre, M.G. and Koltun, S.P. (1985) Formation of ammonia degradation products of aflatoxin $B_1$ in the absence and presence of cottonseed meal. *Journal of the American Oil Chemists' Society,* **62** 656.

Manson, M.M. and Neal, G.E. (1987) The effect of feeding aflatoxin-contaminated groundnut meal, with or without ammoniation, on the development of gamma-glutamyl transferase positive lesions in the livers of Fischer 344 rats. *Food Additives and Contaminants*, **4** 141-47.

McKinney, J.D., Cavanagh, G.C., Bell, J.T., Hoversland, A.S., Nelson, D.M., Pearson, J. and Selkirk, R.J. (1973) Effects of ammoniation on aflatoxin in rations-fed lactating cows. *Journal of the American Oil Chemists' Society*, **50** 79-84.

Norred, W.P. (1981) Excretion and distribution of ammoniated $^{14}$C-labelled aflatoxin $B_1$-containing corn. *Federal Proceedings*, **40** 694.

Open University Business School (1987) Systems concepts and an intervention strategy, Block 3, in *Planning and Managing Change* (ed. Lewis Watson), The Open University, Milton Keynes.

Park, D.L., Lee, L. and Koltun, S.A. (1984) Distribution of ammonia-related aflatoxin reaction products in cottonseed meal. *Journal of the American Oil Chemists' Society*, **61** 1071-74.

Park, D.L., Lee, L.S., Price, R.L. and Pohland, A.E. (1988) Review of the Decontamination of aflatoxins by ammoniation: current status and regulation. *Journal of the Association of Official Analytical Chemists*, **71** 685-703.

Park, D.L. (1993) Perspectives on mycotoxin decontamination procedures. *Food Additives and Contaminants*, **10** 49-60.

Pemberton, A.D. and Simpson, T.J. (1991) The chemical degradation of mycotoxins, in *Mycotoxins and Animal Foods* (eds J.E. Smith and R.S. Henderson), CRC Press, London, pp. 797-813.

Peplinski, A.I., Eckhoff, S.R., Warner, K. and Anderson, R.A. (1983) Physical testing and dry milling of high-moisture corn preserved with ammonia while drying with ambient air. *Cereal Chemistry*, **60** 442-45.

# Appendix    Toxicological research into the effects of some secondary fungal metabolites in food and feeds

G.E. Neal

## A.1    Introduction

For reasons of space the scope of this review has been limited to the possible toxicological effects of only a small number of secondary fungal metabolites that have been found to be contaminants in food and feedstuffs. Even with such a restricted range, it has been necessary to refer to only a small proportion of the existing literature. Although these metabolites are frequently referred to by the generic term 'mycotoxins', the specific toxic properties of many of them and the hazard to human and animal health resulting from exposure to low levels still await rigorous investigation. Others, most notably the aflatoxins and ochratoxins, have been the focus of very extensive toxicological research, resulting in considerable scientific data. In all cases a comprehensive coverage of all aspects of the published work will not be attempted; attention will be centred on those areas of recent research interest.

The assessment of the levels of human and animal exposure to various mycotoxins can be based on different protocols.

As analytical techniques have improved, there has been an increasing capability for the detection and quantitation of progressively smaller amounts of fungal metabolites in foods and feeds. A major problem now in assessing potential human and animal dietary exposure, through analyses of foods and feeds, is the development of improved sampling techniques, because the contamination very frequently arises through localised infection, and hence is not homogeneously distributed throughout the bulk of the stored material.

Another approach to assessing human and animal exposure to these compounds, which is attracting increased attention, is through assays of appropriate biomarkers, for example urinary excretion of the parent compound, or more usually metabolites, or the presence of macromolecular adducts in blood. This is again an area in which increasingly sensitive and specific analytical techniques are being developed. These parameters are of particular importance in terms of their relationship to the subsequent development of pathological responses. Unfortunately at present exposure data based on biomonitoring are available for a very restricted number of mycotoxins.

A further major problem is evaluating the significance, if any, of exposure, particularly over a long period of time, to the low levels of the fungal metabolites that it is now possible to assay. Acute toxicities can often, with reasonable certainty, be ascribed to specific toxins and this frequently results from exposure to comparatively high levels of the mycotoxin. Long-term, low-level exposure might result in chronic pathologies but the correlation between exposure to a particular toxin (or more likely several toxins) at low levels and a subsequent pathology is much more tenuous and difficult to establish. This is perhaps the most challenging area of toxicological research into the hazards presented by exposure to mycotoxins. Two approaches are increasingly contributing valuable data in this area:

- the advent of highly sensitive analytical techniques for assaying human exposure has provided an improved basis for human epidemiological studies, and in particular, prospective studies
- mechanistic biochemical studies in animals, and increasingly in *in vitro* systems, coupled with species differences in sensitivity, can make major contributions to the extrapolation of experimental data to the evaluation of hazards to humans.

These aspects of current research will be considered in this review.

## A.2 Aflatoxins

### A.2.1 In vivo *toxicity*

*A.2.1.1 Animals.* The original identification of the aflatoxins as important naturally occurring toxins resulted from their acutely toxic and carcinogenic effects in sensitive species fed contaminated feedstuffs. In the case of the acutely toxic properties, these were recognised as a result of the investigation into turkey-X disease in domestic flocks in England caused by feeding contaminated groundnut meal. The carcinogenic properties were detected by a subsequent experimental feeding of the contaminated groundnut meal to rats and also by recognising that outbreaks of hepatoma in rainbow trout were the result of feeding cottonseed meal contaminated with aflatoxins. These early observations therefore highlighted the potential hazards of dietary exposure to levels of these toxins existing in naturally contaminated foodstuffs, which could provoke an acutely toxic reaction in sensitive species. The greater potential hazard from prolonged human exposure to the much lower levels, which could provoke a carcinogenic response in sensitive species, was evident. The consignment of Brazilian groundnut meal that gave rise to turkey-X disease contained 10 ppm of aflatoxin $B_1$. Since the 1960s, when the outbreak of turkey-X disease occurred, recognition of sources of aflatoxin contamination, and the factors affecting its production, have received very extensive research attention, which has led to a general lowering of levels of contamination. However, samples of feedstuffs containing levels of aflatoxins in excess of 1 to 2 ppm are still being identified. This level of contamination is capable of presenting a chronic hazard to susceptible species. Since the only alternative is destruction of these consignments of contaminated feeds, considerable attention has been paid to the possible development of techniques for the detoxification of contaminated feedstuffs (Chapter 12). Many of these are based on treatment of the feedstuffs with ammonia. These processes have been demonstrated to result in very substantial reduction of the free aflatoxin content of the meals; greater than 99% destruction of the aflatoxins has been achieved. However, the fate of the aflatoxins in the process still has not been clearly identified and so, given the toxic potencies of the aflatoxins, concern has remained that a decrease in the free aflatoxin content might not necessarily equate to a corresponding reduction in toxicity, in particular, chronic toxicity. Results of studies have been published on this important topic (Chapter 12; Manson and Neal, 1987; Park *et al.*, 1988). In view of the wide spectrum of toxic end-points known, or suspected, for these toxins, including acute and chronic, as well as immunotoxic and perhaps teratogenic effects, it would appear essential to confirm detoxification of treated feedstuffs using an equally wide range of toxicological end-points. In addition, until the fate of the aflatoxins in the detoxification processes is fully understood, there remains the possibility of reversal under particular circumstances, e.g. in the rumen of cattle fed the decontaminated meal.

There have been many experimental animal studies using aflatoxins, too numerous to detail in this review. It has been confirmed in these studies that the liver is a target organ for toxicity in almost all species studied. Toxic effects have also been reported for other organs including kidney, lung, colon and nasal epithelium. Perhaps one of the most important facts to emerge from the experimental animal studies has been the recognition of a wide species variation in sensitivity to these toxins, ranging from the highly susceptible, e.g. avian species, trout and male rats, to the highly resistant, e.g. mice. This has facilitated experimental metabolic studies attempting to identify the basis for these differences. One important objective of this work is to be able to make predictions based on comparative metabolic profiles as to probable human sensitivity.

### A.2.1.2 Humans

That humans are sensitive to acute aflatoxin poisoning, aflatoxicosis, appears to be beyond doubt. There have been several well-documented episodes of acute poisoning in humans, notably one in India in 1974 (Krishnamachari *et al.*, 1975) in which the involvement of aflatoxins was clearly established. In that incident the level of contamination of the maize involved was between 6 and 16 ppm. Dietary exposure resulted in many fatalities. From these data, therefore, it would appear that man is not only susceptible to the acutely toxic effect of aflatoxins but should probably be classified as a moderately sensitive species. Paralleling the results of many animal studies, human males appeared to be more sensitive to aflatoxin than females.

Although acute toxicity in humans would only be expected from the consumption of foodstuffs with exceptionally high levels of contamination, the genesis of liver tumours could result from exposure to low, even very low, levels of the toxin over a period of time. If the same basic aflatoxin $B_1$ bioactivation mechanisms are involved in both acute and chronic toxicities, and since humans are clearly sensitive to the acutely toxic action, it would be anticipated that humans would also be sensitive to the chronic toxic effects of aflatoxins. In agreement with this there has been an increasing body of epidemiological evidence correlating dietary exposure to aflatoxins with the high incidence of primary liver cancer in many Third World countries. There are many excellent reviews on this topic (e.g. Wild *et al.*, 1993). A correlation has been found to exist between the level of aflatoxin exposure and the high incidence of liver tumours in certain areas. A further finding is that high levels of G→T mutations in codon 249 of the P53 suppressor gene correlate with the possible involvement of $AFB_1$ (aflatoxin $B_1$) in the genesis of these tumours (Hsu *et al.*, 1991). This simple correlation, however, is complicated by the equally compelling data connecting the incidence of hepatitis B virus (HBV) with the incidence of primary liver cancer (Nose *et al.*, 1993), which will be considered later in this review.

There have been numerous studies, particularly in developing countries, assaying levels of exposure to aflatoxins in a wide range of human populations. Methods employed have involved biomonitoring assays of albumin $AFB_1$ adducts in serum and aflatoxin metabolites in urine, as well as measuring the aflatoxin content of foodstuffs. For further details on these studies see IARC (1993). The possible relevance of these assays to the development of human disease has been considered in a study examining the correlation between $AFB_1$–serum albumin adduct levels and liver $AFB_1$–DNA adducts in different rodent strains and species. It was found that not only was there a correlation between these levels but that also they related, at least qualitatively, to the relative susceptibilities of the rodent strains and species to $AFB_1$. By comparing the adduct levels in rodents with albumin adduct levels in exposed humans, it was concluded that those humans would have hepatic levels of $AFB_1$–DNA adducts closer to those observed for the $AFB_1$-sensitive rodents and one to two orders of magnitude higher than levels in $AFB_1$-resistant rodent species (Wild *et al.*, 1996). Following the administration of $AFB_1$ to rats and mice, the levels of

$AFB_1$–albumin adducts have also been found to parallel the levels of chromosome aberrations and micronuclei formation in the bone marrow, which again supports a correlation between $AFB_1$–albumin levels and *in vivo* genotoxic events (Anwar *et al.*, 1994).

### A.2.2 Hepatitis B virus and aflatoxins

The presence of both high levels of infection with hepatitis B and exposure to dietary aflatoxins in areas of high incidences of primary liver cancer have been noted in many studies, e.g. in China (Ross *et al.*, 1992) and in Guinea, West Africa (also in association with hepatitis; Diallo *et al.*, 1995). The importance of using biomarkers as indices of exposure to aflatoxins in place of analyses of food has been emphasised by the findings of Qian *et al.* (1994). They carried out a cohort study involving 18 244 middle-aged men in Shanghai, containing 55 cases of hepatocarcinoma (HCC). A much increased relative risk of HCC was found for individuals positive for serum hepatitis B surface antigen and aflatoxin exposure, based on urine analyses for aflatoxin metabolites. The relative risk for HCC was 59.4 for individuals positive for both hepatitis and HCC, demonstrating a high degree of synergism between the two illnesses. However, no strong risk factor was evident when exposure to aflatoxins was assessed on the basis of in-person food frequency interviews combined with surveys of market foods. In a similar study carried out in Singapore, which examined exposure to aflatoxins in groups of control individuals, hepatitis B virus (HBV) carriers and HCC patients, exposure to aflatoxins was found to be widespread but lower than in several other Asian studies. No relationship between the disease status of the subjects and the levels of $AFB_1$ was found. In fact, levels of exposure to $AFB_1$, assessed not by adduct, but by serum analyses, were found to be highest in the control group. The low levels of aflatoxin in these serum samples was suggested as reflecting the stringent monitoring of food levels of $AFB_1$ in Singapore (Chao *et al.*, 1994). Another HBV/$AFB_1$ study carried out in Taiwan again showed an elevated risk of HCC in HBV surface antigen-positive individuals when exposed to $AFB_1$ (Chen *et al.*, 1996). Based on a study in China, the relative hepatic cancer potency for aflatoxin has been evaluated to be 9 mg/kg/day for HBV-negative subjects but 230 for individuals positive for HBV (Bowers *et al.*, 1993).

There have been numerous experimental studies attempting to determine the basis of the synergistic effects between hepatitis virus infection and exposure to aflatoxins in the hepatocarcinogenic process. Many of these studies have centred on possible effects of the virus infection on metabolism of aflatoxin $B_1$ which requires metabolic activation to produce a biological response. In one study, samples of normal human liver, together with samples with hepatitis and cirrhosis, were examined for changed expression of those cytochrome P450 enzymes that might be involved in $AFB_1$ activation

(Kirby *et al.*, 1996). Changed expression was observed. For example, CYP 3A4 expression was induced in HBV-positive livers, adjacent to areas of fibrosis and inflammation but CYP 1A2, another enzyme involved in $AFB_1$ activation, was not affected. Hepatitis C virus (HCV) infection also increased expression of CYP 3A4. In another study in Taiwan involving humans no differences in urinary aflatoxin metabolite patterns were observed between HBV-positive and -negative individuals (Yu *et al.*, 1996). In mice, a species normally resistant to $AFB_1$ carcinogenesis, made transgenic for HBV resulted in an incidence of HCC following the administration of $AFB_1$ (Sell *et al.*, 1991). No adenomas or carcinomas were seen in the transgenic mice not exposed to $AFB_1$. The transgenic mice displayed liver injury secondary to the overexpression of the gene for the large envelope polypeptide of HBVs.

Two cytochrome P450 enzymes of importance in $AFB_1$ metabolism, CYP3a-5 and CYP3A4 have increased expression accompanying the liver injury. There is a possibility that this could have relevance to the human condition (Kirby *et al.*, 1994). Mice made transgenic with the human HBX gene spontaneously develop liver tumours but the administration of $AFB_1$ reduces the period before tumour development. However, in common with other HCC or preneoplastic lesions induced in rodents by the administration of $AFB_1$, no mutations in codon 249 of P53 were detected. Synergism between infection with hepatitis virus and $AFB_1$ administration, in terms of hepatocarcinogenesis, has been reported for several other animal systems. In woodchuck infected also with the virus, a synergism between the virus and $AFB_1$ has been demonstrated (Bannasch *et al.*, 1995). Tree shrews infected with human HBV spontaneously develop HCC but the process is accelerated by administration of $AFB_1$, the virus being integrated into the DNA of the tumours (Yan *et al.*, 1996).

From the human epidemiological data and animal experimentation, synergism between viral infection and exposure to $AFB_1$ is clearly a strong possibility in the genesis of HCC in many species, including man. Exposure to $AFB_1$ or infection with hepatitis virus can act as a complete carcinogen in animal systems and probably in man. $AFB_1$ has been recognised by IARC as a human carcinogen but the increased risk factor presents the greatest hazard to humans. The actual basis for this synergism is still not proven. Changes in the metabolic capacity of the liver have been suggested as important and there is some experimental evidence to support this. However, there is still a possibility that the major factor in the synergism is the capacity of viral infection to produce cell proliferation in the target organ for $AFB_1$, the liver, when the mutational and carcinogenic effects of the $AFB_1$ can be expressed. In the rat, this proliferation can be induced as a result of the acutely toxic property of the $AFB_1$ to which the rat is sensitive. In the mouse, normally resistant to the carcinogenic and cytotoxic effects of $AFB_1$, it is perhaps necessary to induce cell proliferation by another means, e.g. viral infection, in order that the carcinogenic effect of $AFB_1$ can be demonstrated. In this context it is notable that, at the neonate stage, when liver cell proliferation is proceeding naturally, single doses of $AFB_1$ are equally effective in producing HCC in rats and mice (Neal and Judah, unpublished observation).

### A.2.3 Mutational effects

Aflatoxins have been demonstrated to be powerfully mutagenic in *in vitro* systems including the Ames test, but require metabolic activation. In the rat, $AFB_1$ hepatocarcinogenesis has been found to involve mutations of ras genes, principally Ki, with point mutation at codon 12 (Sinha *et al.*, 1988; McMahon *et al.*, 1990). In one study, using sensitive methods of detection, codon 12 Ki-ras mutations were detected in 100% of 10 $AFB_1$-induced hepatocellular carcinomas (Soman and Wogan, 1993). In these studies the principal point mutations observed were G→A transitions with considerably fewer G→T transversions. In humans, for tumours at all sites, there is a high percentage of mutations in the p53 suppressor gene in primary liver cancers. However, for those tumours in which exposure to aflatoxins is believed to play a role, there was a clustering of the mutations on codon 249 and these mutations were predominantly G→T transversions (Hsu *et al.*, 1991; Bressac *et al.*, 1991). The correlation between $AFB_1$ exposure and p53 codon 249 mutations are illustrated in Table A.1.

**Table A.1** Correlation between p53 codon 249 mutations and dietary exposure to $AFB_1$ (after Eaton and Gallagher, 1994)

| Level of $AFB_1$ exposure | | | |
|---|---|---|---|
| High | | Low | |
| Total p53 mutations | Codon 249 mutations | Total p53 mutations | Codon 249 mutations |
| 59/142 | 69/225 | 98/401 | 13/558 |
| 42% | 31% | 24% | 2% |

The original studies correlating codon 249 p53 mutations with exposure to aflatoxins were based on samples from China and South Africa. This correlation has subsequently also been found in HCC samples from other countries, e.g. Mexico (Soini *et al.*, 1996). No clustering of p53 mutations on codon 249 was found in primary liver cancers in countries that have significant incidences of p53 mutations but where exposure to environmental aflatoxins is low. In a study carried out in Taiwan and Japan examining liver tissue from liver cancer patients, 10% of the samples containing

AFB$_1$–DNA adducts had p53 codon 249 mutations, whereas 18% of the samples with no adducts had this mutation. The authors of this study, Hsieh and Atkinson (1995), suggested that in contrast to some other reports their data did not support the hypothesis that codon 249 is a hot spot for aflatoxin mutagenesis as a 'late stage event' in human hepatocellular carcinogenesis.

A question remaining to be resolved is why AFB$_1$ carcinogenesis involves a high incidence of metabolic activation of ras oncogenes in rodents, but mutation of the p53 suppressor gene in humans. *In vitro* experiments using activated AFB$_1$ have demonstrated that the toxin is capable of mutating the human Ha-ras proto-oncogene to its oncogenic form by codon 12 point mutations (Riley *et al.*, 1997). Other studies have demonstrated that the human hypoxanthine guanine phosphoribosyl transferase (HGPRT) gene in β lymphocytes is associated with a mutational hot-spot in exon 3 at a GGGGGG sequence consistent with the affinity of AFB$_1$ for guanine bases (Cariello *et al.*, 1994). The influence of flanking sequences on AFB$_1$ mutagenesis has been demonstrated using two vectors carrying the *E. coli* SupF gene as mutational targets. Surrounding sequences at distances of tens of base pairs influenced the spectrum of mutation (Courtemanche and Anderson, 1994). Concerning the mechanisms of the point mutational changes, there are two principal probabilities: mispairing due to the presence of a bulky AFB$_1$ adduct or incorrect repair of apurinic sites. The primary interaction of metabolically activated AFB$_1$ with DNA results in the formation of AFB$_1$ N-7 guanyl adducts. This is followed either by stabilisation of the unstable AFB$_1$-guanyl adduct by opening of the imidazole ring of guanine forming the AFB$_1$–FAPY adduct or by loss of the AFB$_1$–guanine, leaving an apurinic site. This can be the subject of misrepair through the insertion of an inappropriate base. From experiments in which oligonucleotides with single guanine/AFB$_1$ adducts have been inserted into a phage and then replicated in *E. coli*, it has been concluded that G→T transversions in AFB$_1$-treated cells are due to mispairing with the AFB$_1$ modified bases, and not to the misrepair of apurinic sites (Bailey *et al.*, 1996). These studies also demonstrated that, in contrast to the mutations arising from depurination, which were all targeted to the site of the lesion, in the case of the direct mutagenesis a significant proportion of the mutations targeted to the base 5' to the modified guanine.

### A.2.4 Metabolic aspects

*A.2.4.1 Activating metabolism.* The major metabolic pathways of AFB$_1$ metabolism are illustrated in Figure A.1.

In humans it appears that both CYP 1A2 and 3A4 are capable of metabolising AFB$_1$ to form the reactive metabolite AFB$_1$-8,9-epoxide, with CYP1A2 possibly being responsible for the majority of activation at the low substrate levels that result from the consumption of naturally contaminated

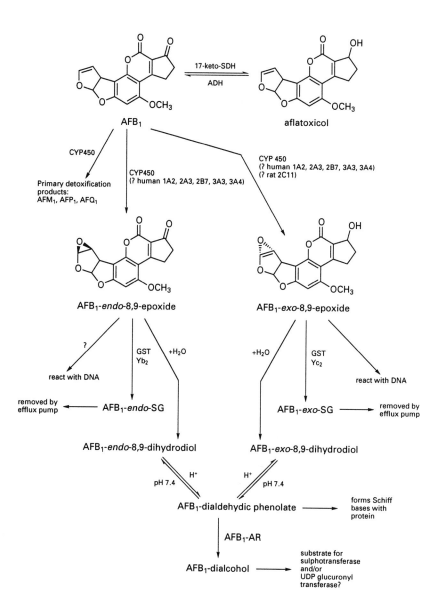

**Figure A.1** Metabolism of AFB$_1$

foods (Gallagher *et al.*, 1996). The suggestion that CYP 1A2 catalyses the formation of the reactive $AFB_1$-8,9-epoxide has been supported by the observation that yeasts expressing human CYP 1A2 when treated with $AFB_1$ display increased mitotic recombination (Sengstag and Wurgler, 1994). In addition, experiments using CYP 1A2 and CYP 3A4-expressing microsomes isolated from suitably transfected lymphoblastoid cells, and exposed to specific inhibitors of the two cytochromes, have demonstrated the capacity of CYP 1A2 to activate low levels of $AFB_1$ (Gallagher *et al.*, 1994). Using human p450s expressed in *E. coli* it has been reported that CYP 3A4 metabolises $AFB_1$ exclusively to the exo-epoxide whereas CYP 1A2 produces both exo- and endo-epoxides (Ueng *et al.*, 1995). Only the exo-epoxide is capable of reacting covalently with DNA. In a study using normal and tumorous human liver tissue from Thailand, metabolic activation of $AFB_1$ was found to correlate with the level of expression of CYP 3A3/4 and, to a lesser extent, with CYP 2B6 (Kirby *et al.*, 1993). There was a reduced expression of the major CYS p450 in the tumour tissue compared with the control tissue, a situation that parallels that observed in the rat model system involving the induction of pre-neoplastic and neoplastic lesions with $AFB_1$. This reduction of CYP 450s in the human tumour tissue was accompanied by a decreased capacity for the formation of $AFB_1$ tris-diol in incubations of microsomes with $AFB_1$, reflecting a decreased activation of $AFB_1$ to the epoxide (tris acts as an alternative acceptor for Schiff's base formation with $AFB_1$-dialdehyde; Figure A.1). Interestingly, there was an increased capacity of the microsomes from the tumours to produce aflatoxin $P_1$, a metabolite found to correlate with HCC in a study in China (Ross *et al.*, 1992). In studies using other human tissues, it has been found that in bowel tissue in explant culture, exposed to $AFB_1$, the pattern of formation of $AFB_1$–DNA adducts was similar to the distribution of CYP 3A4. The correlation was rendered more apparent following the induction of CYP 3A4 with dexamethazone (Kolars *et al.*, 1994). The question as to which CYS p450, 1A2 or 3A4 play the more significant role in activation of $AFB_1$ to the DNA-reactive exo-epoxide appears to be still a matter for debate.

Mechanisms of activation of $AFB_1$ other than that catalysed by CYP 450 have also been examined. In the human lung a major role for activation by lipoxygenase and prostaglandin H synthase has been described (Donnelly *et al.*, 1996). The activation of $AFB_1$ by mechanisms not involving p450 in the lung is of interest because of the possible involvement of exposure to aflatoxins in the genesis of some human lung tumours. It is noteworthy that in mice, a species that is normally resistant to the induction of liver tumours by $AFB_1$ due to the presence of mechanisms protective against p450-activated $AFB_1$, lung tumours can be induced by $AFB_1$ in the A/J strain. It has also been found that lipoxygenase isolated from human placenta and liver can activate $AFB_1$ (Roy and Kulkarni, 1997; Datta and Kulkarni, 1994).

*A.2.4.2 Detoxification mechanisms.* The male rat is highly sensitive to $AFB_1$ toxicity, whereas the mouse is resistant. However, the relative presence of CYP 450 enzymes capable of activating $AFB_1$ in the livers of the two species does not correlate with the difference in sensitivity. Indeed the reverse is the case. The mechanism behind the difference in sensitivity is the presence in the mouse liver of a constitutively expressed alpha class GST with a high capacity for conjugating $AFB_1$-epoxide to GSH (Hayes *et al.*, 1992). This enzyme has a highly homologous counterpart in the rat (GSTs containing the $Yc_2$ subunit) but this subunit is only expressed in the neonate, and to a very limited extent in the adult female, or in preneoplastic and neoplastic liver tissue or after induction with certain inducing substances, particularly antioxidants (Hayes *et al.*, 1991). Recently another $AFB_1$ detoxifying enzyme has been described, $AFB_1$ aldehyde reductase (dE) (Judah *et al.*, 1993). This enzyme prevents the binding of $AFB_1$ dihydrodiol in the dialdehydic form to proteins (Figure A.1). The pattern of expression of this enzyme is similar to that for GST $Yc_2$ expression. Both GST $Yc_2$ and AFAR are cytosolic enzymes. In the sheep a microsomal GST with activity towards $AFB_1$ has been described. To date this enzyme has not been further characterised (Larsson *et al.*, 1994).

*A.2.4.3 Chemoprotection.* Many substances have been found to afford protection against $AFB_1$ toxicity in animals. This has led to attempts to protect human populations at risk from environmental exposure to high levels of exposure to these toxins. At the metabolic level, since aflatoxins require activation to exert potent biological effects, two main methods of protection would appear possible. A reduction in the level of activation or an increased level of detoxification. From a consideration of the biochemical mechanisms underlying natural species differences in sensitivity between mice and rats, sensitivity or resistance seem to depend principally on the level of detoxifying metabolism. It would therefore appear that a monofunctional induction of phase II detoxifying metabolism would be the best stratagem. Many inducers, however, are bifunctional, inducing both primary and secondary metabolism. The use of these as chemoprotective agents raises the possibility that induction of specific primary metabolic pathways while protective against one toxin might actually potentiate the toxicity of another.

A wide range of compounds has been found to be protective against $AFB_1$-induced toxicity in experimental animals. This includes BNF (Santhanam *et al.*, 1996), curcumin (Firozi *et al.*, 1996), selenium (Shi *et al.*, 1994), chlorophyllin (Breinholt *et al.*, 1995a), indole-3-carbinol (Takahashi *et al.*, 1995a), vitamins A and C (Yu *et al.*, 1994), allyl sulphides (Habermignard *et al.*, 1996), oltipraz (Primiano *et al.*, 1995), green tea (Qin *et al.*, 1997) and BHA and BHT (Williams and Iatropoulos, 1996). The mechanisms involved are varied.

Induction of GSTs containing the $Yc_2$ subunit with high activity towards $AFB_1$ epoxide has been found to be an important mechanism in chemoprotection against $AFB_1$ toxicity in the rat (Hayes *et al.*, 1991). This applies particularly to resistance induced by ethoxyquin and oltipraz. An oltipraz prophylactic trial in humans exposed to high levels of $AFB_1$ was based on the results of rodent experiments. However, to date there is no firm evidence that mechanisms involved in resistance in the rat are inducible in man (Buetler *et al.*, 1996). It appears possible that if there is a successful outcome to the human oltipraz trial it will not be due to the same mechanism of resistance as that operating in the rat. Experiments using human hepatocytes in culture have suggested that oltipraz might afford protection by an inhibition of $AFB_1$ activation through CYP 1A2 and 3A4 (Langouet *et al.*, 1995). This stratagem, however, raises the possibility of the induction of adverse effects through inhibiting metabolism of endogenous substrates of these cytochromes. Protective mechanisms against $AFB_1$ toxicity other than induction of $Yc_2$ and AFAR have been identified. Chlorophyllin protects by complexing with the toxin (Breinholt *et al.*, 1995b). Indole-3-carbinol protects against $AFB_1$ toxicity in the trout due to both inhibition of $AFB_1$ activation and scavenging of the $AFB_1$-epoxide (Takahashi, 1995a), and at the levels present in cruciferous vegatables, induction of CYP 1A1 is unlikely to play a significant role (Takahashi *et al.*, 1995b). BNF protects in the rat by both enhancing the formation of a less toxic, hydroxylated, metabolite (aflatoxin $M_1$) as well as increasing detoxifying secondary metabolism (Stresser *et al.*, 1994).

### A.3  Ochratoxin A

*A.3.1*  In vivo *toxicity*

*A.3.1.1 Animals.* Exposure to ochratoxin A (OTA) though the ingestion of naturally contaminated feedstuffs has been clearly identified as the cause of a disease in pigs called mycotoxic porcine nephropathy (MPN). Possibly in some cases this is in association with ingestion of citrinin or fungal quinones such as viomellein. This disease has been identified in many European countries. The widespread contamination of animal feedstuffs, including a range of cereals, with OTA is evidence for the frequency of an equally widespread exposure of animals to the toxin. This is confirmed by the results of surveys of OTA residues present in tissues of farm animals, e.g. kidneys and blood (IARC, 1993). Kidneys show renal changes characteristic of MPN and the presence of OTA in these tissues in pigs at the time of slaughter (Krogh, 1992). The blood content of OTA was also correlated with the level of contamination of the feed. However, female pigs fed 1 mg OTA/kg in the diet for two years had progressive nephropathy but did not exhibit renal failure (Elling, 1979).

The widespread contamination of a variety of grains or other feedstuffs with OTA, together with the fact that all single-stomach animals investigated, including rodents, dogs, pigs and birds, exhibit renal damage when exposed to OTA, make it probable that exposure to naturally contaminated feedstuffs has been involved in a highly significant incidence of renal disease in domestic animals. Ruminants are believed to be resistant to OTA toxicity because the toxin is largely eliminated in the forestomach by protozoal and bacterial enzymes. This hypothesis is supported by the observation that young ruminants, still functioning as single-stomach animals, are susceptible to OTA toxicity. The data supporting the correlation between natural exposure to OTA and MPN is illustrated in Table A.2.

**Table A.2**  Exposure to ochratoxin A (OTA) and occurrence of mycotoxin porcine nephropathy (MPN) (adapted from Krogh, 1992)

| Country | No. of MPN kidneys examined | % containing OTA | Range of OTA (µg/kg) |
|---------|-----------------------------|------------------|----------------------|
| Denmark | 60 | 35 | 2–68 |
| Sweden | 129 | 25 | 2–104 |
| Hungary | 122 | 39 | 2–100 |

The kidney pathology in MPN is degeneration of the proximal tubules followed by atrophy of the tubular epithelium. Poultry have been identified in Denmark as having kidney lesions probably associated with exposure to OTA-contaminated feedstuffs. The lesions were characterised by a degeneration of the proximal and distal tubules and interstitial fibrosis (Elling *et al.*, 1975).

As already noted, all single-stomach animals examined have been found to develop renal disease as a result of OTA exposure. OTA may have carcinogenic, genotoxic, immunotoxic or teratogenic properties depending on the dose, with dogs and pigs being highly sensitive to oral dosing (IARC, 1993). There is a species-dependent range in the acute toxicity of OTA, varying from 3.4 to 30.3 mg/kg in the reported $LD_{50}$ (Chapter 7, Table 7.4).

Although on the evidence of *in vitro* mutagenicity assays it was originally thought that OTA was non-genotoxic, there is now increasing evidence that this is not the case. OTA has been found to be carcinogenic in rodent studies. Male mice fed a diet containing 40 mg OTA/kg diet for 44 weeks and killed on week 49 demonstrated a significant incidence of hepatocellular carcinoma and hyperplastic liver nodules, as well as a significant increase in the incidence of renal cell tumours (Kanisawa and Suzuki, 1978). A similar study in which male DD mice were given a diet containing 25 mg/kg OTA for 70 weeks also showed the development of a significant incidence of renal cell tumours with none present in the controls. There was also a significant increase in the incidence of hepatomas (Kanisawa, 1984). Several other studies have confirmed the fact that OTA is both a renal and hepatic carcinogen in mice. Other OTA-induced effects have been noted in mice. Oral vitamin C was able to moderate the damage (Bose and Sinha, 1994).

Rats have also been found to be sensitive to the carcinogenic effects of OTA. Groups of Fischer rats given doses of 21 to 210 µg/kg bodyweight by gavage, five days per week for 103 weeks were found to have renal cell tumours in both males and females, with the incidences increasing in a dose dependent manner (US National Toxicology Program, 1989).

In a short-term 90 day study in rats given 2 mg OTA/kg of diet, increased levels of enzymes originating from the brush border of the proximal convoluted tubules were found in the urine, indicating a toxic response in this tissue (Kane et al., 1986).

A further possible source of hazard, in addition to ingestion of contaminated foods, is suggested by the finding that OTA was efficiently absorbed from the lungs of rats given an intratracheal administration of 50 mg OTA/kg bodyweight (Breitholtz Emanuelsson et al., 1995).

OTA has been reported to induce immunotoxic, teratogenic and embryotoxic effects. In one study pregnant mice were treated intraperitoneally with 3 mg OTA/kg on day 10 of gestation and the offspring culled at six weeks of age. It was observed that pre-natal exposure to OTA resulted in microcephaly in the offspring and that there was a significant decrease in weight of the brain but not of the body. The decreased brain weight was accompanied by an increased density of neurones (Miko et al., 1994). In a study in which possible embryotoxic or immunotoxic effects of OTA were examined, female Balb/c mice were exposed to OTA in the diet of doses of 30 or 200 mµg/kg before or during gestation. It was found that the OTA exposure of the dams did not influence the reproductive outcome, but that there was a decrease in the percentages of splenic CD4+ and CD8+ cells (Thuvander et al., 1996b) in the offspring of the high dose group. There was also an increase in CD4+ sub-population in the thymus. The proliferative response of splenic or thymic lymphocytes to mitogens was not significantly altered as a result of the treatment with OTA. The authors concluded that although exposure of dams to relatively low levels of dietary OTA alters absolute and relative numbers of lymphocyte sub-populations in lymphoid organs, it does not result in any immune suppression in the offspring. However, in another study by the same group in mice, it was found that a single dose exposure of dams to 500 mµg OTA/kg bodyweight on day 16 of gestation resulted in a decreased proliferation of splenic and thymic lymphocytes in response to mitogens in the offspring at 15 days of age, with lower percentages of mature CD4+ cells and higher percentages of immature double positive CD4+ CD8+ cells (Thuvander et al., 1996a). In another study of possible immunotoxic effects of OTA female Balb/c mice were given a 6250 or 2600 mμg OTA/kg diet for 28 days. Antibody production in response to sheep red blood cells was suppressed in a dose-related manner. After a 90 day exposure to OTA there was a decreased proportion of mature CD4+ and CD8+ thymic lymphocytes, and the mitogenic response to concanavalin A was reduced. The authors concluded that sub-chronic oral exposure to OTA affects certain immune functions in mice at exposure levels that may be found in contaminated food (Thuvander *et al.*, 1995). Work has also been carried out on possible immunotoxic effects of OTA in rats. In one study laboratory rats were given a single dose of OTA (10 to 1250 μg/kg bw) on day 11 of lactation. Possible effects on cell numbers in the spleen and thymus, and on the mitogen responses of lymphocytes, were evaluated in the suckling offspring on day 14 of lactation. The proliferative response of splenocytes to concanavalin A was significantly stimulated in pups from dams given 10 or 50 mμg OTA, and the response of thymocytes to this mitogen was also stimulated in the 50 mμg OTA dose group. When exposure to OTA was both pre- and post-natal (50 μg OTA/kg bw for 5 days a week, e.g. 2 weeks before mating, during gestation and then 7 days a week until weaning), the results demonstrated a decrease in mitogen-induced proliferation only in the splenocytes of pre-natally exposed offspring, but not in those groups receiving both pre- and post-natal treatment or post-natal treatment only. The results indicated that whereas pre-natal exposure to relatively low doses of OTA may induce immunosuppression, exposure of offspring to OTA via the milk actually stimulates the proliferative responses of lymphocytes to polyclonal activation (Thuvander *et al.*, 1996c). It is evident that the effect of exposure to OTA on the immune system is not a simple one.

*A.3.1.2 Humans.* Paralleling the evidence for the natural exposure of animals to OTA, based on analyses of blood, there is a correspondingly extensive literature indicating exposure of humans, based on the same criteria. These data cover a number of countries and have used a variety of analytical techniques. The following are just a few examples of recent studies.

A survey in southern Italy, of 65 samples from both healthy and subjects with kidney disorders, showed a mean concentration of 0.53 ng OTA/ml serum in the healthy group. In the group with the kidney disorders, the highest mean concentration (1.4 ng OTA/ml serum) was detected in the sub-set receiving dialysis (Breitholtz Emanuelsson *et al.*, 1994).

A survey carried out in Tunisia indicated a range of contamination of 0.7 to 7.8 ng OTA/ml serum for the general population and 12 to 55 ng OTA/ml for individuals suffering from chronic renal failure (Maaroufi *et al.*, 1995).

A recent study in Hungary showed that OTA concentrations in 355 samples varied between <0.2 to 10 ng OTA/ml serum, but 75% of the samples contained 0.2–1.0 ng/ml. 6.8% of the samples, which exceeded 1.0 ng

OTA/ml, indicated a dietary intake in excess of the recommended 'virtually safe dose' (Solti *et al.*, 1997).

The major focus of interest in the chronic exposure of humans to OTA is the possible connection between this and the aetiology of Balkan endemic nephropathy (BEN), a chronic tubular-interstitial renal disease. Epidemiological studies have shown that in areas where high OTA levels are reached in food, and the blood of the population, there is a high incidence of nephropathy and renal tumours. The presence of DNA adducts in the kidneys of animals exposed to OTA, and similar adducts in renal tissue and tumours from regions where BEN is endemic, have provided a molecular epidemiological basis for a correlation between the two phenomena (Simon, 1996). Karyomegaly in the proximal and distal tubular epithelial cells, a frequent feature of the human disease, is indicative of DNA damage. Evidence has also been forthcoming for the involvement of OTA in renal disease in Tunisia, a region of high human exposure to OTA (Maaroufi *et al.*, 1996).

Limited data from Yugoslavia, involving more than 600 samples from inhabitants of two villages, one recognised as being endemic for BEN and the other not, has not provided unequivocal evidence in support of OTA involvement in this disease (Table A.3).

**Table A.3**  OTA in the blood of inhabitants of two Yugoslavian villages (from Hult *et al.*, 1982)

| OTA (ng/g serum) | Village endemic for BEN | | Village not-endemic for BEN | |
|---|---|---|---|---|
| | No. of positive samples | % positive | No. of positive samples | % positive |
| 1–2 | 11 | 2.6 | 4 | 1.8 |
| 3–5 | 11 | 2.6 | 7 | 3.2 |
| 6–10 | 2 | 0.5 | 6 | 2.7 |
| > 11 | 1 | 0.2 | 0 | 0 |
| Total | 25 | 5.9 | 17 | 7.8 |

There are few cases in the literature reporting acute poisoning in humans from OTA, which is perhaps surprising considering the widespread distribution of this mycotoxin in foodstuffs throughout the world. One such possible case was acute renal failure in an Italian farmer's wife following working for eight hours in a granary, previously closed for several months. Renal biopsy of the woman revealed acute tubular necrosis. An OTA-producing strain of *Aspergillus ochraceus* was isolated from the wheat (Simon, 1996).

### A.3.2 Metabolic aspects

Pathways of OTA metabolism are illustrated in Figure A.2. It appears probable that OTA is both directly toxic and that other toxicities result from metabolism. *In vitro* studies, including primary cultures of hepatocytes,

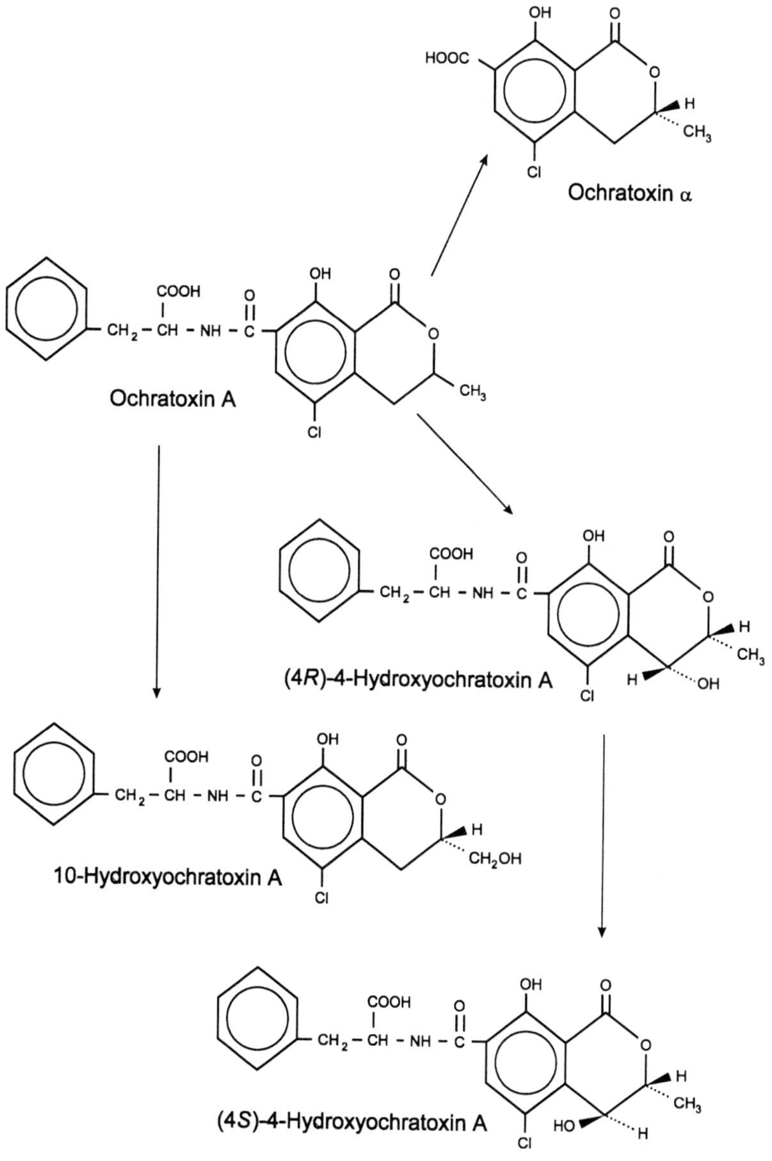

**Figure A.2**  Metabolism of OTA

have provided evidence that toxicological effects may be linked to biotransformation processes. *In vitro* incubations of liver microsomes from rats
treated with a range of P450 inducers have been used to study effects on the
metabolism of OTA to 4(*R*)-4-hydroxy-ochratoxin A (4*R*), the major
metabolite, and 4(*S*)-4-hydroxyochratoxin A (4*S*), the minor metabolite
(Omar *et al.*, 1996). Pretreatment of rats with phenobarbital (PB), dexam-
ethasome (DEX), 3-methyl cholanthrene (3MC) and isosafrole (ISF),
increased 4*R* formation. PB, DEX, 3MC, ISF and clofibrate also induced 4*S*
formation. Isoniazid (NA) primarily induced 4*S* formation. Studies using the
inhibitors metyrapone and alpha-naphthoflavone, as well as monoclonal
antibodies against various P450s, suggested that at least the P450 isoforms
1A1, 1A2, 11B1, 111A1 and 111A2 are involved in 4*R* formation. Induction
of 11B1 by pretreatment with PB protects against OTA nephrotoxicity and
so may be viewed as a detoxication mechanism. Vero cells (a monkey kid-
ney-derived cell line) metabolise OTA to the chlorinated dihydroiso-
coumarin moiety of OTA (OT alpha), 4*S*-hydroxy and 4*R*-hydroxy OTA
during a 24 hour incubation (Grosse *et al.*, 1995). [32]P postlabelling showed
the formation of some OTA-induced adducts similar to those found in the
kidneys of OTA-treated mice. Structure–activity toxicity studies in a
prokaryotic system, an *in vitro* eukaryotic cell system (HeLa cells) and in
rats and mice, *in vivo*, using OTA, its opened lactone ring form and several
analogues have indicated that the acute toxicity of the mycotoxin is attributable to its isocoumarin moiety. The lactone carbonyl group may also be
involved in its toxicity. There is a considerable body of evidence that OTA
inhibits protein synthesis *in vivo* and *in vitro* at the elongation step by competing with phenylalanine for its specific tRNA. OTA is a structural analogue of L-β-phenylalanine and treatment with this amino acid very
efficiently counteracts the inhibition of protein synthesis induced by OTA
(Creppy *et al.*, 1979). The dechlorinated derivative (OTB) is much less toxic
than OTA.

Biodistribution studies have demonstrated that the kidney has the highest tissue burden of OTA. This toxin is transported in the kidney via the
*para*-amino hippurate sulphate and succinate transporters. Following a single oral dose of 2 mg OTA/kg bw to mice, DNA adducts were found in kidney, liver and spleen. Administration of indomethacin or aspirin to mice
before OTA reduces the level of DNA adducts. This suggests prostaglandin
H synthase may be involved in the production of active OTA metabolites
(Obrerchtpflumio *et al.*, 1996).

The acute effects of OTA administered intraperitoneally to mice can be
prevented by the concomitant injection of phenylalanine (Creppy *et al.*,
1980). This is presumably due to a competition between the two compounds
for binding to phenylalanine tRNA. A number of other compounds have
been examined for their capacity to inhibit OTA nephrotoxicity. Another

structural analogue of OTA, the artificial sweetener aspartame, has been found to be very effective in this respect (Creppy *et al.*, 1995). Treatment with OTA results in lipid peroxidation, suggesting that the lesions induced by the mycotoxin could be related to oxidative pathways. Superoxide dismutase and catalase (20 mg/kg bw) injected subcutaneously into rats every 48 h, one hour before OTA administration (289 µg/kg every 48 h), for 3 weeks are reported to prevent most of the nephrotoxic effects induced by OTA, including proteiuria and creatinuria. The results indicated that superoxide radicals and hydrogen peroxide are probably involved in the *in vivo* nephrotoxic effects of OTA (Baudrimont *et al.*, 1994).

The role of metabolism of OTA in mutagenic and carcinogenic effects has been studied using NIH/3T3 cells stably transfected with human cytochrome P450 enzymes, together with a shuttle vector containing a lac Z gene, to act as a mutation reporter. The mutation frequency was elevated in cells expressing CYP 1A1, CYP 1A2, CYP 2C10 and CYP 3A4, but not CYP 2B6 or CYP 2E1 expressing cells (De Groene *et al.*, 1996a). In subsequent studies using these cells it was determined that the mutations induced in the lac Z gene involved extensive deletions (De Groene *et al.*, 1996b).

DNA strand breaks are induced by OTA in cultures of primary rat hepatocytes (De Groene *et al.*, 1996b). Other studies have demonstrated the DNA damaging capabilities of OTA (Follmann *et al.*, 1995). OTA administration can cause single strand breaks in DNA in rat kidney and liver, at a level corresponding to that found in foodstuffs contaminated at a low level (2 mg/kg) (Creppy *et al.*, 1995). OTA induces DNA adducts in a dose- and time-dependent manner in rats and mice with the highest adduct levels of the organs studied being in the kidney, followed by the liver and spleen. The half-life of the adducts was longest in the kidney (Pfohl-Leszkowicz *et al.*, 1993a). OTA gives rise to micronuclei in ovine seminal vesicle cells (Wild *et al.*, 1996).

Interestingly, some tumours in kidneys and bladders from patients living in areas associated with BEN using [32]P postlabelling techniques have been found to contain DNA adducts similar to those obtained from the kidneys of mice following OTA treatment (Pfohl-Leszkowicz *et al.*, 1993b).

## A.4  Fumonisins

### A.4.1  In vivo *toxicity*

*A.4.1.1 Animals.* Exposure to feedstuffs naturally contaminated with fumonisins has been clearly identified as the causative agent in the incidence of equine leucoencephalomalacia (ELEM), a pathology of the brain in horses. It has subsequently been established experimentally, using cultures of *F.*

*proliferatum* containing principally fumonisins $B_2$ or $B_3$ at levels of 75 mg/kg diet fed to ponies, that ELEM was observed after 150 days of feeding. The liver was also found to be affected. Rabbits dosed with 1.75 mg fumonisin $B_1$/kg bw per day developed brain lesions similar to ELEM, indicating that the sensitivity to the toxin in the genesis of this lesion was not limited to horses (Bucci *et al.*, 1986) The American Association of Veterinary Laboratory Diagnosticians has recommended that diets containing levels of fumonisins in excess of 5 mg/kg should not be fed to horses.

Fumonisins have also been implicated in the development of lung oedema in piglets. Maize containing fumonisins at a level of 92 mg/kg induced lung oedema in piglets after 5 to 7 days (Osweiler *et al.*, 1992). Other studies in pigs, fed diets containing 0.1, 1.0 and 10 ppm of fumonisin $B_1$ in the diet, showed decreased weight gain, males being more affected than females. Food intakes, however, were increased over those of controls during the first four weeks (Rotter *et al.*, 1996). There have been reports implicating dietary fumonisins in poultry diseases (Bryden *et al.*, 1987).

It appears from animal data, mainly involving feeding to rats, that fumonisins are not strong initiators of carcinogenesis. A level in the diet of 250 ppm fed for three weeks was necessary to initiate cancer (Gelderblom *et al.*, 1994). In studies in which male Fischer rats were fed diets containing 0.1% fumonisin $B_1$ for 26 days, followed by a partial hepatectomy to stimulate cell division and a promoting regime of feeding AAF and $CCl_4$, focal changes were observed containing elevated levels of mitoses together with proliferation of the bile ducts (Gelderblom *et al.*, 1992). The phenotypic changes observed in the hepatic nodules induced in rat liver by feeding fumonisins include expression of *gamma*-glutamyl transpeptidase, a marker enzyme associated with pre-neoplastic nodules induced by a variety of hepatocarcinogens (Gelderblom *et al.*, 1992). Rats fed diets containing low levels of fumonisins were found to lose weight initially, which, however, may have been due to diet refusal (Gelderblom *et al.*, 1994). It is interesting that similar diet refusal effects are observed when rats are fed diets containing significant levels of other mycotoxins, including aflatoxins. The same diets, only lacking the mycotoxin content, appear to be readily accepted by the rats (Neal and Judah, unpublished observations).

In longer term feeding studies with fumonisin the development of hepatocarcinogenesis in rats is accompanied by a significant incidence of cholangic carcinoma (Gelderblom *et al.*, 1991). Since hepatocarcinogenesis in rats by fumonisins is accompanied by toxic hepatitis and cirrhosis, it has been suggested that although poor initiators, fumonisins may be more powerful promoters, acting at dietary levels much lower than those required for initiation and complete carcinogenesis. This would correlate with the fact that fumonisins have been found to be negative in Ames tests (Park *et al.*, 1992), *in vitro* rat hepatocyte DNA repair assays (Gelderblom *et al.*, 1989) and micronucleus tests (Gelderblom *et al.*, 1995).

There are no data in the literature on whether fumonisins are developmental or reproductive toxins in farm animals or humans at the levels encountered in naturally contaminated foodstuffs. Developmental toxicity has been noted in Syrian hamsters (Floss *et al.*, 1994). Studies on rats have failed to demonstrate significant reproductive effects of doses at levels that are minimally toxic (Voss *et al.*, 1996). Studies in which cultured rat embryos were exposed to a range of concentrations of fumonisin $B_1$ showed inhibition of growth and development at concentrations of 0.28 mμM and above of this fumonisin. The authors concluded that rat embryos are highly sensitive to $FB_1$ toxicity (Flynn *et al.*, 1996).

*A.4.1.2 Humans.* Human exposure through the ingestion of contaminated food has been estimated in several countries. In Canada between 1991 and 1995 consumption averaged 0.109 μg/kg bw/day (Kuiper-Goodman *et al.*, 1995) and in the Transkei, South Africa, 14 μg/kg bw/day (Thiel *et al.*, 1992). Exposure through inhalation of dust and spores at work is likely to be a significant route of exposure for some workers as it is known that *Fusarium* spores contain fumonisins (Tejada-Simon *et al.*, 1995). Despite very high levels of human exposure to these mycotoxins there are no details in the literature of any resulting toxicities. It appears, therefore, that although there are animal data of toxicities at low levels of exposure, man is not very sensitive to the acutely toxic effects.

One of the principal concerns in terms of hazards to human health is the possible involvement of exposure to fuminosins in the development of oesophageal cancer. Such a possibility has been indicated by epidemiological studies in South Africa, where there are high incidences of oesophageal cancer in areas of high contamination of the staple foodstuff, maize, with fumonisins (Rheeder *et al.*, 1992). In these areas it was found that contamination of food with other mycotoxins was low. Studies in areas of China with high incidences of oesophageal cancer have shown correlations with exposure to fumonisins (Chu and Li, 1994). In certain areas of northern Italy, where there is one of the highest incidences of oesophageal cancer in Europe, locally grown maize forms a substantial portion of the diet. It has been found to be contaminated with fumonisins and possibly to constitute a significant risk factor to health (Visconti *et al.*, 1996).

*A.4.2 Mechanisms of toxicity*

There is a strong structural similarity between fumonisin $B_1$ and sphinganine, which has led to the hypothesis that $FB_1$ exerts its toxic effect through a disruption of sphingolipid metabolism or by inhibiting a function of sphingolipids. This hypothesis has been supported by considerable experimental evidence for a role of impaired sphingolipid function in cellular damage both *in vitro* and *in vivo* (Riley *et al.*, 1994a). The fumonisins are potent inhibitors of sphinganine N-acetyl transferase, an enzyme involved in sphingolipid biosynthesis and turnover. Normally free sphingosine and sphinganine are present in cells and tissues only in trace amounts (Riley *et al.*, 1994b). Fumonisin $B_1$ toxicity results in changes in this situation. For example, in horses fed fumonisins, elevated levels of serum sphinganine and altered sphinganine/sphingosine ratios were observed (Wang *et al.*, 1992).

In non-human primates (Vervet monkeys) given diets containing low (0.3 mg/kg bw/day) and high (0.8 mg/kg bw/day) levels of fumonisin, serum sphingosine levels were not altered significantly but sphinganine levels were significantly elevated. As a consequence the sphinganine/sphingosine ratio was elevated, from a control level of 0.43 to 1.72 and 2.57 in the low- and high-dosed animals, respectively (Shephard *et al.*, 1996). Similar changes were observed in urine samples and in studies of rat liver and kidney exposed for 20 h to $FB_1$ (Norred *et al.*, 1996). However, in contrast to the sphingolipid change observed in the liver, changes in kidney slices were less than those reported as taking place *in vivo*, suggesting that some of the *in vivo* changes in the kidney might be the result of changes in other tissues (Norred *et al.*, 1996).

### References

Anwar, W.A., Khalil, M.M and Wild, C.P. (1994) Micronucleus, chromosomal aberrations and aflatoxin–albumin adducts in experimental animals after exposure to aflatoxin B₁. *Mutation Research*, **322** 61-67.

Bailey, E.A., Iyer, R.S., Stone, M.P., Harris, T.M. and Essigmann, J.M. (1996) Mutational properties of the primary aflatoxin B₁–DNA adduct. *Proceedings of the National Academy of Sciences of USA*, **93** 1535-39.

Bannasch, P., Khoshkhov, N.I., Hacker, H.J., Radaewa, S., Mrozek, M., Zillmann, U., Koppschneider, A., Haberkorn, U., Elgas, M., Tolle, T., Roggendorf, M. and Toshkov, I. (1995) Synergistic hepatocarcinogenic effect of hepadna virus infection and dietary aflatoxin B₁ in woodchucks. *Cancer Research*, **55** 3318-35.

Baudrimont, I., Betbeder, A.M., Gharbi, A., Pfohlleskowicz, A., Dirheimer, G. and Creppy, E.E. (1994) Effect of superoxide dismutase and catalase on the nephrotoxicity induced by the subchronic administration of ochratoxin A in rats. *Toxicology*, **89** 101-11.

Bose, S. and Sinha, S.P. (1994) Modulation of ochratoxin-produced genotoxicity in mice by vitamin C. *Food and Chemical Toxicology*, **32** 533-37.

Bowers, J., Brown, B., Springer, J., Tollesfson, L., Lorentzen, L., Lorentzen, R. and Henry, S. (1993) Risk assessment for aflatoxin: an evaluation based on the multistage model. *Risk Analysis*, **13** 637-42.

Brienholt, V., Hendriks, J., Pereira, C., Arbogast, D. and Bailey, G. (1995a) Dietary chlorophyllin is a potent inhibitor of aflatoxin B₁ hepatocarcinogenesis in rainbow trout. *Cancer Research*, **55** 57-62.

Breinholt, V., Schimerlik, M., Dashwood, R. and Bailey, G. (1995b) Mechanisms of chlorophyllin anti-carcinogenesis against aflatoxin B₁: complex formation with the carcinogen. *Chemical Research in Toxicology*, **8** 506-14.

Breitholtz Emanuelsson, A., Minervini, F., Hult, K. and Visconti, A. (1994) Ochratoxin A in human serum samples collected in southern Italy from healthy individuals, and individuals suffering from different kidney disorders. *Natural Toxins*, **2** 366-70.

Breitholtz Emanuelsson, A., Fuchs, R. and Hult, K. (1995) Toxicokinetics of ochratoxin A in rats following intra-tracheal administration. *Natural Toxins*, **3** 101-103.

Bressac, B., Kew, M., Wands, J. and Ozturk, M. (1991) Selective G to T mutations of p53 gene in hepatocellular carcinoma from Southern Africa. *Nature*, **350** 429-31.

Bryden, W.L., Love, R.J. and Burgess, L.W. (1987) Feeding grain contaminated with *Fusarium gramineum* and *Fusarium moniliforme* to pigs and chickens. *Australian Veterinary Journal*, **64** 225-26.

Bucci, T.J., Hansen, D.K. and La Borde, J.B. (1996) Leukoencephalomalacia and hemorrhage in the brain of rabbits gavaged with mycotoxin, fumonisin $B_1$. *Natural Toxins*, **4** 51-52.

Buetler, T.M., Bammler, T.K., Hayes, J.D. and Eaton, D.L. (1996) Oltipraz-mediated changes in aflatoxin $B_1$ biotransformation in rat liver: implications for human chemointervention. *Cancer Research*, **56** 2306-13.

Cariello, N.F., Cui, L. and Skopek, T.R. (1994) *In vitro* mutational spectrum of aflatoxin $B_1$ in the human HGPRT gene. *Cancer Research*, **54** 4436-41.

Chao, T.C., Lo, D., Bloodworth, B.C., Gunasegaram, R., Koh, T.H. and Ng, H.S. (1994) Aflatoxin exposure in Singapore. Blood aflatoxin levels in normal subjects, HBV carriers and primary H.C.C. patients. *Medicine, Science and Law*, **34** 289-98.

Chen, C.J., Wang, L.Y., Lu, S.N., Wu, M.H., You, S.L., Zhang, Y.J., Wang, L.W. and Santella, R.M. (1996) Elevated aflatoxin exposure and increased risk of hepatocellular carcinoma. *Hepatology*, **24** 38-42.

Chu, F.S. and Li, G.Y. (1994) Simultaneous occurrence of fumonisin $B_1$ and other mytoxins in mouldy corn collected from the People's Republic of China in regions with high incidences of oesophageal cancer. *Applied Environmental Microbiology*, **60** 847-52.

Courtemanche, C. and Anderson, A. (1994) Shuttle vector mutagenesis by aflatoxin $B_1$ in human cells. Effects of sequence context in the SupF mutational spectrum. *Mutation Research*, **306** 143-51.

Creppy, E.E., Schlegel, M., Roschenthaler, R. and Dirheimer, G. (1979) Action of ochratoxin A on cultured hepatoma cells, reversion of inhibition by phenylalanine. *FEBS Letters*, **104** 287-90.

Creppy, E.E., Schlegel, M., Roschenthaler, R. and Dirheimer, G. (1980) Phenylalanine prevents acute poisoning by ochratoxin A in mice. *Toxicology Letters*, **6** 77-80.

Creppy, E.E., Baudrimont, I. and Betbeder, A.M. (1995) Prevention of nephrotoxicity of ochratoxin A, a food contaminant. *Toxicology Letters*, **83** 869-77.

Datta, K. and Kulkarni, A.P. (1994) Oxidative metabolism of aflatoxin $B_1$ by lipoxygenase purified from human term placenta and intrauterine conceptual tissues. *Teratology*, **50** 311-17.

De Groene, E.M., Hassing, I.G.A.M., Blom, M.J., Seinen, W., Fink-Gremmels, J. and Horbach, G.J. (1996a) Development of human cytochrome P450-expressing cell lines: application in mutagenicity testing of ochratoxin A. *Cancer Research*, **56** 299-304.

De Groene, E.M., Jahn, A., Horbach, G.J. and Fink-Gremmels, J. (1996b) Mutagenicity and genotoxicity of the mycotoxin, ochratoxin A. *Environmental Toxicology and Pharmacology*, **1** 21-26.

Diallo, M.S., Sylla, A., Sidibe, K., Sylla, B.S., Trepo, C.R. and Wild, C.P. (1995) Prevalence of exposure to aflatoxin and hepatitis B and C viruses in Guinea, West Africa. *Natural Toxins*, **3** 6-9.

Donnelly, P.J., Stewart, R.K., Ali, S.L., Conlan, A.R., Reid, K.R., Petsikas, D. and Massey, T.E. (1996) Biotransformation of aflatoxin $B_1$ in human lung. *Carcinogenesis*, **17** 2487-94.

Eaton, D.L. and Gallagher, E.P. (1994) Mechanisms of aflatoxin in carcinogenesis. *Annual Review of Pharmacology and Toxicology*, **34** 135-72.

Elling, F. (1979) Ochratoxin A-induced mycotoxic porcine nephropathy: alterations in enzyme activity in tubular cells. *Acta Pathologica et Microbiologica Scandinavica*, Section A, **87** 237-43.

Elling, P., Hald, B., Jacobsen, C. and Krogh, P. (1975) Spontaneous causes of toxic nephropathy in poultry associated with ochratoxin A. *Acta Pathologica et Microbiologica Scandinavica*, Section A, **83** 739-41.

Floss, J.L., Casteel, S.W., Johnson, G.C., Rottinghaus, G.E. and Krause, G.F. (1994) Developmental toxicity of fumonisin in Syrian hamsters. *Mycopathologia*, **128** 33-38.

Flynn, T.J., Pritchard, D., Bradlaw, J.A., Eppley, R. and Page, S. (1996) *In vitro* embryotoxicity of fumonisin B$_1$ evaluated with cultured post implantation staged rat embryos. *In Vitro Toxicology*, **9** 271-79.

Follmann, W., Hillebrand, I.E., Creppy, E.E. and Bolt, H.M. (1995) Sister chromatid exchange frequency in cultured isolated porcine urinary bladder epithelial cells (PUBEC) treated with ochratoxin A and alpha. *Archives of Toxicology*, **69** 280-86.

Firozi, P.F., Aboobaker, V.S. and Bhattachary, R.K. (1996) Action of curcumin on the cytochrome P450 system catalysing the activation of aflatoxin B$_1$. *Chemico-Biological Interactions*, **100** 41-51.

Gallagher, E.P., Wienkers, L.C., Stapleton, P.L., Kunze, K.L. and Eaton, D.L. (1994) Role of human microsomal and human complimentary DNA-expressed cytochromes P450 1A2 and P450 3A4 in the bioactivation of aflatoxin B$_1$. *Cancer Research*, **54** 101-108.

Gallagher, E.P., Kunze, K.L., Stapleton, P.L., and Eaton, D.L. (1996) The kinetics of aflatoxin B$_1$ oxidation by human c-DNA-expressed and human liver microsomal cytochromes P450 1A2 and 3A4. *Toxicology and Applied Pharmacology*, **141** 595-606.

Gelderblom, W., Marasas, W., Thiel, P., Semple, E. and Farber, E. (1989) Possible non-genotoxic nature of active carcinogenic components produced from *Fusarium moniliforme*. *Proceedings of the American Association for Cancer Research*, **30** 144.

Gelderblom, W.C.A., Kriek, N.P.J., Marasas, W.F.O. and Thiel, P.G. (1991) Toxicity and carcinogenicity of the *Fusarium moniliforme* metabolite fumonisin B$_1$ in rats. *Carcinogenesis*, **12** 1247-51.

Gelderblom, W.C.A., Semple, E., Marasas, W.F.O. and Farber, E. (1992) The cancer initiating potential of the fumonisin B mycotoxins. *Carcinogenesis*, **13** 433-37.

Gelderblom, W.C.A., Cawood, M.E., Snyman, S.D. and Marasas, W.F.O. (1994) Fumonisin B$_1$ dosimetry in relation to cancer initiation in rat liver. *Carcinogenesis*, **15** 209-14.

Gelderblom, W.C.A., Snyman, S.D., Abel, S., Lebepe-Mazur, S., Smuts, C.M., van der Westhuizen, L. and Marasas, W.F.O. (1995) Hepatotoxicity and carcinogenicity of the fumonisins in rats: a review regarding mechanistic implications for establishing risk in humans, in *Fumonisins in Food* (eds L. Jackson, J.W. De Vries and L.B. Bullerman), New York, Plenum Press, pp. 279-96.

Grosse, Y.M., Baudrimont, I., Castegnaro, M., Betbeder, A.M., Creppy, E.E., Dirheimer, G. and Pfohlleszkowicz, A. (1995) Formation of ochratoxin A metabolites and DNA adducts in monkey kidney cells, *Chemico-Biological Interactions*, **95** 175-87.

Habermignard, D., Suschetet, M., Berges, R., Astorg, P. and Siess, M.H. (1996) Inhibition of aflatoxin B$_1$ and N-nitrosodiethylamine induced liver pre-neoplastic foci in rats fed naturally occurring allyl sulphides. *Nutrition and Cancer*, **25** 61-70.

Hayes, J.D., Judah, D.J., McClellan, L.I. and Neal, G.E. (1991) Contributions of the glutathione S-transferases to the mechanisms of resistance to aflatoxin B$_1$. *Pharmacology and Therapeutics*, **50** 443-72.

Hayes, J.D., Judah, D.J., Neal, G.E. and Nguyen, T. (1992) Molecular cloning and heterologous expression of a cDNA encoding a mouse glutathione S-transferase Yc subunit possessing high catalytic activity for aflatoxin B$_1$-8,9-epoxide. *Biochemical Journal*, **285** 173-80.

Hsieh, D.P.H. and Atkinson, D.N. (1995) Recent aflatoxin exposure and mutation at codon 249 of the human p53 gene. Lack of association. *Food Additives and Contaminants*, **12** 421-24.

Hsu, I.C., Metcalf, R.A., Sun, T., Welsh, J.A., Wang, N.J. and Harris, C.C. (1991) Mutational hotspot in the p53 gene in human hepatocellular carcinomas. *Nature*, **350** 427-28.

Hult, K., Plestina, R., Habazin-Novak, V., Radic, B. and Cedvic, S. (1982) Ochratoxin A in human blood and Balkan endemic nephropathy. *Archives of Toxicology*, **51** 313-21.

IARC (1993) *Some Naturally Occurring Substances: Food Items and Constituents Heterocyclic Aromatic Amines and Mycotoxins*, IARC monographs on the evaluation of carcinogenic risks to humans, vol. 56, IARC, Lyon.

Judah, D.J., Hayes, J.D., Yang, J.C., Lian, L.Y., Roberts, G.C.K., Farmer, P.B., Lamb, J.H. and Neal, G.E. (1993) A novel aldehyde reductase with activity towards a metabolite of aflatoxin $B_1$ is expressed in rat liver during carcinogenesis and following the administration of an anti-oxidant. *Biochemical Journal*, **292** 13-18.

Kane, A., Creppy, E.E., Roschenthaler, R. and Dirheimer, G. (1986) Changes in urinary and renal tubular enzymes caused by sub-chronic administration of ochratoxin A in rats. *Toxicology*, **42** 233-43.

Kanisawa, M. (1984) Synergistic effect of citrinin on hepato renal carcinogenesis of ochratoxin A in mice, in *Toxigenic Fungi, their Toxins and Health Hazard* (eds H. Kurata and Y. Ueno), Japanese Association of Mycotoxicology, Tokyo, pp. 245-54.

Kanisawa, M. and Suzuki, S. (1978) Induction of renal and hepatic tumors in mice by ochratoxin A, a mycotoxin, *GANN*, **69** 599-600.

Kirby, G.M., Wolf, C.R., Neal, G.E., Judah, D.J., Henderson, C.J., Srivatanakul, P. and Wild, C.P. (1993) *In vitro* metabolism of aflatoxin $B_1$ by normal and tumorous liver tissue from Thailand. *Carcinogenesis*, **14** 2613-20.

Kirby, G.M., Chemin, I., Montesano, R., Chisari, F.V., Lang, M.A. and Wild, C.P. (1994) Induction of specific P450s involved in aflatoxin $B_1$ metabolism in hepatitis B virus transgenic mice. *Molecular Carcinogenesis*, **11** 74-80.

Kirby, G.M., Batist, G., Alpert, L., Lamoureux, E., Cameron, R.G. and Alaouijamali, M.A. (1996) Overexpression of cytochrome P450 isoforms involved in aflatoxin bioactivation in human liver with cirrhosis and hepatitis. *Toxicologic Pathology*, **24** 458-67.

Kolars, J.C., Benedict, P., Schmiedlinren, P. and Watkins, P.B. (1994) Aflatoxin $B_1$-adduct formation in rat and human small bowel enterocytes. *Gastroenterology*, **106** 433-39.

Krishnamachari, K.A.V.R., Bhat, R.V., Nagarajan, V. and Tilak, T.B.G. (1975) Hepatitis due to aflatoxicosis. *Lancet*, **i** 1061-63.

Krogh, P. (1992) Role of ochratoxins in disease causation. *Food Chem. Toxicol.*, **30** 213-24.

Kuiper-Goodman, T., Scott, P.M., McEwan, N., Lombaet, G.A. and Ng, W. (1995) Approaches to the risk assessment of fumonisins in corn-based foods in Canada, in *Fumonisins in Food* (eds l. Jackson, J.W. De Vries and L.B. Bullerman), Plenum Press, New York, pp. 369-93.

Langouet, S., Coles, B., Morel, F., Becquemont, L., Beaune, P., Guengerich, F.P., Ketterer, B. and Guillouzo, A. (1995) Inhibition of CYP1A2 and CYP3A4 by oltipraz results in reduction of aflatoxin $B_1$ metabolism in human hepatocytes in primary culture. *Cancer Research*, **55** 5574-79.

Larsson, P., Busk, L. and Tjalve, H. (1994) Hepatic and extra-hepatic bioactivition and GSH conjugation of aflatoxin $B_1$ in sheep. *Carcinogenesis*, **15** 947-55.

Maaroufi, K., Achour, A., Hammami, M., El May, M., Betbeder. A.M., Ellouz, F., Creppy, E.E. and Bacha, H. (1995) Ochratoxin A in human blood in relation to nephropathy in Tunisia. *Human and Experimental Toxicol.*, **14** 609-14.

Maaroufi, K., Achour, A., Zakhama. A., Ellouz, F., May, M., Creppy, E.E. and Bacha, H. (1996) Human nephropathy related to ochratoxin A in Tunisia. *Journal of Toxicology*, **15** 223-37

Manson, M.M. and Neal, G.E. (1987) The effect feeding an aflatoxin conataminated ground-nut meal, with or without ammoniation, on the development of gamma-glutamyl transferase positive lesions in the livers of Fischer F344 rats. *Food Additives and Contaminants*, **4** 141-47.

McMahon, G., Davis, E.F., Huber, L.J., Kim, Y.S. and Wogan, G.N. (1990) Characterisation of c-Ki-ras and N-ras oncogenes in aflatoxin $B_1$-induced rat liver tumors. *Proceedings of the National Academy of Sciences of USA*, **87** 1104-1108.

Miko, T., Fukui, Y., Uemura, N. and Takeuchi, Y. (1994) Regional difference in the neurotoxicity of ochratoxin A on the developing cerebral cortex in mice. *Developmental Brain Research*, **82** 259-64.

Norred, W.P., Riley, R.T., Meredith, F.I., Bacon, C.W. and Voss, K.A. (1996) Time and dose-response effects of the mycotoxin, fumonisin $B_1$ on sphingoid base elevations in precision-cut rat liver and kidney slices. *Toxicology In Vitro*, **10** 349-58.

Nose, J., Imazeki. F., Ohto, M. and Omata, M. (1993). Gene mutation and 17p allelic deletion in hepatocellular carcinoma from Japan. *Cancer*, **72** 355-60.

Obrechtpflumio, S., Grosse, Y., Pfohl-Leszkowicz, A. and Dirheimer, G. (1996) Protection by indomethacin and aspirin against genotoxicity of ochratoxin A, particularly in the urinary bladder and kidney. *Archives of Toxicology*, **70** 244-48.

Omar, R.F., Gelboin, H.V. and Rahimtula, A.D. (1996). Effect of cytochrome P450 induction on the metabolism and toxicity of ochratoxin A. *Biochemical Pharmacology*, **51** 207-216.

Osweiler, G.D., Ross, P. F., Wilson, T.M., Nelson, P.E., Witte, S.T., Carson, T.L., Rice, L.G. and Nelson, H.A. (1992) Characterisation of an epizootic of pulmonary edema in swine associated with fumonisin in corn screenings. *Journal of Veterinary Diagnostic Investigation*, **4** 53-59.

Park, D.L., Lee, L.S., Price, R.L. and Pohland, A.E. (1988) Review of the decontamination of aflatoxins by ammoniation: current status and regulation. *Journal—Association of Official Analytical Chemists*, **71** 685-703.

Park, D.L., Rua, S.M., Mirocha, C.J., Abd-Alla, E.A.M. and Weng, C.Y. (1992) Mutagenic potentials of fumonisin-contaminated corn following ammonia decontamination procedure. *Mycopathologica*, **117** 105-108.

Pfohl-Leszkowicz, A., Grosse, Y., Kane, A., Creppy, E.E. and Dirheimer, G. (1993a) Differential DNA adduct formation and disappearance in three mice tissues after treatment by the mycotoxin, ochratoxin A. *Mutation Research*, **289** 265-73.

Pfohl-Leszkowicz, A., Grosse, Y., Castegnaro, M., Nicolov, I.G., Chernozemski, I.N., Bartch, H., Betbeder, A.M., Creppy, E.E. and Dirheimer, G. (1993b) Ochratoxin A-related DNA adducts in urinary tract tumours of Bulgarian subjects, in *Postlabelling Methods for Detection of DNA Adducts* (eds D.H. Phillips, M. Castegnaro and H. Bartch), IARC Scientific Publication No. 124, IARC, Lyon, pp. 141-48.

Primiano, T. Egner, P.A., Suter, T.R., Kelloff, G.J., Roebuck, B.D.O. and Kensler, T.W. (1995) Intermittent dosing with oltipraz: relationship between chemoprevention of aflatoxin-induced tumorigenesis and induction of glutathione S-transferases. *Cancer Research*, **55** 4319-24.

Qian, G.S., Ross, R.K., Yu, M.C., Yuan, J.M., Gao, Y.T., Henderson, B.E., Wogan, G.N. and Groopman, J.D. (1994) A follow-up study of urinary markers of aflatoxin exposure and liver cancer risk in Shanghai, People's Republic of China. *Cancer Epidemiology, Biomarkers and Prevention*, **3** 3-10.

Qin, G., Gopalankriczky, P., Su., J., Ning, Y. and Lotlikar, P.D. (1997) Inhibition of aflatoxin $B_1$-induced initiation of hepatocarcinogenesis in the rat by green tea. *Cancer Letters*, **112** 149-54.

Rheeder, J.P., Marasas, W.F.O., Thiel, P.G., Syndenham, E.W., Shephard, G.S. and Van Schalkwyk, D.J. (1992) *Fusarium moniliforme* and fumonisins in corn in relation to human oesophogeal cancer in Transkei. *Phytopathology*, **82** 353-57.

Riley, R.T., Hinton, D.M., Chamberlain, W.J., Bacon, C.W., Wang, E., Merrill, A.H. and Voss, K.A. (1994a) Dietary fumonisin $B_1$ induces disruption of sphingolipid metabolism in Sprague Dawley rats: a new mechanism of nephrotoxicity. *Journal of Nutrition*, **124** 594-603.

Riley, R.T., Wang, E. and Merrill, A.H. (1994b) Liquid chromatographic determination of sphinganine and sphingosine: use of the free sphinganine to sphingosine ratio as a biomarker for consumption of fumonisins. *Journal—Association of Official Analytical Chemists International*, **77** 533-40.

Riley, J, Mandel, H.G., Sinha, S., Judah, D.J. and Neal, G.E. (1997). *In vitro* activation of the human Harvey-ras proto-oncogene by aflatoxin $B_1$. *Carcinogenesis*, **18** 905-10.

Ross, A.K., Yu, M.C., Henderson, B.E., Yan, J.M., Qian, G.S., Tu, J.-T., Gao, Y-T., Wogan, G.N. and Groopman, J.D. (1992) Aflatoxin biomarkers. *Lancet*, **340** 119.

Rotter, B.A., Thompson, B.K., Prelusky, D.B., Trenholm, H.L., Stewart, B., Miller, J.D. and Savard, M.E. (1996) Response of growing swine to dietary exposure to pure fumonisin $B_1$ during an 8 week period. *Natural Toxins*, **4** 42-50.

Roy, S.K. and Kulkarni, A.P. (1997) Aflatoxin $B_1$ epoxidation catalysed by partially purified human liver lipoxygenase. *Xenobiotica*, **27** 231-41.

Santhanam, K., Ho, L., Gopalankriczky, P. and Lotlikar, P.D. (1996). A mechanism of inhibition of aflatoxin $B_1$ hepatocarcinogenesis by beta-naphthoflavone pre-treatment of rats. *Experimental Molecular Medicine*, **28** 135-40.

Sell, S., Hunt, J.M., Dunsford, H.A. and Chisari, F.V. (1991) Synergy between hepatitis B virus expression and chemical hepatocarcinogenesis in transgenic mice. *Cancer Research*, **51** 1278-85.

Sengstag, C. and Wurgler, F.E. (1994) DNA recombination induced by aflatoxin $B_1$ activated by cytochrome P450 1A enzymes. *Molecular Carcinogenesis*, **11** 227-35.

Shephard, G.S., Van Der Westhuizen, L., Thiel, P.G., Gelderblom, W.C.A., Marasas, W.F.O. and Van Schalkwyk, D.J. (1996). Disruption of sphingolipid metabolism in non-human primates consuming diets of fumonisin containing *Fusarium moniliforme* culture material. *Toxicology*, **34** 527-34.

Shi, C.Y., Chua, S.C., Lee, H.P. and Ong, C.N. (1994) Inhibition of aflatoxin $B_1$–DNA binding and adduct formation by selenium in rats. *Cancer Letters*, **82** 203-208.

Simon, P. (1996) Ochratoxin and kidney disease in the human. *Journal of Toxicology*, **15** 239-49.

Sinha, S., Webber, C., Marshall, C.J., Knowles, M.A., Procter, A., Barrass, N.C. and Neal, G.E. (1988) Activation of ras oncogene in aflatoxin induced rat liver carcinogenesis. *Proceedings of the National Academy of Sciences of USA*, **85** 3673-77.

Soini, Y., Chia, S.C., Bennett, W. P., Groopman, J.D., Wang, J.S., De Benedetti, V.G.M., Cawley, H., Welsh, J.A., Hansen, C., Bergasa, N.V., Jones, E.A., Di Bisceglie, A.M., Trivers, G.E., Sandoval, C.A., Calderon, I.E., Munozespinosa, L.E. and Harris, C.C. (1996) An aflatoxin-associated mutational hot-spot at codon 249 in the p53 tumor suppressor gene occurs in HCC from Mexico. *Carcinogenesis*, **17** 1007-12.

Solti, L., Salamon, F., Barnavetru, F., Gyongyosi, A., Szabo, E. and Wolfling, A. (1997) Ochratoxin content of human sera determined by a sensitive ELISA. *Journal of Analytical Toxicology*, **21** 44-48.

Soman, N.R. and Wogan, G.N. (1993) Activation of the c-Ki-ras oncogene in aflatoxin $B_1$-induced hepatocellular carcinoma and adenoma in the rat: detection by denaturing gradient gel electrophoresis. *Proceedings of the National Academy of Sciences of USA*, **90** 2045-49.

Stresser, D.M., Bailey, G.S. and Williams, D.E. (1994) Indole-3-carbinol and beta naphthoflavone induction of aflatoxin $B_1$ metabolism and cytochromes P450 associated with bioactivation and detoxication of aflatoxin $B_1$ in the rat. *Drug Metabolism and Disposition*, **22** 383-91.

Takahashi, N., Dashwood, R.H., Bjeldawes, L.F., Williams, D.E. and Bailey, G.S. (1995a) Mechanisms of indole-3-carbinol anti-carcinogenesis: inhibition of aflatoxin $B_1$–DNA adduction and mutagenesis by I-3-C acid condensation products. *Food and Chemical Toxicology*, **33** 851-57.

Takahashi, N., Stresser, D.M., Williams, D.E. and Bailey, G.S. (1995b) Induction of hepatic CYP 1A by indole-3-carbinol in protection against aflatoxin $B_1$ hepatocarcinogenesis in rainbow trout. *Food and Chemical Toxicology*, **33** 841-50.

Tejada-Simon, M.V., Marovatsanga, L.T. and Pestka, J.J. (1995) Comparative detection of fumonisins by HPLC, ELISA and immunochemical localisation in *Fusarium* cultures. *J. Food. Protection*, **58** 666-72.

Thiel, P.G., Marasas, W.F.O., Sydenham, E.W., Shephard, G.S. and Gelderblom, W.C.A. (1992) The implications of naturally occurring levels of fumonisins in corn for human and animal health. *Mycopathologia*, **117** 3-9.

Thuvander, A., Breitholz Emanuelsson, A. and Olsen, M. (1995) Effect of ochratoxin A on the mouse immune system after sub-chronic exposure. *Food and Chemical Toxicology*, **33** 1005-11.

Thuvander, A., Breitholtz Emanuelsson, A., Brabencova, D. and Gadhasson, I. (1996a) Prenatal exposure of Balb/C mice to ochratoxin A: effect on the immune system in the offspring. *Food and Chemical Toxicology*, **34** 547-54.

Thuvander, A., Dahl, P. and Breitholtz Emanuelsson, A. (1996b) Influence of perinatal ochratoxin A exposure on the immune system in mice. *Natural Toxins*, **4** 174-80.

Thuvander, A., Funseth, E., Breitholtz Emanuelsson, A., Hallen, I.P. and Oskarsson, A. (1996c) Effect of ochratoxin A on the rat immune system after perinatal exposure. *Natural Toxins*, **4** 141-47.

Ueng, Y.F., Shimada, T., Yamazaki, H. and Guengerich, F.P. (1995) Oxidation of aflatoxin $B_1$ by bacterial recombinant human cytochrome P450 enzymes. *Chemical Research in Toxicology,* **8** 218-25.

US National Toxicology Program (1989) *Toxicology and Carcinogenesis. Studies of Ochratoxin A (cas No 303-47-9) in F344/N rats (Gavage studies),* BTP TR 358: DHHS Publ. No. (NIH) 89-2813, Research Triangle Park, North Carolina.

Visconti, A., Boenke, A., Solfrizzo, M., Pascale, M. and Doko, M.B. (1996) European intercomparison study for the determination of the fumonisin content in 2 maize materials. *Food Additives and Contaminants,* **8** 909-27.

Voss, K.A., Bacon, C.W., Norred, W.P., Chapin, R.E., Chamberlain, W.J., Plattner, R.D. and Meredith, F.I. (1996) Studies on the reproductive effects of *Fusarium moniliforme* culture material in rats and the biodistribution of [$^{14}$C] fumonisin $B_1$ in pregnant rats. *Natural Toxins,* **4** 24-33.

Wang, E., Ross, P.F., Wilson, T.M., Riley, R.T. and Merrill, A.H. (1992) Increases in serum sphingosine and sphinganine and decreases in complex sphingolipids in ponies given feeds containing fumonisins, mycotoxins produced by *Fusarium moniliforme. Journal of Nutrition,* **122** 1706-16.

Wild, C.P., Hasegawa, R., Barraud, L., Chutimataewin, S., Chapot, B., Ito, N. and Montesano, R. (1996) Aflatoxin–albumin adducts: a basis for comparative carcinogenesis between animals and humans. *Cancer Epidemiology, Biomarkers and Prevention,* **5** 179-89.

Wild, C.P., Jansen, L.A.M., Cova, L. and Montesano, R. (1993) Molecular dosimetry of aflatoxin exposure; contribution to understanding the multifunctional etiopathology of primary hepatocellular carcinoma with particular reference to hepatitis B virus. *Environmental Health Perspectives,* **99** 115-22.

Williams, G.M. and Iatropoulos, M.J. (1996) The inhibition of the hepatocarcinogenicity of aflatoxin $B_1$ in rats by low levels of the phenolic antioxidants butylated hydroxy anisole and butylated hydroxytoluene. *Cancer Letters,* **104** 49-53.

Yan, R.Q., Su, J.J., Huang, A.R., Gan, Y.C., Yang, C. and Huang, G.H. (1996) Human hepatitis virus and hepatocellular carcinoma: experimental induction of HCC in tree shrews exposed to hepatitis virus, and $AFB_1$. *Journal of Cancer Research and Clinical Oncology,* **122** 289-95.

Yu, M.W., Zhang, Y.J., Blaner, W.S. and Santella, R.M. (1994) Influence of vitamins A, C and E and beta-carotene on aflatoxin $B_1$ binding to DNA in woodchuck hepatocytes. *Cancer,* **73** 596-604.

Yu, M.N, Lien, J.P., Lian, Y.F. and Chen, C.J. (1996) Effect of multiple risk factors for hepatocellular carcinoma on formation of aflatoxin $B_1$–DNA adducts. *Cancer Epidemiology, Biomarkers and Prevention,* **5** 613-19.

# Index

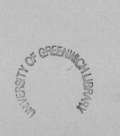